Acknowledgements

Once again, there are many people to thank. First must be my fiancée, Dr. Simone Reuter, for her tested patience and critical eye. A long list of individuals assisted me in updating the text for this edition by verifying the accuracy of my information. I thank you all once again.

The author would also like to thank the following, all of whom supplied figures: Prof. Roger L. Brown, University of Wisconsin (Fig. 26); Assoc. Prof. Joel W. Goldwein, University of Pennsylvania School of Medicine (Fig. 32); Prof. A.M. House, Memorial University of Newfoundland (Fig. 15); Dr. Iain Kewley, CompuServe UKPROF SysOp (Fig. 8); Paul Lynas, The Current Science Group (Fig. 39); Kristi Reilly, VocalTec (Fig. 33); Asst. Prof. Keith E. Willard, University of Minnesota (Fig. 11); and the US National Library of Medicine (Fig. 35). Figures 12, 28, and 29 were captured with the help of Dr. David Brooks. Line illustrations were expertly drawn by Samantha Armstrong.

Many thanks go to the team at Oxford University Press, and to the proprietors of *Il Vincio* in Tuscany, whose outstanding hospitality displaced a very stubborn writer's block. A special note of thanks to the Chesterfield Vocational Training Scheme for General Practice, and to my friends and colleagues at Ashgate Hospice in Chesterfield for their support during the writing of this edition.

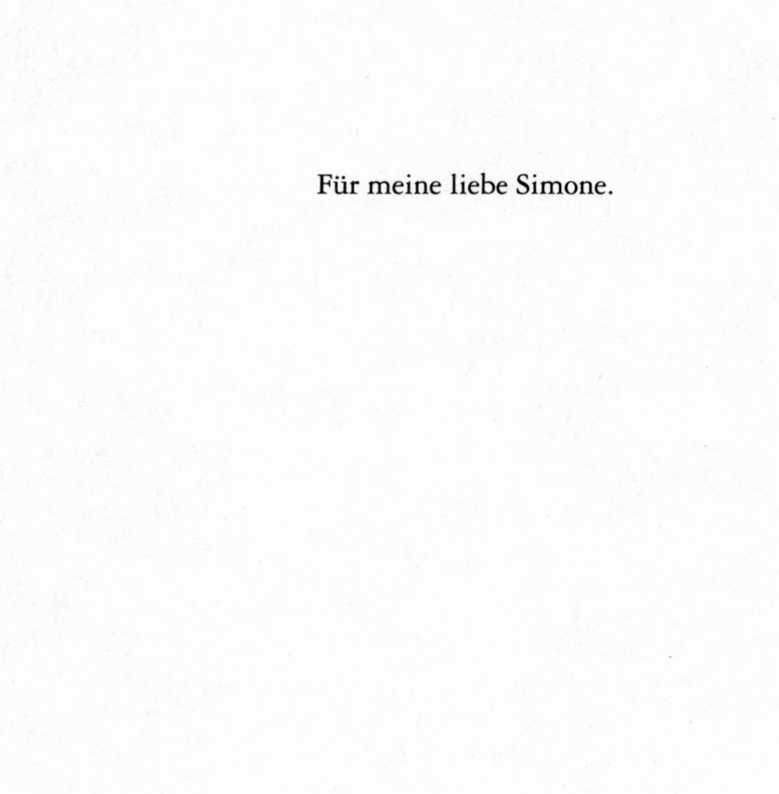

Für meine liebe Simone.

Preface

Since the conception of the first edition of *Medicine and the Internet* in November 1994, the face of the Internet has aged. Evolution has produced a superior being—a truly interactive **World-Wide Web** that has arguably positioned all but e-mail on the verge of extinction. But for all its myriad offerings, the Internet boils down to just two things—communication, and information—both of which lie at the core of medical practice.

This book introduces doctors and medical students to communications tools and health care information available on the Internet and other online services. Other health professionals will find much of the material in this book relevant to their own requirements for an introduction to online resources and terminology. If you are uncertain about the usefulness of online resources in clinical practice or study, this book will help make up your mind.

Doctors are among the growing number of people who are using modems. A **modem** is a device used to send information from one computer to another over telephone lines. Computers can be linked together to form **networks** so that they can exchange information on a regular basis. Using a modem you can connect to one of these networks and access the information stored on the computers that make up the network. Part One of this book covers getting started with computers, modems, and communications programs.

Sometimes computerized information consists of electronic forums where you can read and post **electronic mail** (e-mail). Sometimes it consists of libraries of programs and other files. Those who offer this sort of facility are said to provide an **online service**, as your modem connects to that service over telephone lines. Part Two of the book tells you how to join an online service, what to expect, what is expected of you, and looks briefly at examples of health-oriented services.

Individual online services are, however, limited in content by comparison with the Internet. The **Internet** is the name for the global network of computer networks and online services providing worldwide communications and linking together many diverse resources. In Part Three, the Internet is introduced, including information on how to get connected and why you might want to do so.

The Internet can be very daunting to new users in search of information or wanting to contact like-minded colleagues. One of the secrets of success is knowing where to look before you go looking. Part Four gets you started by examining the tools you are likely to encounter.

Most readers will already be familiar with the MEDLINE bibliographic database. Part Five describes how to do a MEDLINE search without ever going to the library.

After using the Internet for a while, some may want to harness it to better serve their personal needs, or those of their colleagues and clients. Part Six guides you through becoming an information provider.

This book doesn't avoid jargon. It is well worth the effort of familiarizing yourself with terms in common usage. Without this familiarity, you will encounter many difficulties in understanding the language you will come across online, including that used by those whom you ask for help. Learning the language (like the Latin of gross anatomy) makes universal communication possible. Throughout the book jargon is clearly identified by **bold** type as it is introduced, and if a meaning is not clear from its context you will find an additional explanation in the Glossary.

Some Internet services—**Archie**, **Gopher**, **Telnet**, and **WAIS**—could almost be ignored by many users. They are described in this book, however, as not all users have the luxury of WWW-based access to the Internet, and those with slow Internet connections will find non-graphical utilities less demanding. Our patients already have access to online health information (databases, discussion groups, mailing lists) and support forums. In the UK, **NHSnet** and **JANET** make the Internet available to both the clinical and academic communities. Through an introduction to these and other services, health professionals will learn how individuals and health care organizations can access databases and other forms of electronic information quickly and at little cost.

This book is not a 'picture album' annotating Web sites in detail (there is no better way to ensure a book will quickly date). In following the successful formula of the first edition, it serves as both guide and reference, imparting to the reader all the 'know how' necessary for independent exploration. Careful attention to the organization of information ensures readers can quickly locate relevant facts, and means this text is ideally suited as a course manual.

February 1997 B.C.M.

bruce@cybertas.demon.co.uk

How to use this book

Each of the six main Parts of the book contains a number of chapters, and Parts One through Four are proceeded by an overview chapter. Chapters are broken into manageable sections that serve to answer a certain question or emphasize individual topics.

Because the Internet is too dynamic to be mirrored on paper, the book points to up-to-date online lists and sources of further information whenever possible. The Oxford University Press's World-Wide Web pages (p.301) make it easier to locate these and other important online resources. These online addresses appear in a different type-style, separated from the main body of text, like this:

<URL:http://www.oup.co.uk/scimed/medint/>

Technical notes and various tips and traps are indicated by marginal icons as follows:

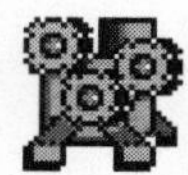

Technical note: how it works in more detail. You are not obliged to read these sections, but the curious can be satisfied.

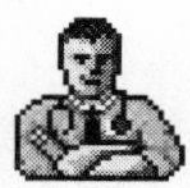

Tip-or-trap advice: practical guidance to help both novice and veteran get the most out of the online experience.

Quick Reference Cards (see inside cover flaps) can be customized so that important details (such as e-mail addresses and key resources) are close at hand.

If you are new to computers, telecommunications, or the Internet you might decide to read this book from beginning to end. Alternatively, you are free to read the Parts or chapters in any order, in accordance with your interests and familiarity with the contents.

Contents

PART TWO - GOING ONLINE

List of contributors

Electronic communication with patients

Beverley Kane MD
Chair, American Medical Informatics Association Internet Working Group
Demonstration Projects Committee
Apple Computer Inc., Cupertino USA
E-mail: bkane@apple.com

Telemedicine and the Internet

Richard Wootton DSc PhD
Professor, Institute of Telemedicine and Telecare
Queen's University, Belfast UK
E-mail: r.wootton@qub.ac.uk

Running a medical mailing list

Ian Purves MBBS MRCGP DCCH DRCOG
Director, Sowerby Unit for Primary Care Informatics
Newcastle University, Newcastle UK
E-mail: ian.purves@ncl.ac.uk
Mike Bainbridge BMedSci BM BS MRCGP
Telematics Officer, British Computer Society Primary Health Care Specialist Group
Applied Intellect, Derby UK
E-mail: mikebain@phcsg.demon.co.uk
Ian Trimble BMedSci BM BS MPhil MRCGP
General Practitioner
Sherwood Health Centre, Nottingham UK
E-mail: trims@sherwood.demon.co.uk

Developing for the WWW

Richard Charkin MA
Chief Executive Officer
The Current Science Group, London UK
E-mail: richard@cursci.co.uk
Paul Lynas
Executive Assistant
The Current Science Group, London UK
E-mail: paull@cursci.co.uk

Medical specialty resources (Appendix)

Eric Rumsey MA MLS
Reference Librarian and Webmaster
Hardin Library for the Health Sciences, University of Iowa USA
E-mail: eric-rumsey@uiowa.edu

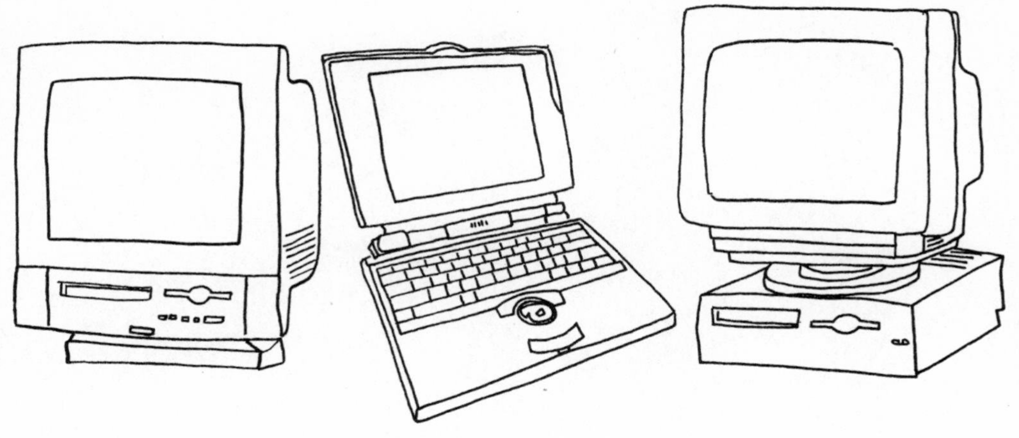

PART I

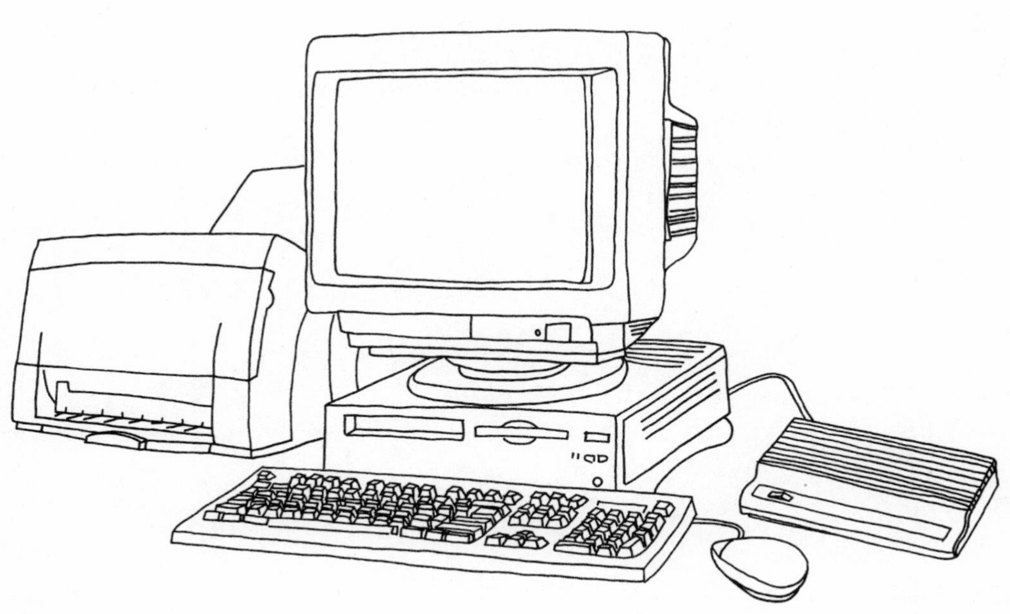

CHAPTER ONE
Getting Started

It is still surprising how many of us feel an aversion to computer technology. How many times have you heard a colleague say, 'I don't understand computers!'? Often they mean 'I'm not willing to spend a little time learning how to use one'. In this Part, we examine the basic set-up needed for medical telecommunications.

Starting at the beginning

In modern usage, the term **computer** describes an electronic machine that uses well-defined instructions to manage information. Early computers were large and awkward, but miniaturization of components means today's versions can easily fit on top of your desk or even in your lap. This technology has become affordable in recent years, and a computer is an integral part of the work space of many offices and homes. In this respect, these machines are truly deserving of their common acronym—the **PC**, or *personal* computer. While digital watches and microwaves are technically computers too, they are designed for specific operations, such as telling the time or cooking food. PCs, however, are multipurpose machines; they can be instructed to perform tasks varying from letter-writing to playing games. Each set of instructions for doing a particular thing (such as controlling a communication link) is called a **program** or **software**. Software comes in two broad categories: operating-system software and **application** software. Operating-system software is explained in Chapter Two. Application software refers to programs used for a particular purpose: software used for writing a letter is a word-processing application. Other applications include communications, databases, and graphics. The machine itself is **hardware**, made of metals and plastics, and must interpret these software instructions. Other physical items, such a disks and printers, are also classed as hardware.

If you plan to go **online** from your home or office you are likely to use a PC. If you have access to a university computing centre you might use a PC or a workstation—a computer connected to a network that allows many people (or **users**) to use the network at once. Users can sit at their own terminals (monitor and keyboard) and work independently of each other, although sharing a connection to a powerful computer called a server. Even more powerful are 'supercomputers', some of which are linked together to form the backbone of the Internet (see Chapter Eleven). Communication between computers (and their users) is fundamental to the concept of network-based resources.

What do I need to get started?

Before beginning your exploration of medicine online you will need a computer. We will first take a look at the hardware and software components of a computer system to ensure that your cheque book gives its informed consent. See Chapter Two.

The second requirement is a modem. '**Modem**' is an acronym for *mo*dulator/*dem*odulator, which describes its role in the modulation (conversion) of computer-generated (digital) signals to telephone (analogue or sound) signals and back. This digital information takes the form of **binary code**—strings of 0s and 1s which computers and mathematicians understand. Thus, when two computers with modems are connected, one of them (the sending modem) translates the binary data into sound signals for transmission along the phone line, while the other (the receiving modem) converts the sound signal back into binary data so it can be used on the receiving computer. See Chapter Three.

To control the modem we use lists of instructions in the form of **communications software**. Once a modem is installed or set somewhere and connected to the computer, you are ready to **load** and set up your communications software so it can control your modem. Before we discuss configuring (setting up) communications software (Chapter Seven), we will have a look at features you should take into account if you need to obtain this software, and explain some concepts concerning its use. See Chapter Four.

When you've finished this Part you should:

be able to read a computer advertisement and

- know what is meant by Pentium 120 MHz, 16 MB RAM, 1.2 GB hard disk, with a quad-speed CD-ROM drive and 15" SVGA display

understand that modems

- convert computer language to sound and back over telephones
- require hardware handshaking for high-speed connections
- use data-compression protocols to speed up file transfers
- use error-correction protocols to make sure a message is received intact

know what communications software is and understand

- the concept of terminal emulation, and the client–server relationship
- the basic difference between ASCII (text) files and binary (program) files
- what file-transfer protocols are, and that there are two basic types.

CHAPTER TWO

Choosing a computer system

Despite the lack of indisputable evidence that the 'computerization' of general practice (Sullivan and Mitchell 1995) and NHS hospitals (Lock 1996) has provided the anticipated benefits, computers have numerous applications in health care settings (see Table 1). Anecdotally at least they can be productivity tools of significant potential for individual clinicians and academics. Medical utilization of online services and the Internet is the topic of this book, although information about other uses of computers in medicine is increasingly easy to find (see *Bibliography*).

Choice of computer hardware and software and a commitment to familiarization are factors in the degree of productivity afforded by any system. This is why it is appropriate for doctors to develop a basic working knowledge of the technologies involved. This is the first of three chapters in this Part covering, in turn, concepts in computing, modems, and communications software.

Would you understand a newspaper advertisement for a 'WonderPC' 120 MHz Pentium, 16 MB RAM, 1.2 GB hard disk, with a quad-speed CD-ROM drive and 15" SVGA display? Pick yourself up off the floor and read on. The components of a computer system such as these can be daunting to the new user. This section covers essential elements that you will need to consider if you intend to purchase a new machine (or upgrade an old one). You don't need the fastest or latest available set-up: new products and technologies are appearing all the time and it won't be possible to buy top-of-the-line equipment unless money is no object.

The system unit

The **system unit** is the box that contains the microprocessor and other electronic components involved in managing such things as memory, graphics, and sound. The system unit is what makes personal computers *personal*: a monitor and keyboard on their own are known as a **terminal**. At the back of the system unit (Fig. 1) there are various **ports** (connectors for cables) for attaching **peripherals** (add-on equipment) such as printers and modems.

A choice of microprocessor

The **microprocessor** ('chip' or central processing unit/**CPU**) is the computer's equivalent of a brain, giving it control over other parts of the computer. Until relatively recently, most new PCs used microprocessors numbered in '80x86' manner from Intel and other

TABLE 1 Using computers in medical practice

Task		Type of software/facility required*
Accounts/financial affairs		Spreadsheet. Dedicated business management software. Some practice administration systems.
Assisting with diagnosis		Diagnostic decision support tools, e.g. DXplain.
Audit		Clinical audit/information system. Some practice administration systems.
Clinical coding		Clinical audit/information system. Read Codes, ICD-10, etc.
Communicating with colleagues		Communications software. Fax software.
Continuing medical education (CME)/ computer-assisted learning		CME credits can be earned from disk and CD-ROM-based problem-solving tools, e.g. Scientific American Medicine's DISCOTEST.
Deciding on treatment		Therapeutic decision support software, e.g. online Cochrane database of clinical trials.
Diary/contact management		Personal information manager (PIM) software.
Distance learning/telemedicine		Videoconferencing software/hardware.
Electronic medical records (EMR)		Dedicated EMR system may incorporate case notes, automated recall, referral letters, repeat prescriptions, etc.
Illustrations/diagrams		Paint (using mouse movements as a pen/brush) and/or draw (mathematically calculated lines/shapes) programs. Medical 'clip-art' collection (ready-made images).
Information retrieval		Communications software (for online services, the Internet). CD-ROM-based multimedia textbooks or database collections (including full-text medical journals).
Medical imaging		Specialized imaging systems.
Patient education		Patient handouts can be generated by computer; educational software is available on disk and CD-ROM (e.g. from the Mayo Clinic).
Planning treatment		Dedicated planning systems, e.g. for radiotherapy. Virtual reality software/hardware and 3-D software for simulations.
Practice administration		Dedicated practice administration system (may be integrated with EMR).
Presentations/slide production		Presentation software e.g. Microsoft PowerPoint.
Research		Database, e.g. Microsoft Access. Spreadsheet (for simple maths and charting), e.g. Microsoft Excel Statistical software, e.g. Pro-Stat. Bibliographic/literature management software, e.g. EndNote Plus. Search software, e.g. Grateful Med.
Result reporting		Hospital network systems.
Sending/receiving faxes		Fax software.
Writing	letters, medical reports, papers/articles, CVs, information leaflets, handouts, overheads	Word processor (simple), e.g. Microsoft Word. Desktop publishing package (advanced), e.g. Adobe PageMaker. Dictionary, e.g. Stedman's Medical Dictionary. Presentation software, e.g. Microsoft PowerPoint can be useful for overhead/handout production.

* See Bibliography for pointers to more information.

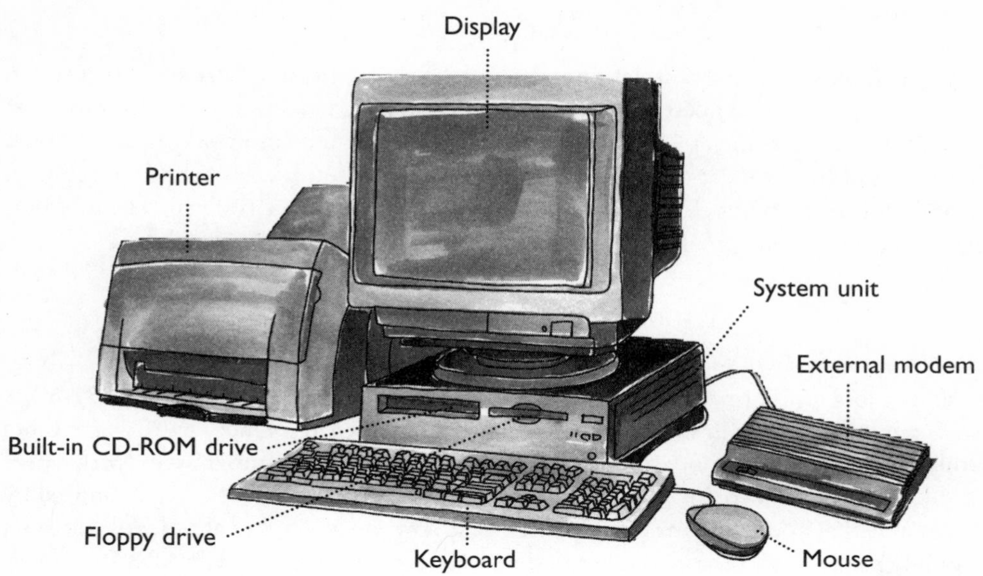

Fig. 1 A basic PC set-up. The monitor sits on top of the system unit with built-in CD-ROM and floppy disk drives. Ports at the rear of the unit provide for the addition of peripheral devices such as a printer or modem, as well as the keyboard and mouse.

manufacturers, including the '80486' (or 486) in several 'SX' and 'DX' variations. Notebook PCs sometimes use a power-saving 'SL' chip. Lower-end Apple **Macintosh** (Macs) and Amiga computers use Motorola CPUs numbered in '680x0' fashion. In both instances, the higher the number of the CPU, the more advanced the design. Microprocessors with an SX or LC in their naming scheme don't have a 'floating point unit' (also known as a maths **coprocessor**). A coprocessor boosts the speed of a computer, particularly when it is used for complex graphics and mathematical calculations.

Both Intel '80x86' and Motorola '680x0'-type chips have been virtually phased out by newer microprocessors. The **Pentium** from Intel is based on CISC (Complex Instruction Set Computing) technology, like the 486 it has virtually displaced. Personal computers with a **PowerPC** chip (from the Apple, IBM, and Motorola alliance) appeared in March 1994, based on Reduced Instruction Set Computing (RISC) technology. Hailed as the 'next generation' microprocessor type, RISC-based processors from other manufacturers have since become available.

In general, the more advanced the CPU, the longer it is likely to serve you. Purchasers of new machines should be considering a PowerPC or Pentium-based system, rather than a 680x0 or 486 CPU.

Clock speed

All chips 'think' or process information at a particular speed, measured in megahertz (MHz). This is called the **clock speed** or frequency. As an example, a given type of microprocessor (e.g. a Pentium) working at 120 MHz is faster than a Pentium chip working at 75 MHz. If two types of chip work at the same clock speed, such as a 386 and a 486 both at 33 MHz, the 486 will be the faster chip. If you see an advertisement for a 'P100', you can interpret this as a Pentium-type processor that 'runs' at 100 megahertz.

Random access memory (RAM)

It's all very well having a brain, but to show it off you need to be able temporarily to remember lots of information at once. The amount of random access memory (**RAM**) is like a count of neurones in short term memory: the more RAM memory there is, the more numbers you could remember simultaneously. RAM, measured in **megabytes** (MB, where 1024 **kilobytes** [KB] equals 1 MB, and 1000 MB equals 1 **gigabyte** [GB]), is limited by the amount that your machine can support—and how much you can afford. All software, including the programs that actually run the computer, must be loaded into RAM memory in order to work. The more RAM you have, the more programs you can load into this 'work space' and use at the same time. One can think of RAM as 'working memory'. RAM is erased every time you shut down the computer, whether intentionally or accidentally when the computer **crashes**. You can buy extra RAM which slots into the circuit board holding the processor.

As programs are getting more memory hungry, 8 MB of RAM has become the absolute minimum to consider in a new machine. A Power Macintosh or PC running Windows 95 will perform better still if it is equipped with 16 MB of RAM (or more).

Read only memory (ROM)

ROM chips contain unchangeable instructions built in by the manufacturer which tell the computer what to do when it is turned on, or 'booted'. These instructions are specific to each type of computer, and allow it to carry out hardware and operating system checks during the **startup** process. Sometimes part of the operating system itself (see below) is built into these chips.

Cache memory

A **cache** is a special memory space acting as a repository for those bits of information that the processor uses frequently. Rather than fetch information from the hard disk (see below), this allows the processor to keep certain information such as pieces of software code close at

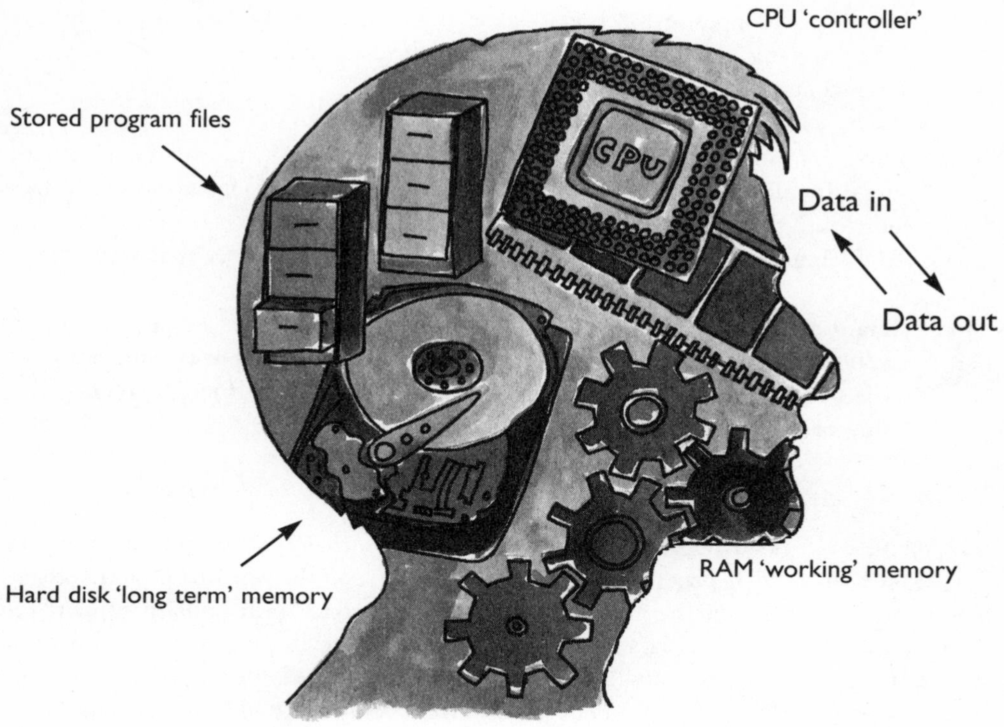

Fig. 2 How computers work. Programs that the computer uses are stored in 'long term memory' (on the hard disk). When needed they are loaded into 'working memory' (RAM). The CPU oversees the operation of the program in RAM, and directs the presentation of information back to the user (data output—to the screen or printer) along with the organization of new information (data input—from the keyboard and mouse).

hand. The effect of this is to speed up the operations that the processor directs as it controls the various components of the computer. You can speed up your PC by adding a secondary cache.

Storage space

The **hard disk** provides a place to store software programs along with any information that you have been working with in RAM and want to keep. The relationship between the hard disk, RAM, and the CPU is illustrated in Fig. 2. Saving your work on a disk is similar to recording a movie on video tape on your video cassette recorder.

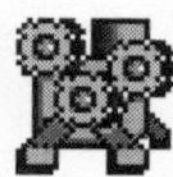

The term 'hard' refers to the fact that these disks consist of layered platters of inflexible metal. Particles on the surface of these disks are magnetized as the disk spins so that a magnetic pole in one direction indicates a 1, whilst a pole in the opposite direction indicates 0. In this way binary data, including the programs used to start up and operate the computer, is stored as a series of magnetic 0s and 1s.

You can store a lot more information on a hard disk than in RAM. Information on a hard disk is more difficult to erase accidentally than data in RAM memory, although it does take longer to open the stored item (called the 'access time'). Hard disks come in two main varieties: 'IDE' (Intelligent Drive Electronics) and 'SCSI' (Small Computer System Interface).

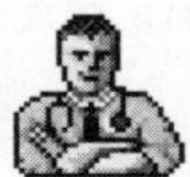

Hard disks tend to fill more quickly than you would think, especially if you've been online for a while and have accumulated an impressive medical file library of your own. Try to afford at least 500 MB, although you can upgrade to a higher capacity disk later on.

Video circuitry

Video circuits and video memory (**VRAM**) determine how many colours your monitor can display, the size of the display the computer can support, and the **resolution** of the image (how many dots make up the picture). Most machines come with built-in support for adequate colour and display sizes, but a video **upgrade card** can increase the number of colours, the image resolution, and/or the size of display your machine can use. A computer equipped with 1 MB of VRAM, in effect the current standard, will be able to display at least 256 colours on a 14 or 15 inch screen (see below). 'Local bus video' is sometimes promoted in advertisements: this means that the CPU can control video memory directly, speeding up graphics. PC video cards are used in conjunction with a software **driver**.

Expansion options

If for financial reasons you are committed to buying a system with a minimal specification, you may also wish to consider the expansion capability of the machine. A machine with several expansion options may allow you to add on extras such as additional memory or a graphics card, or to upgrade the CPU at a later date.

Removable disks

Although hard disks are built into the system unit, you can also store information on disks that can be carried around. These disks are therefore referred to as 'removable media'. Floppy disks and CD-ROMs are common examples of removable media.

Floppy disks

A **floppy disk** (flexible, inside a plastic case) is a portable storage disk that is 'read' by a floppy disk drive. The most common disks in use today are 3.5 inch 'double density' floppy disks storing 800 KB and 'high density' floppy disks storing 1.4 MB of data. You can use these disks to easily transfer data between computers that are not networked (connected together by cables). Commercial software is often shipped on this media, which is then **installed** on to the hard drive where it can be accessed at a faster speed.

CD-ROM and multimedia

CD-ROM stands for Compact Disk-Read Only Memory, which means that it is a compact disk (like an audio CD) containing data that can be read by the computer, but *not written to* in the same way as you can save data to a floppy disk. If you wish to use CD-ROM, you will need a CD-ROM drive or player. This may already be fitted into your computer, or available as an add-on later. Dual or double-speed drives, running at twice the speed of the original design, soon gave way to quad-speed drives. Eight-speed drives are now becoming available. CD-ROM can store about 650 megabytes of data.

Aside from games, **multimedia** encyclopedias, software, and photographic collections, there is an increasing range of medical titles appearing on CD-ROM such as the *Oxford Textbook of Medicine*, interactive demonstrations, and bibliographic databases. Many drives also allow you to play music CDs. Because CD-ROMs are cheaper to mass-produce and have a higher capacity than floppy disks, some computing magazines give them away on the cover, and ever more software is being distributed on this medium.

Virtually all CD-ROMs, and increasingly the Internet, make use of sound (with or without video). Although standard on the Macintosh, PCs require a **sound card** to enable audio playback. If you have a choice, specify a sound card that is compatible with 'SoundBlaster', the *de facto* standard. A '16-bit' card will produce CD-quality sound (with an appropriate set of speakers). Listening to Grieg's *In the Hall of the Mountain King* while waiting for a slow-loading World-Wide Web page to be displayed reduces boredom!

The keyboard and mouse

A computer **keyboard** resembles that of a typewriter only in that it is used to type in letters and numbers. A few extra keys can be configured to automate certain tasks quickly, called 'keyboard short-cuts', or 'function keys'. Others make up a numeric keypad like the buttons on a calculator, and arrow keys let you move the **cursor** on the screen. Still others perform tasks specific to computers. Anything you type is translated into binary code so that it can be stored and manipulated by the computer.

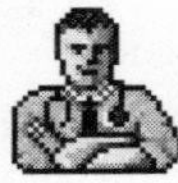

Although they have a fairly standard layout, keyboards differ in terms of ergonomics and feel, so try-before-you-buy if you can.

A **mouse** consists of a ball that is rolled across a flat surface to direct a pointer around the screen. Moving the mouse with your hand produces a corresponding movement of the pointer on your screen. Mouse buttons can be used in combination with mouse movements to 'point and click' on something such as an **icon** (mini pictures representing programs and files) or **scroll bar**, 'drag and drop' things around in **windows**, or use a **pull-down menu** to select a command. The keyboard and mouse are the most common ways of giving your instructions to the computer. Portable computers often use trackballs (an 'upside-down mouse'), trackpads (where your finger moves the pointer), or similar devices.

Display monitor

At the heart of most **monitors** is a cathode ray tube (CRT), just like in television sets. Most colour monitors use a metal sheet punctured by round holes through which coloured phosphors emit dots of light (the 'shadow mask'). The proximity of these dots to each other is called the **dot pitch**. Trinitron monitors (commonly supplied with Macs) use fine vertical wires instead of a metal sheet, so we speak of 'stripe' pitch instead. A dot/stripe pitch of at least 0.28 mm produces a reasonably crisp image.

A 14 or 15 inch screen size (measured diagonally) is adequate for the majority of users: most software titles are accommodated by these dimensions. Colour makes many tasks more pleasant such as navigating on the World-Wide Web (see Chapter Eleven). **Greyscale** (shades of grey) is second best and more prevalent in portable machines, while monochrome screens are almost redundant.

Differently coloured individual dots (**pixels**) make up the image displayed on the screen. Screen resolution describes the number of horizontal and vertical dots or pixels making up the display area. Video Graphics Array (**VGA**) is a PC graphics standard capable of displaying 256 colours on a screen with a resolution of 640 x 480 pixels. Super VGA provides higher resolution displays with more colours and larger screen sizes. An **SVGA** resolution of 800 x 600 pixels is popular on PCs, while Macs commonly use a 640 x 480 resolution. Some Macs do use adapted VGA monitors, but unlike VGA on a PC they can display more than 256 colours. Monitors are sometimes capable of changing their resolution (e.g. 640 x 480 or 1024 x 768) and, because this changes the speed of the display, are labelled 'multisync' or **multiscan**. Too high a resolution on a small screen can result in text which is too small to read comfortably.

An annoying flicker can occur as the screen is 'redrawn' (refreshed) many times a second, particularly on higher resolution displays that use a redraw technique called 'interlaced scanning'. The number of frames per second is called the **refresh rate** and measured in hertz. Flicker is less likely with a refresh rate of at least 72 Hz at all resolutions and non-interlaced scanning.

Many factors influence the sharpness of the image such as focus (especially in the corners of the screen), colour convergence, and the finish on the screen itself. Avoid monitors that produce unacceptable image distortion or moiré patterns. Trinitron screens produce a characteristic flat image (the corners of the screen don't bow out).

Monitors with a tilt-and-swivel base let you position the display to suit your preferences. Consider also the position and type of controls available for adjusting monitor settings. Commonly the monitor is sold with the system unit, but sometimes you will have the option of a separate purchase.

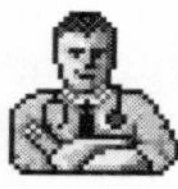

The safest way to buy a monitor is to compare your choices side-by-side in a computer store. In terms of clarity of image and size of display, you get what you pay for. This may be something you will stare at for some time, so don't skimp on quality.

Remember that your monitor's capabilities (number of colours, resolution, size of display) may be restricted by the video circuitry in your computer (see above).

Printing

Despite the dream of a paperless office, most people can't cope without a **printer** in order to make paper or 'hard copies' of their documents. If you've been trawling the Internet for information on treatment of ovarian cancer for a computer-deprived colleague, you will need to get what you find out of the computer and on to paper. The three principal types of printer in order of increasing quality and cost are *dot matrix*, *ink jet*, and *laser*. Other factors to consider in your choice include speed, requirement for colour or black-and-white output, image resolution (an ink jet at 360 dots per inch approximates laser quality), noise, running cost, paper handling, and its 'footprint' (how much desk space it takes up).

Software

What do you want the computer to do?

The most important thing in buying a computer is choosing application software that will do the job effectively and efficiently. Even if you plan on using the computer mainly for telecommunications, it is wise to consider what other uses you could make of the machine (see Table 1, p.6). Many home users will buy an 'integrated' software package because it offers several functions at minimal cost. This often consists of a word processor (for writing letters, reports), spreadsheet (accounting, numerical data entry), paint module (for freehand graphics), drawing module (for precise lines), database (storing related data), and communications module (for talking to other computers). These 'works' packages are often pre-loaded on new machines, although not usually the latest versions.

Don't feel that every task on your list can only be performed by an expensive commercial package: there are usually free or 'shareware' (try-before-you-buy, for a small fee) alternatives available that are perfectly adequate. You can obtain these legally from colleagues, mail-order outfits, computer magazines, or online services. If you have specialist requirements, such as a certain computer-assisted learning package, buy your software first and then a machine to run it. Most quality software comes with a tutorial, and a number of companies produce training videos or run an introductory course.

What are operating systems?

The abbreviation 'PC' is usually applied to personal computers made by a variety of manufacturers (e.g. Compaq, Packard Bell, Dell, etc.) to be mostly compatible with an original design by IBM. Other designs, such as the Amiga and Apple Macintosh are not **IBM-compatibles** (or 'clones'). That is, they cannot use software designed for use with IBM-compatible PCs. The reason for this incompatibility relates to the fact that these machines use different operating systems running on different CPUs.

An **operating system** is the set of special programs and routines a computer uses to perform basic tasks like starting up and managing files. More specific tasks, such as word processing, are handled by different *application* programs that call on the routines in the operating system software to accomplish their special functions. You could think of the operating system as being analogous to the nervous system in the human body. It controls all the other systems that let us perform everyday tasks like digestion or movement. Operating-system software is usually pre-installed on the computer when you buy it (see Table 2).

A PC ordinarily runs **DOS** (such as MS-DOS from Microsoft), **OS/2** (from IBM), or **Microsoft Windows** software (commonly Windows 3.1, Windows for Workgroups 3.11, or Windows 95). A PC running the DOS operating system alone can run only DOS application programs. Windows (including Windows 95) can run DOS programs in addition to its own Windows programs. OS/2 can run DOS, Windows and native OS/2 programs simultaneously. **UNIX** is an operating system for larger multi-user computers likely to be encountered on campus and in dealings with the Internet, but not often on a personal computer. The Macintosh and Amiga also have unique operating systems. The Amiga is

TABLE 2 Operating systems

Operating system (OS)	Company	Notes
JavaOS	Sun Microsystems	An OS designed to run Java applets directly on network computers (NCs)†.
MS-DOS	Microsoft	An 8-bit* command-line OS developed for the first IBM PCs.
Windows 3.1	Microsoft	A graphical interface program for DOS. Windows 3.1 programs are easier to use but run more slowly than those written for DOS only.
Windows for Workgroups	Microsoft	As Windows 3.1, but with built-in networking.
Windows 95	Microsoft	A mostly 32-bit OS for PCs which provides interface improvements and no longer depends on DOS (although it can run DOS and Windows 3.1 software.)
Windows NT	Microsoft	A memory-hungry 32-bit version of Windows designed to run on multi-user computers. Does not rely on DOS.
OS/2 Warp	IBM	A 32-bit alternative to DOS/Windows that will run Windows programs, but few programs are available specifically for OS/2.
Mac OS	Apple	A 32-bit OS for the Macintosh.
UNIX	Various	A 32-bit OS designed to run on powerful multi-user computers. Versions exist for all major platforms. X Windows provides a window-based interface.

† See p.207.

* An 8-bit OS processes 8 units of information at a time; a 32-bit OS can work with four times as much data and is therefore more powerful. Bits are explained on p.21.

primarily a home computer and although it can be used to connect to online services, for reasonable compatibility in other medical applications your choice is really between an IBM-PC compatible and a Macintosh.

Windows 95 from Microsoft no longer operates as an add-on graphical interface to DOS, but is an integrated window-based operating system. The Macintosh operating system (**Mac OS**) will work on both PowerPC-based machines, and older 680x0-based Macs. The Windows NT, Windows 95, Mac OS, and OS/2 operating systems now have built-in support for Internet connections.

It does not really matter what type of computer/operating system you use to view World-Wide Web pages (p.197) on the Internet. Most Internet software looks and works pretty much the same across the range of operating systems. Furthermore, because the basic software behind the Internet (Chapter Twelve) is understood by practically all types of operating system, it is easy to get information from one type of computer to another.

The integration of Sun Microsystems' Java technology into future versions of major operating systems may change the way some applications are currently dependent on a particular operating system/hardware platform. By building a 'Java Virtual Machine' into operating systems, programs written in Java (applets) will work on machines running Macintosh, Windows, and UNIX operating system software. The 'picoJava' microprocessor, a hardware alternative to the Java Virtual Machine, will run Java applets directly and is expected to appear in network computers (NCs). For more details about Java and NCs, see p.207.

Future releases of Macintosh and Windows operating systems are expected to bring the familiarity of the World-Wide Web interface (p.197) to everyday file-management tasks. Both these developments could see that the actual operating system running on your computer almost becomes irrelevant.

PC versus Macintosh

Most people using modems to connect to the Internet use a PC or a Mac. Macs and PCs running Microsoft Windows use pull-down menus and icons, and are said to provide a **graphical user interface**, or GUI (the alternative is a **command-line interface**, as used by DOS and UNIX). The Mac OS is cleaner and more intuitive than Windows, making the Mac an easier machine for new users. The gap is closing, however, and both systems can be learned quickly; but basic tasks like installing new software, naming files, using icons, and adding peripherals are still simpler on the Mac. The biggest advantage of the PC is its historical market dominance with many companies producing 'clone' PCs, whereas Apple Computer did not license their technology until early 1995.

Because of this dominance, more software titles are available for PCs than for Macs. As software written for one operating system/hardware **platform** will not necessarily be available for another, your choice of application software may restrict you to either a PC or a Mac.

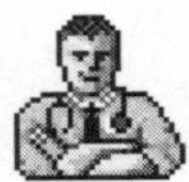

If the software you want is available for both Mac and PC, go to a supplier and compare the machines side-by-side, and talk to an advocate of each platform. Compatibility is a major consideration: will you be exchanging files with a like machine at work or home?

On more powerful Macs you can run Microsoft Windows under **emulation** (software translation of instructions for one operating system into instructions for another, a typically slow process). Some Macs can be fitted with a 'DOS Compatibility Card', creating a hybrid Mac/ PC in hardware. Macs can read and write PC disks as standard, and if you are attracted to the Mac but need to use the occasional PC program, this degree of cross-platform compatibility could be a satisfactory solution.

But choosing a machine isn't as simple as that. The application software itself can have hardware requirements additional to the operating system with which it can be run, such as available memory and hard-disk size, the power of the CPU, the presence of a coprocessor, a CD-ROM drive, etc. Some of these factors can also influence the speed at which communications software works. Be sure to take this into account when you define the minimum hardware configuration that will perform the tasks you require.

Notebook versus desktop

A **notebook** computer, the book-sized successor to the portable and laptop, has a distinct advantage: it can go where you go. You can get the same power in a notebook as you can in a bigger **desktop** machine. Portability, however, creates engineering difficulties, and you will have to pay for the genius of those who solve such problems.

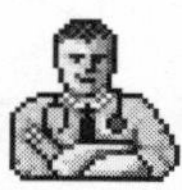

Unless you really need portability, opt for a desktop computer.

If you do want to take a modem-equipped notebook on call with you for between-patient Internet access, there are extra considerations specific to these machines. Inherently compact screens reduce the size of the display and in many cases the quality (unless you plug in an external monitor, but then its no longer portable!). Notebook computers use either active or passive matrix displays. 'Active matrix' technology (including the thin film transistor or **TFT**) produces a sharp image but at a premium. Cheaper 'passive matrix' screens (including the **dual scan** type) are characterized by less clarity and contrast, disappearance of the moving cursor ('submarining'), and a restricted viewing angle. A further cost of a more advanced screen in notebook computers is battery life. Notebooks can be used while simultaneously recharging the battery, but battery quality varies.

Because of battery drainage and compact design the ability to add internal accessories is limited. Most notebooks can be used with externally powered devices such as modems, and sometimes plug-in credit card-sized **PC card** (formerly PCMCIA) devices. Some can slide in to a 'docking station' attached to a larger monitor and other devices, giving you the double benefit of portability and desktop practicality.

An even smaller alternative to a notebook is the 'palmtop computer' or '**personal digital assistant**' (PDA). Able to fit in a coat pocket, these devices feature miniature keypads or an electronic stylus/pen. An increasing range of medical utility and database software is available, and several devices can be connected to a pocket-sized modem for online access.

Optional extras

Remember to budget for certain optional extras and consumables such as ink and paper for the printer, a copy holder, mouse mat, floppy disks, CD-ROMs, games (for the children!), diagnostic software or hard-disk utilities (to keep the computer healthy), external speakers, a backup system (to protect against the loss of important files), a scanner (to copy images or text into the computer), insurance, software upgrades, maintenance, sound cards, notebook replacement batteries, virus-protection software, more memory, a multi-extension power lead, security (hardware or software), and file-compression software (p.44)—for example.

How to buy

You will usually buy a new computer from a reseller, high-street dealer, or mail-order company. Resellers are more likely to be able to give you specialist advice than sales people in a high-street store. Mail-order companies offer variable support, and you can't view what you're buying first, but they are usually the cheapest option. Many vendors have special deals on certain combinations of equipment or configurations, and it may be worthwhile examining these. Computing magazines often include buying advice ranging from things to consider before you buy, to what to do if there is a problem with your purchase, in addition to reviewing current 'best buys'.

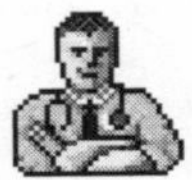

Choosing a system with several expansion options may provide better value in the longer term, ensuring that your hardware can keep up with your software requirements. *No* system will remain 'current' for more than a few years: this is a fact in the computer industry.

Once you have made your purchase, you can set up your system and familiarize yourself with it by following the instructions in the manuals that come with it. If you are a computer novice, you may want to invest in a book that will educate you on the specific quirks of your type of computer or operating system. Any good book store has a computing section, and you can peruse many choices of title to find one that suits your needs.

Bibliography

Lock, C. (1996). What value do computers provide to NHS hospitals? *BMJ*, **312**, 1407–10.

Sullivan, F. and Mitchell, E. (1995). Has general practitioner computing made a difference to patient care? *BMJ*, **311**, 848–52.

Lee, N. and Millman, A. (1996). *ABC of medical computing*. BMJ Publishing Group, London.

Osheroff, J.A. (ed.) (1995). *Computers in clinical practice: managing patients, information, and communication*. American College of Physicians, Philadelphia.

British Journal of Healthcare Computing and Information Management, available from: BJHC Limited, 45 Woodland Grove, Weybridge, Surrey KT13 9EQ, UK.

M.D. Computing, available from: Springer-Verlag New York Inc., 175 Fifth Avenue, New York NY 10010, USA.

CHAPTER THREE
Choosing a modem

As mentioned in Chapter One, a modem is a device that translates computer data (binary code) to and from sound for transmission over telephone lines. The following headings serve to guide you in your choice of modem from the many makes available. Remember, however, that by law you are obliged to buy a modem that has been ratified by the British Approvals Board for Telecommunications (BABT) if you intend to use it in the UK. Shop around, bearing in mind that a well-known manufacturer is more likely to offer technical support. The quality of manuals for both the modem itself and communications software supplied with it are also important considerations. Take into account the warranty.

Hayes compatibility

The industry standard for modems is Hayes compatibility: Hayes have been manufacturing modems for some time, and support for the **Hayes AT command set** ensures that a modem of any make can perform the tasks asked of it (the 'AT' stands for 'attention'). The letters, numbers, and symbols that make up the AT command set are used to control the protocols and features to be used when a modem connects to another modem. A Hayes-compatible modem can be connected, using an appropriate cable, to any computer with a **serial-communications port** (i.e. a socket for external modems and other peripherals).

Types of modem

There are three main types of modem: internal, external, and PC card modems. Internal modems, in the form of a plug-in card inside the computer, are designed to be fitted into a specific platform (e.g. PC or Mac) but take up less space and don't require an external power supply. External modems, encased in a plastic box connected to a computer, can easily be swapped from one computer to another, and many feature flashing lights that let you know what is happening—or what isn't. Some are so small that they make ideal 'pocket' companions for notebook computers. The third type is the smallest. PC card modems are the size of a credit card, and slot in to the PC card slot commonly found in notebook computers (p.17). **Cable modems**, using TV cable networks for data transmission, have been developed more recently (p.136).

The need for speed

Modulation protocols govern the basic speed of a connection before the application of data compression and other variables, which is measured as **bits per second** (bps). A **bit** is the smallest unit of data used by a computer: a 0 or 1—the elements of binary code.

TABLE 3 Important modem protocols

Protocol	Speed (bps)	Note
V.22bis	2400	Slow, used by older modems.
V.32	Up to 9 600	Low-end high-speed connection.
V.32bis	Up to 14 400	Widely available high-speed connection. Practical minimum for using Internet WWW.*
V.34	Up to 28 800	Current ratified top speed over ordinary phone lines. Current standard for Internet access.
(Unofficial)	Up to 33 600	Enhanced V.34, not ratified or widely supported.
MNP5	n/a	2:1 data compression (and MNP4 error correction).
V.42bis	n/a	4:1 data compression.
MNP4	n/a	Older error-correction protocol.
V.42	n/a	More recent error-correction protocol.

* World-Wide Web.

Modulation protocols are standardized by a United Nations agency called ITU-T (International Telecommunication Union, formerly the CCITT); the more important protocols are listed in Table 3.

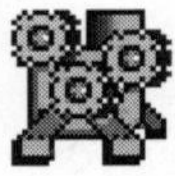

Modem speeds are sometimes given as a **baud** rate, an outdated term describing the number of signal events transmitted per second using a single frequency change. Bits per second and baud are not necessarily equivalent since today's modems transmit a variable number of bits per signal event using multiple frequencies, so if someone talks about baud ask them what they mean.

There are a number of proprietary protocols too, such as HST (US Robotics); PEP (Telebit); and Express 96 (Hayes). Proprietary modulation requires a modem of the same make in order to achieve a high-speed (9600 bps or greater) connection, although some also support ITU-T protocols, so you can connect to them at high speed (such modems are known as 'dual standard'). It would be unwise to buy a modem that supported only a proprietary protocol.

Since time costs money, one can quickly run up some rather expensive phone bills with a slow modem, additional to those imposed by the online service (if applicable). This factor will soon exceed the cost of the modem itself. One caveat: a link between two modems will be only as fast as the slowest of the two, since one will drop down to the highest shared speed. All fast modems are capable of dropping their speed to connect to slower ones ('automatic speed fallback'). Thus, be realistic in your choice: there's little gained by paying for a 28 800 bps modem if you'll only be connecting to a 9600 bps bulletin board. Of course if you do buy such a device, it may be a long wait until the rest of the world catches up, by which time these modems will be significantly cheaper.

Reading bulletin-board messages online isn't really faster using a high-speed modem: extra speed becomes apparent when **downloading** (retrieving) files. Internet connections, however, generally require a high-speed modem: even 14 000 bps can be frustratingly slow at times, and using the World-Wide Web (see Chapter 26) at 9600 bps is barely tolerable. Today, a modem with **V.32bis** (see Table 3) is a good buy only if you really can't afford **V.34**. Even a 2400 bps modem will suffice, however, if you intend only to read and send occasional e-mail on a bulletin board (BBS) and not transfer large files. Do remember, though, it's easy to get hooked and you will soon lust for speed.

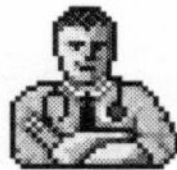

Most people would advise that you buy the fastest modem you can afford. Think of this as an investment, however. A 28 800 bps modem, for example, may not always provide you with the improvement you might expect over a 14 400 bps modem. Often the bottleneck is the Internet itself—not the top speed of your modem (although this can be a bottleneck as well). Future improvements in the Internet's data-carrying capacity (bandwidth) should enable users to take better advantage of the hardware we are using today.

Handshaking

Handshake or 'flow control' is jargon for the regulation of the rate of flow of data between your modem and computer (and between the two modems either end of a link). Flow control ensures that the modem never has to wait for data, and nor is it swamped by too much data at once. Flow control can take place using *software* or **XON/XOFF handshaking** in which case control signals are included in the transmitted data, although modems achieve higher connection speeds through **hardware handshaking** (or 'RTS/CTS', using certain pins on the RS-232 serial port). This is more reliable and requires a special cable to connect computer and modem. Make sure your modem comes with the appropriate cable (note that Mac and PC modem cables are different too).

What are compression protocols for?

Look at the supported **compression protocols** when making your choice: using data compression it is possible to get transfer rates equal to a 38 400 bps link using a 9 600 bps

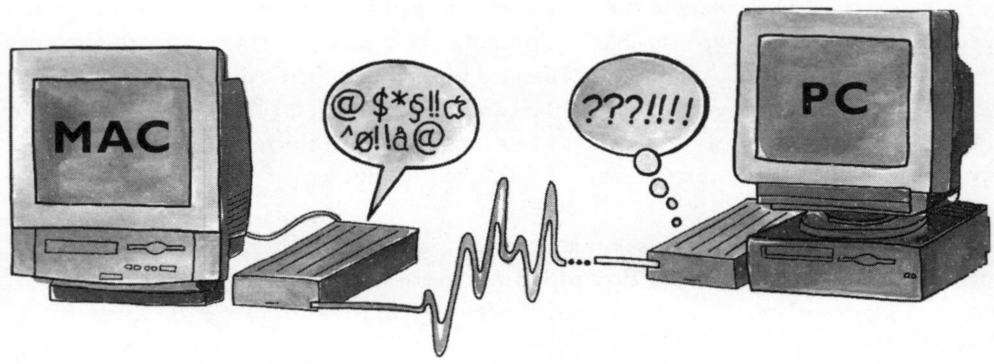

Fig. 3 Speaking the same language. A modem at either end of a telephone line allows digital information (the 0s and 1s of binary code) to be converted into analog sound for transmission—and back again. Both modems must understand the same protocols, or conversation will be impossible.

modem—at least in *theory*. As with modulation protocols, compression (and error-correction) protocols can be invoked only if they are supported by *both* modems in the link (see Fig. 3). Data compression involves the sending modem compacting the data to reduce transmission time, and the receiving modem decompressing it again. When downloading files from a bulletin board (BBS), **MNP5** data compression can halve transfer time in the case of text files, and ITU-T **V.42bis** can quarter it. Neither protocol is of much use when a file has already been compressed, by a program such as Stuffit or WinZip, as these programs are more efficient. Using MNP5 in this instance can even make files larger! (V.42bis can detect compressed files). Because compressing data may introduce errors, some form of error correction is required. But there are other sources of error in modem transmissions, and these are overcome by specific error-correction protocols.

What does error correction do?

Noisy phone lines, among other factors, can introduce errors into data transmitted along them. This problem is worse if you are making a long distance call. **MNP4** and ITU-T **V.42** are examples of **error-correction protocols**, which filter out bits of data that shouldn't be there (literally). Proprietary protocols also exist, such as 'ARQ' hardware error checking from US Robotics. A modem with ITU-T V.42 can error control when connected to a modem supported by MNP4. Error correction is recommended during online chat (see Chapter Six), and when sending messages to a bulletin board. It is less important during file transfers, since file-transfer protocols usually have built-in error checking—see Chapter Four, p.31. These protocols can slightly improve transfer times because of the way error correction organizes data before sending it.

Communications software

When you connect to an online service, transfer times may be limited not only by the speed of their modem, but also by the characteristics of the software you use to connect with. For example, the speed at which you are able to collect and read mail may differ from that of file downloads.

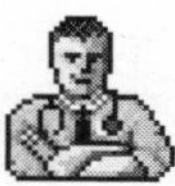

Good modems come with communications software which includes modem drivers (configuration instructions) for that particular modem.

A good strategy is to talk with users of various packages, and read magazine reviews to decide what would best suit your needs. For further guidance, refer to Chapter Four.

S-Registers

You may see this term listed in a modem specification sheet. Like a computer, a modem stores basic settings, such as 'answer the phone after one ring', in a certain area of memory which is not erased when the power is switched off. S-Register commands are similar to the Hayes AT command set and allow you to change these settings. They serve the same function as the 'preferences' file created by many application programs, where certain settings are maintained until they are deliberately changed. You don't normally have to worry about these.

Fax capability

Nearly all modems sold today come with the capacity to send and receive faxes. Getting the software working reliably still seems to be a bit of a task, but it can be done! Your computer is transformed into a *limited* fax machine: a letter typed in Microsoft Word, for example, complete with your digitized signature and letterhead graphic, can be converted to a high-quality fax. Fax modems cannot transmit documents that are already on paper—a scanner will solve this problem.

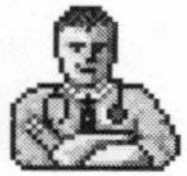

It is possible to 'sign' faxes sent from your screen. Have a colleague fax a copy of your signature to the computer (or use a digital scanner). Using 'cut-and-paste', the image can be placed within a document.

Any fax-capable modem you purchase should support the 'Group 3 Protocol', which is the standard common to all fax-capable devices.

CHAPTER FOUR
Communications software basics

In this section we discuss choosing a communications software package for general use. In addition, the important difference between transferring text files and binary files is explained. Although the type of software looked at here can be used for certain types of Internet access, Internet communications software is covered elsewhere (see Parts Three and Four).

Terminal emulation

A **terminal emulator** is a type of communications software that provides a simple interface to allow communication between two or more computers. A terminal consists of a monitor and keyboard physically linked to a central computer-system unit. Communications software can 'emulate' such a physical terminal connection over ordinary telephone lines, or over cabling directly linking two personal computers together. When using terminal emulation to 'talk' with another computer, terminal software displays messages that are sent back to your computer from the one you are communicating with. It also controls the sending of anything you type to the remote **host** (i.e. the distant computer that is hosting the communications session). The other principal use of terminal emulation software is supporting file transfers over telephone or direct links, meaning two or more people can swap information and programs without ever meeting each other (see below). These facilities are at the heart of the bulletin-board concept.

An easy way to obtain terminal emulation programs is to get a 'shareware' (try-before-you-buy) program from a friend, a user group, online service, or mail order software company. Popular examples are ProComm for the PC and ZTerm for the Macintosh. The alternative is to invest in a commercial package which will, for the most part, offer little over its shareware cousins.

Frequently, you will be asked to complete a terminal-preferences questionnaire when you first log on to a particular online service. This is necessary because of the way terminal emulation works; when you use this software, you are in effect emulating a certain type of terminal that would usually be connected to the computer playing host to you. The different types of terminal are characterized by such things as the number of rows and columns on their screens, which key will indicate a **Delete** or **Backspace** command, the use of graphics and special characters, how a screen full of information is cleared, and how the cursor is controlled. Some types of terminal that you may come across are given in Table 4. Emulation of an ANSI terminal is illustrated in Fig. 4.

TABLE 4 Common types of terminal emulation

Terminal type	Note
TTY	'Teletype' is the basic type of terminal, capable of displaying ASCII characters but no graphics. Formatting of text is simple.
ANSI	American National Standards Institute terminal emulation. Uses an ASCII sequence beginning with the escape character to control cursor movement, text attributes (e.g. bold, blink), simple colour graphics, and keyboard settings. If not enabled you will see only plain text. If the service called is run on a PC this type would be a good choice.
VT series	Versions of Digital Equipment (DEC) terminals, the most basic being VT52, with VT100, VT102, VT220, VT320, and VT420 adding control sequences. If the service called is run on a UNIX or DEC machine, VT100 is an industry standard and would be a good choice.
RIP	Uses graphical elements stored on the callers machine to draw colour screens rapidly. Also permits mouse input.

Client software

A **client** program is operated by a user, and provides an interface to a **server** (a machine hosting an online service) which directs the sharing of the resources it controls among a number of users/clients. Client software is specific to one type of online service. For example, CompuServe produce their own particular client program, designed to work only with their server software (the programs running the service). Client and server programs always work together, with the client issuing requests and the server fulfilling them. So long as the server software can understand the requests made by a client program, it does not matter if a user has a different type of computer from that of the server. The rules for such an understanding are defined in a 'client–server protocol'. A 'networking protocol', such as TCP/IP (see Chapter Twelve), sometimes transports the client–server protocol across the physical link between machines.

Client software is more sophisticated than a basic terminal emulator. Commands are still being sent back-and-forth, but behind the facade of an easier-to-use graphical interface. This is similar to the relationship between DOS and Windows (pre-Windows 95), where Windows acts as a buffer between the user and the ugly workings of DOS prompts and commands. While graphical elements like windows, icons, progress bars, and pull-down menus are attractive, you will still need a basic terminal emulation program so you can try out other online services. Client software is often available free of charge, although certain commercial services request that you pay for it as part of your membership package.

Basic file types and file-transfer protocols

The two basic types of file you will encounter when using an online service or the Internet are ASCII files and binary files.

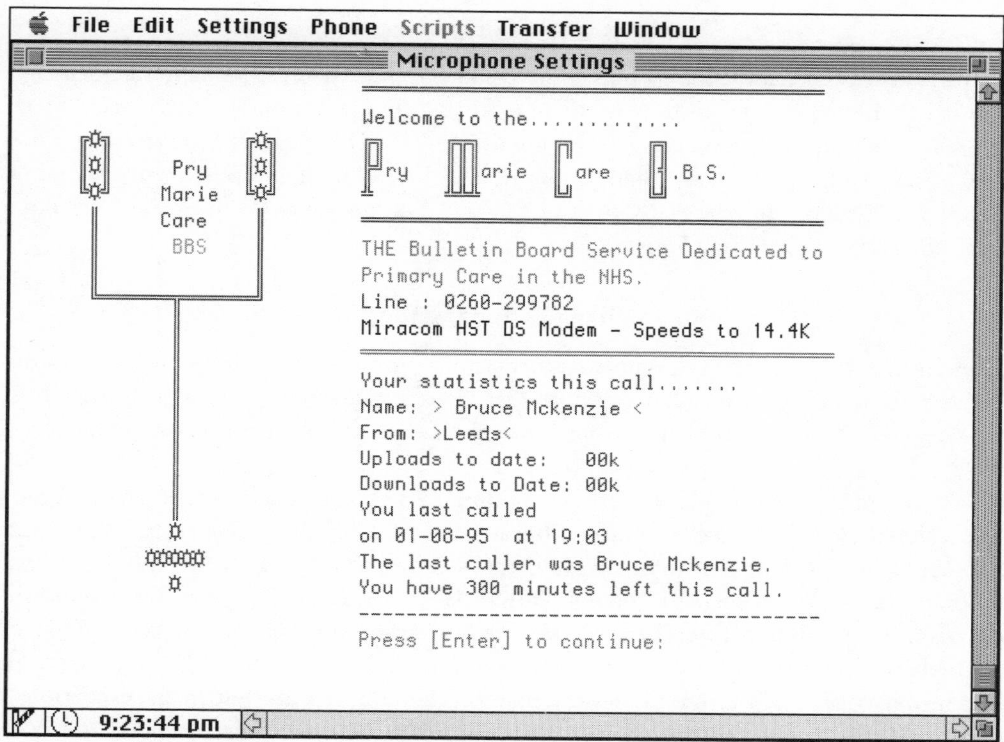

Fig. 4 Terminal emulation. This bulletin board supports the emulation of an ANSI terminal, allowing the display of simple colour and graphics. [Reproduced with permission.]

What is ASCII?

Chapter Two introduced the idea that all information stored on a computer is represented in terms of 0 and 1, or 'binary code'. Early in the history of personal computers these binary digits (i.e. 'bits') were grouped together in lots of seven, creating 128 possible combinations of 0 and 1 (2 to the power of 7). Each combination was known as an 'ASCII code', an acronym for **American Standard Code for Information Interchange**. As the name indicates, these codes were devised as a standard for exchanging information between computers (although there are several international variants of US-ASCII now). Because a string of 7 numbers doesn't mean much to most people, each code is represented by a simple symbol that carries some meaning—a **character** like the letter '**a**', or a full stop. For example, the character '**B**' represents the code 1000010. Once codes had been assigned to upper- and lower-case letters, numbers, punctuation, and other familiar 'typewriter' symbols (the 'printable set'), the remaining codes were taken up with 'control codes' (such as **Backspace** and **Carriage Return**). The full set of 128 characters is known as the **ASCII character set**.

What is an ASCII or text file?

To the eye, ASCII data contains only simple characters with very basic arrangements of words into blocks of text. In fact, **text file** is frequently used synonymously with **ASCII file**, even though a text file may (rarely) contain non-ASCII characters. An ASCII/text file contains *only* ASCII characters, and will appear on any type of computer with the same characters displayed in essentially the same layout. Simple '**Read Me**' files and electronic mail, for example, fall into this category.

What is a binary file?

Modern personal computers group together 8 bits (in one of two states) at a time and, because 2 to the power of 8 is 256, can store 256 different characters. The first 128 characters are relegated to the ASCII character set across the range of computer operating systems.

However, the lack of a standard for the remaining 128 codes led computer manufacturers to develop their own unique '**extended character sets**'. Most are used to represent various lines and graphics symbols. On the IBM PC they became 'PC-graphics characters' whereas, for example, on a Mac keyboard **Option-Shift-K** produces the Apple logo from the Macintosh character set. The International Organization for Standardization has defined its own version of the extra codes (often incorrectly called 'extended ASCII') in ISO 8859-1 (known as 'Latin alphabet No. 1'). Program files and many of their documents (with a few exceptions) use all 256 possible characters and are called **binary files** to distinguish them from ASCII files.

Why is the difference important?

There are two main reasons why binary files should be distinguished from ASCII files. Firstly, because binary files created for one type of computer may contain characters unique to that computer's character set, they may not be readable on a different type of machine. While every word processor has an option to read ASCII text files, binary files are more complex. Some binary programs adopt certain **cross-platform** standards for their files, such as the Graphics Interchange Format and some word-processor files. These help ensure that they can be used on a different computer types without prior modification. Other binary files can be used on different type of computer providing that the receiving computer has 'translation' software. Thus, a Microsoft-Word file created on a PC can be read by a Mac user with the Mac version of Word, or alternatively a program like ClarisWorks which has a Word-format translator. Another group of binary files comprises those that are of no use at all on any computer but the one they were created on.

Mac files actually comprise two principal parts (so-called data and resource forks), both critical to Mac files (with exceptions, like text files and GIF images). Sometimes Mac files have to pass through non-Mac computers or online services that don'trecognize this unique structure. Mac communications programs, by default, ensure that files are converted into a single binary file using the **MacBinary** file format for uploading, and automatically split into separate forks again when downloaded. If you see a file ending in the suffix **.bin** it is a MacBinary file and no use to you unless you have a Macintosh.

The second reason for users being aware of the difference between binary and ASCII files relates to the way they are handled by file-transfer protocols.

File-transfer protocols

File-transfer protocols describe certain rules for handling file transfers between computers. The two types of file-transfer protocols are those that use 7-bit characters and those that use 8-bit characters (data bits) to transfer information. The common individual protocols are listed in Table 5. The file-transfer protocol used on the Internet, FTP, is discussed separately in Chapter Twenty one.

Because the ASCII character set contains only 7-bit characters, ASCII or 'text' transfer protocol is commonly used (inappropriately) to describe file transfers using only 7-bit characters. If sending a text file or message, the '**ASCII file-transfer protocol**' will do.

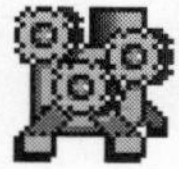

ASCII codes describing printable characters are the same on all platforms, but operating systems differ in the way they indicate the end of a line using ASCII control codes. For example, the Mac OS interprets 'line feeds' in files originating on a DOS system as a box, indicating that it does not use them in the same way. Such differences are usually automatically corrected for during an ASCII file-transfer, which poses no problem for text-only files.

Protocols like **Zmodem**, **Xmodem**, and **Ymodem** (see Table 5), on the other hand, work with 8-bit characters. These protocols are collectively termed **binary file-transfer protocols**, so-named because 'binary files' contain 8-bit characters. Binary protocols transfer characters several at a time as a 'packet'. These packets are reassembled into the original file on the receiving computer *without correction* by the operating system, as happens with ASCII transfers. Since they incorporate error checking, binary protocols instruct the sending modem to re-send any packet that the receiving modem has not received correctly. The sending modem will execute a limited number of retries before it terminates the file transfer.

TABLE 5 Summary of common file-transfer protocols

File-transfer protocol	Notes
ASCII	Works only for text transfers, such as sending and receiving e-mail. No error correction therefore noisy lines may result in data loss, especially at high speed, if not using your modem's built-in error correction.
Kermit	Old, little used but most platforms support it. Can transfer binary files over 7-bit communications links.
Xmodem	Widespread error-correcting protocol. Transfers one file at a time.
Ymodem (Xmodem-1K)	Xmodem derivative with larger data blocks. Transfers one file at at time.
Ymodem (Batch)	As Ymodem but allows simultaneous file transfers.
Ymodem-g	Variant of Ymodem (Batch) with no error correction. Fast but requires MNP4, V.42, or similar error control.
Zmodem	Resumes download after interruption. Fast. Allows simultaneous file transfers and wildcards (e.g. *.txt sends all text files).

Binary protocols often achieve error correction using 'checksums' or 'Cyclical Redundancy Checks' (CRCs), with the latter being more reliable but increasing the size of the transmitted file.

Zmodem is a widely supported and useful protocol, so if the terminal emulation software you are considering does not support it, you should probably look elsewhere.

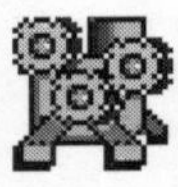

Error-correcting (i.e. binary) file-transfer protocols may be used in conjunction with a modem's own error-correction protocols (i.e. MNP5 and V.42bis—p.24), and likewise must be supported at the sending and receiving end of the connection.

You cannot download or upload a binary file using a 7-bit file transfer protocol because all the 8-bit non-ASCII characters within it would be misinterpreted, rendering it unusable. Binary file-transfer protocols *do* understand 8-bit characters and therefore transmit binary files intact. You can also use a binary transfer-protocol to transfer ASCII text files (although it won't be modified to suit your operating system).

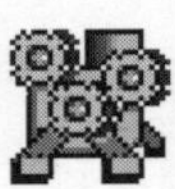

Note that all binary files can be converted into text files for transfer as electronic mail. This is called 'ASCII encoding' and is discussed in Chapter Seventeen. **Kermit** is an especially clever binary file-transfer protocol that can be used to transfer binary files over 7-bit systems by encoding the 8-bit data into 7-bit packets for transmission.

Summary

The two basic types of file are ASCII files and binary files. ASCII (text) files can be read on any type of computer. Binary (program) files contain non-ASCII data and often require a specific program or operating system to be used so they can be read.

A binary file-transfer protocol should always be used to transfer binary files. The so-called ASCII file-transfer protocol can handle text files without problems, but using it to transfer binary files will corrupt them (unless they are specially encoded).

Other features of communications software

Scripting

Some packages and client programs supply you with a scripting option. A 'script' is a list of instructions that tells the modem how to behave when you dial a particular online service. It can navigate a path via several networks to connect to the desired host computer, automate the **log-on** process, give control to another program, or automatically collect messages and **log off** (disconnect). In this regard, scripts can save time by allowing you to read your messages **offline** (when you have disconnected). Some services offer utilities that improve and greatly simplify this facility in the form of **offline readers**, such as BulkRate for FirstClass or Navigator for CompuServe.

Macros

Macros can likewise save precious seconds online by assigning a string of text to a key or key combination that you specify (such as **F-6**, or **Command-Shift-I**). You can use macros to automate the typing of such things as an alternative initialization string (see below), your user name or signature, or storing Hayes commands that change the configuration of your modem (such as switching 'auto answering' on/off).

Phonebooks

A phonebook will allow you to store frequently dialled numbers, or even better, the configuration details that are particular to each service such as terminal type. A variation of this is the settings document created by some programs.

Scroll-back buffer

A scroll-back buffer (also called a review buffer) stores in memory a record of the most recent dialogue between the two connected computers, allowing you to review instructions, messages, or menu options. It is also useful to be able to 'cut' from this and other text files, and 'paste' the text into a message to save retyping.

Keyboard buffer

The keyboard buffer is useful primarily for online discussions such as a two-way 'chat' on a bulletin board (p.47). In the keyboard buffer window you can type a few sentences and ensure they are correct. Usually you then press the **Enter** key so what you have typed will be sent out all in one go, rather than character-by-character as typed.

Capture log

You may also like to save the continually updated data in the scroll-back buffer to a more permanent text file on disk. This is called a capture log, and can later be edited or stored like any other file. In order to keep down the cost of your telephone calls, you can use this facility to capture messages without reading them until you have closed the modem connection.

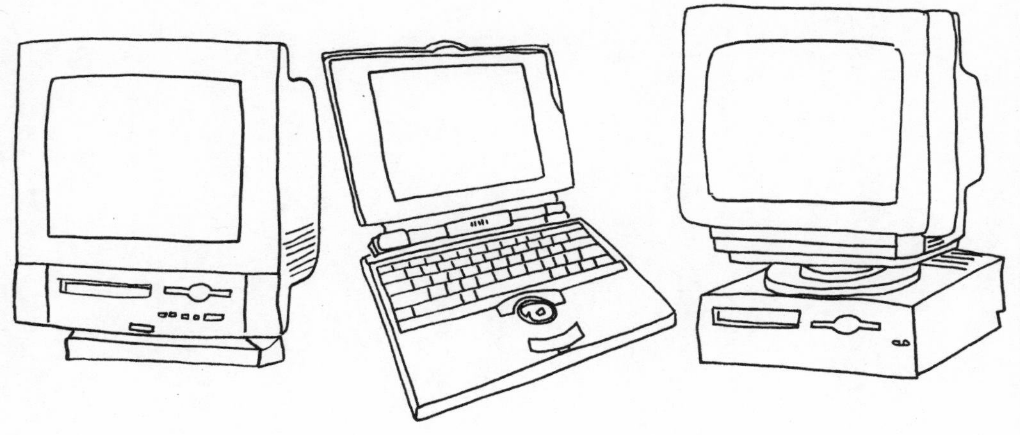

PART 2

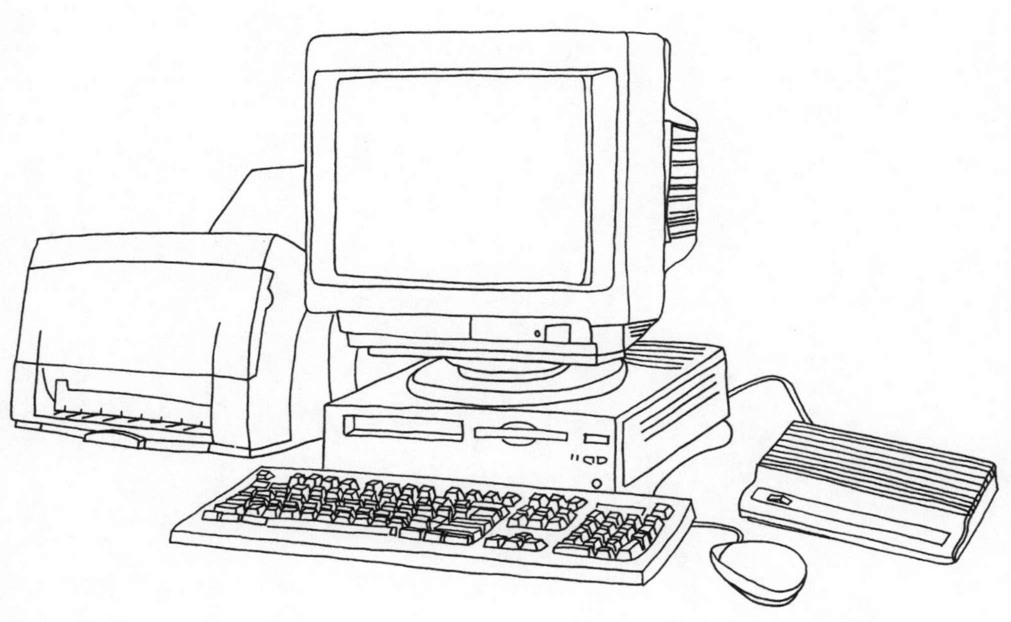

CHAPTER FIVE
Going online

For the purposes of this Part, 'going **online**' refers to the act of connecting to a bulletin board service or commercial online service. Although one also goes online when connecting to the Internet, this is discussed elsewhere (see Parts Three and Four).

Bulletin-board services

A bulletin board is a forum where callers can read and post messages relating to certain topics. A **bulletin-board service** (BBS), however, is not limited to messages. Most offer file libraries like their commercial cousins (see below), but their resources are not normally sufficient to provide online reference databases. A number of these services make CD-ROMs available online. The simplest BBSs run server software which callers interact with by typing in commands and menu choices. Others have a graphical user interface. BBSs are usually hosted on a single computer with one or two modem lines, operated by amateurs from home and without profit (Fig. 5). BBS administrators are also known as **sysops**, as in *sys*tem *op*erator. A few BBSs are set up by various organizations for a specific purpose, such as support, or to foster communication between members of a learned organization.

Small BBSs sometimes link up by modem to a neighbouring service on a regular basis to exchange messages. This 'pass-the-parcel' way of communicating (known technically as 'store-and-forward') forms the basis of the **FidoNet** and **OneNet** networks. An increasing number of BBSs are also able to exchange Internet e-mail and Usenet news (p.138).

Commercial online services

At some uncertain point, a BBS becomes sufficiently distinct to be called something else. Commercial **online services** have a number of general characteristics when compared with a typical BBS.

- They comprise a large network of computers, rather than a single machine.
- They normally have many modem lines allowing users to connect via a local call, sometimes by way of a third-party network.
- Some services are international, meaning you can use them without making a long distance call when travelling.
- They are profit-generating, and as a result cost more to use.
- They make available a greater volume and variety of material than smaller privately run services, including comprehensive databases such as MEDLINE.

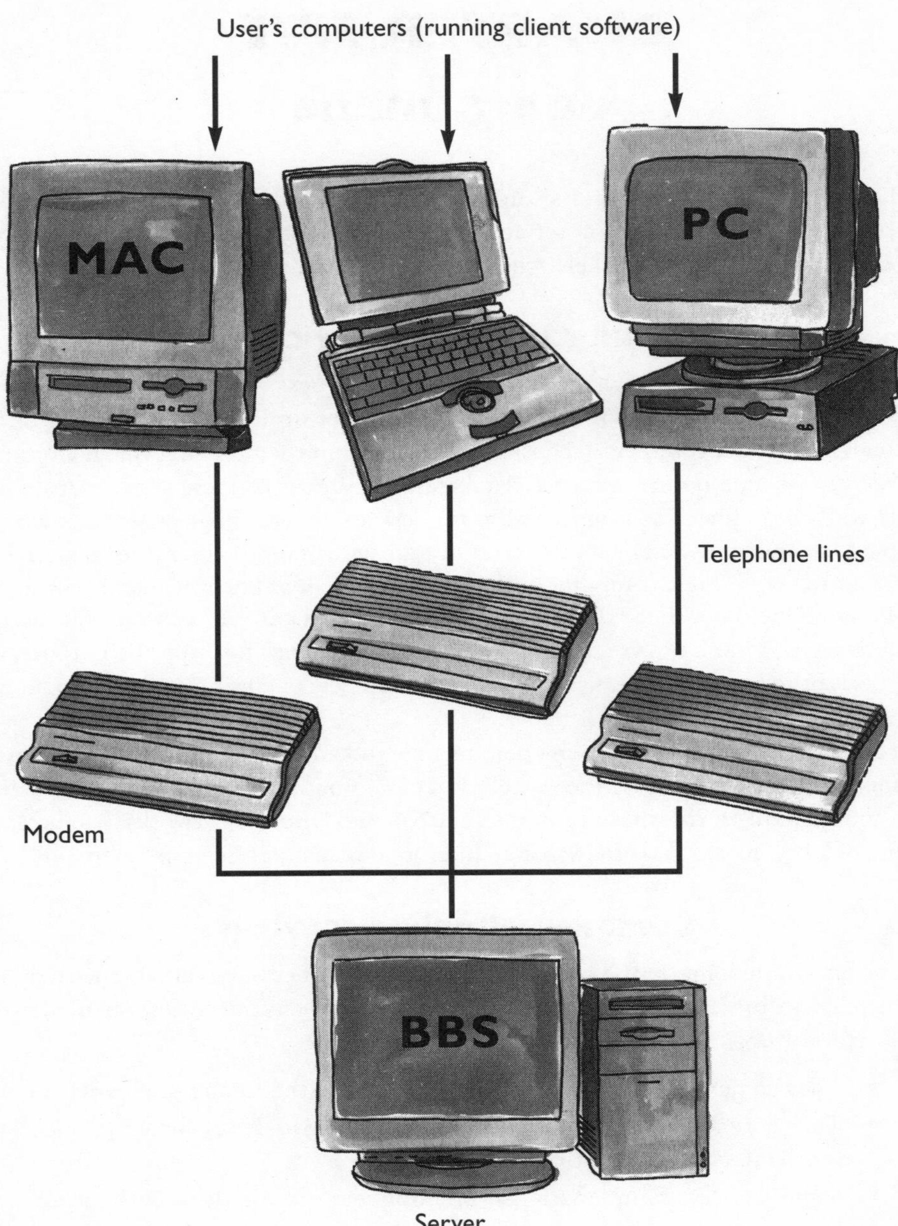

Fig. 5 How a bulletin board works. One or more users connect to the server using a modem. The server is a computer running software that allows it to fulfil the requests made by each user, such as reading messages and downloading files. CD-ROMs, such as a MEDLINE database or image collection, can be made available online.

A host of commercial online services are available such as America Online, Compulink Information eXchange (CIX), CompuServe, Delphi, and Prodigy. The largest commercial service in the world is the US-based America OnLine (AOL), followed closely by the CompuServe Information Service (CIS). Both AOL and CIS are available to UK and other European callers. CIS is a more established service and the variety of its medical content is exemplified in Chapter Ten.

Where to start?

If you are starting out with computers and modems you may already have discovered that telecommunicating is somewhat trickier than using a word processor.

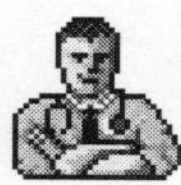

This author recommends learning about online services by joining one with an easy-to-use graphical interface.

The skills that you will learn through using the service—sending and receiving electronic mail, retrieving files, handling file suffixes, and participating in forums, etc.—will all prove invaluable when you come to tackle the Internet.

Further, many smaller BBSs and the larger services offer some form of Internet connectivity. This has the advantage of allowing you to learn about the Internet in a *familiar* and friendly environment with the support of other users. Jumping head-first into the Internet without some basic experience in using an online service can lead to confusion. Online services are not alike, so find one that suits you.

Getting help

All bulletin boards and commercial online services provide some sort of member assistance. In its simplest form, this can involve sending a message to the sysop. At the other extreme some services offer new user forums, online manuals and help files, printed user guides and manuals, and even books describing how to get the most out of their service. Of these choices, the most satisfying solution is often to pose a question in a relevant online forum and wait for more experienced users to reply. The online community is generally altruistic!

A number of bulletin boards are associated with 'user groups'. These groups are composed of both experienced and novice users, and often hold local meetings or send out newsletters sharing advice and offering assistance. Computing magazines commonly list user-group details.

Another option is to become a member of the British Computer Society (BCS). Among its specialist groups are the Primary Health Care Specialist Group (PHCSG), Medical London, Medical Northern, Medical Scotland, and Nursing. All these groups provide forums for discussion and support. The BCS can be contacted on 01793 417417, or you can send Internet e-mail to **membenq@bcs.org.uk**.

When you've finished this Part you should:

in relation to online services,

- know something of the different characters of bulletin-board services and commercial online services, and also of their similarities
- be able to indentify the file type and/or program needed to decompress a file by its' suffix

be capable of

- configuring your communications software and modem in order to get online

understand

- your responsibilities with respect to online etiquette, patient confidentiality, data security, and the acknowledgement of electronic authorship

be aware of

- the variety of online medical services and resources that exist even before considering those on the Internet.

CHAPTER SIX
Using a bulletin-board service

Before looking at the actual process of getting connected to an online service, it is worth reviewing what to expect once you have logged on. The sorts of computer files you might come across (whether you are connecting to a bulletin board or to the Internet) are also introduced here. Whether or not the service uses a graphical interface (see Fig. 6) or a command-line interface (like DOS), most have a number of common features.

The most prevalent type of online service is the bulletin board. A 'bulletin-board service' (BBS) is a computer system set up to enable users to dial in over phone lines with a modem, talk to one another by leaving messages, send each other files using the BBS as a common 'pick-up point', and 'download' (retrieve by modem) software that they would otherwise have to post on floppy disk. BBSs are often run by independent administrators who are involved because it's fun, and charge a very modest (or no) fee. Some services, such as AOL and CompuServe, are large commercial organizations who offer wider variety, more conferences, and larger software archives, and in the process make a profit. However, using such services is not unlike using a smaller BBS.

Some people like to conceptualize an online service as a sort of 'electronic town', or 'virtual community'. This analogy is derived from the electronic equivalents of services that you would find in a real town: a post office (electronic mail); library (file archive); news stand (electronic digests); community centres (sometimes heated discussions); cafes (casual online chat); and medical centre (where doctors lurk); etc.

Public messages

Public messages are sent by a user to an area on the BBS where they are readable by all users, such as a **conference** (online discussion, or forum) area. For some, such conference areas form the most significant part of the BBS; they provide an opportunity to ask other users for assistance, to share news and reviews, and to meet fellow callers. Participating can simply involve opening a new message, addressing it, giving it a name, typing the message, and sending or 'posting' it.

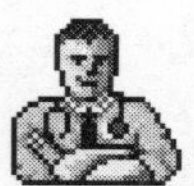

If composing a well thought-out reply to a message on a bulletin board (or even just posing a question), it is cheaper to compose the message 'offline'.

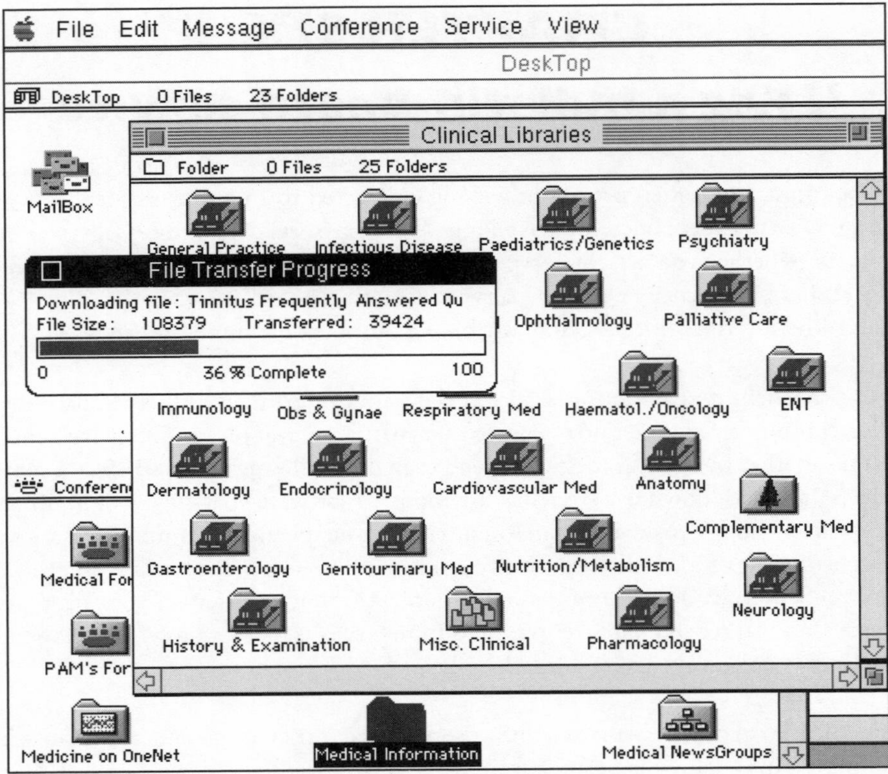

Fig. 6 A FirstClass bulletin board. A graphical interface, incorporating icons and pull-down menus, brings exceptional ease to navigating online conferences and file areas.

Some client programs, such as the CompuServe Information Manager, enable you to compose messages offline easily. An alternative way is to save the message as a text file and copy it into memory; when online, paste it into the body of a new message. Simple BBS software, however, may require you to indicate line ends within a message manually using the **Enter** or **Return** key (unlike word processors which automatically 'wrap' the text on to the next line). Offline message-reader programs automatically collect messages in pre-specified forums, and save them to disk for reading after logging off.

The nature of conference areas on a BBS will vary depending on the interests of the users of that BBS. You may find areas relating to messages from the administrator, areas discussing software and hardware, special-interest areas such as health, finance, news headlines, press releases, etc. Some BBSs carry conferences which are not simply local to that service, but shared among similar bulletin boards (e.g. FidoNet and FirstClass, p.47), or Internet conferences (called 'newsgroups', p.99).

Private messages

Private messages are similar to public messages, except that they are invisible to the majority of users, and readable only by one or more individuals you specify. To facilitate the reception of private mail, each user will have his or her own 'mailbox', appearing as a menu item or special folder depending on the BBS software. You will know when you have new mail, because the bulletin board software will tell you when you log on, or flag your mailbox in some way.

'Private', however, means your mail is not visible to the wider online community: it *does not* mean it can be read only by the recipient. Indeed, the administrator of a BBS will reserve the right to access these messages, although he or she would not have reason to do so. The same applies to the sending of e-mail through the Internet (see Chapter Nine).

Download areas

Not all software comes with a price tag, and not all software that does is sold through retailers. Commercial software is obviously under copyright, and its distribution through online services is in violation of copyright law (see also p.62). The main classes of downloadable software are **shareware** (fully working or partially disabled programs to 'try-before-you-buy'), **freeware** (the author does not request any money), and **public domain** programs. These types of software are explained further in Chapter Eight.

Downloadable files are often grouped by the BBS into separate areas such as games, applications, utilities (programs that aid the working of other programs), text files, sounds, graphics, etc. Obviously, much of this software is going to be of use to you only if it is compatible with the computer platform you are using (i.e. PC, Macintosh, Amiga, etc.). Graphics and text files are readable by virtually every platform, if not directly then via a program that modifies the file so it can be read or displayed on your machine.

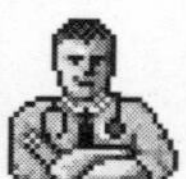

Remember that ASCII (text) files can be used on any type of computer, but the same may not be true of program (binary) files (see p.30). Before you download a binary file, make sure you can use it on your computer.

Often when you initiate a file download you will be given a choice of file-transfer protocol by the BBS software (see below). Once you have selected one, there will be a command required to proceed with the download, and then usually some indication that the download is taking place. Sometimes you need to tell your own communications program to begin receiving the file, depending on what file-transfer protocol you are using.

Some communications programs, such as those supporting the Zmodem file-transfer protocol (p.31), provide for the resumption of a file transfer at a later date, if for some reason the modem connection is lost. This means that rather than download the file from scratch, you can finish off receiving a partially downloaded file. To save time online, some services allow you to start downloading a file, and while this is happening you will be able to read your e-mail or peruse the messages in the conference area.

Understanding file suffixes

A **file suffix** is usually a three-letter acronym beginning with a full stop at the end of a file name, such as **.DOC**. PCs typically indicate the type of program that created the file by using such a suffix. Sometimes the suffix will have fewer than three letters, e.g. **.au**, or more than three, such as **.html**. In the context of an online service, suffixes fall into one of three groups: file *compression*, *encoding*, and *miscellaneous*. The concept of encoding was briefly mentioned in Chapter Four, and is discussed in greater detail in Chapter Eighteen. The miscellaneous group includes cross-platform file types such as text (**.txt**) and graphics formats (like **.jpg** and **.gif**), executable PC programs (**.EXE**), and various document formats. See Table 6, opposite.

Common suffixes in the group indicating **file compression** are shown in Table 7, along with an example program required to expand them (usually there is a choice). Compressed files have been altered by a special program that attempts to reduce the size of a file, replacing frequently occurring elements with a smaller string of binary code. Smaller files take up less storage space on a computer, and take less time to download. Not all files on an online service will be compressed, but larger ones usually are and repositories for them are called 'file archives'. Once you have downloaded a compressed file you cannot use it until it has been 'decompressed' or 'expanded' with special software. The file suffix allows us to determine which expansion program is needed to convert the file back into a usable document or program. An exception to the need for an expansion program is a file ending with the suffix **.SEA** or **.EXE**: this indicates that the file will automatically expand when you open it, or 'execute' (open) it at the DOS prompt or under Windows.

If the BBS you are calling is run on a Macintosh, you would encounter a different set of suffixes than you would if calling a PC-based system. The programs needed to expand files on a given service should be available for downloading from that service; if not, you will find them on magazine cover disks. Some expansion programs, such as Stuffit Expander from Aladdin Systems (PC and Mac versions), will decompress many types of archived file.

TABLE 6 File formats on the Internet and online services*

Category and file suffix		File format and requirements for viewing
Applications	.class	An executable Java applet: a Java-aware Web browser or operating system.
	.doc	A non-specific word processor file: open in a word processor.
	.eps	Encapsulated PostScript (EPS) file format: print to laser printer.
	.exe	A self-executing binary PC program.
	.bin	Macintosh file in MacBinary format. Handled by Stuffit Expander.
	.hqx	Macintosh BinHex format for encoding binary files into ASCII.† Mac files are often archived in this format. Handled by Stuffit Expander.
	.pdf	Adobe Portable Document Format (PDF): view with Acrobat Reader or Web browser (with appropriate plug-in.)
	.rtf	Rich Text Format (RTF): most word processors.
	.tar	UNIX tar format archive: TARREAD (PC) or Tar (Mac), for example.
Audio	.aif	Audio Interchange File Format (AIFF): a sound utility.
	.au	Sun Audio format (includes μ-law): a sound utility.
	.snd	Macintosh System 7 sound file: double-click to play on a Mac.
	.wav	Windows Wave format: a Wave-aware Web browser, or a sound utility.
Images	.gif	Graphics Interchange Format (GIF): many graphics utilities and Web browsers. (Also known as CompuServe Image Format.)
	.jpg	Joint Photographic Experts Group (JPEG) graphics format: many graphics utilities and Web browsers.
	.tif	Tagged Image File Format (TIFF): many graphics utilities.
Text	.html (or .htm)	Hypertext Markup Language (HTML) format: any Web browser.
	.txt	Plain ASCII text file: any text editor or word processor.
Video	.avi	Video for Windows Audio Video Interleave (AVI) format: any Video for Windows-aware application.
	.mov	QuickTime video: any QuickTime-aware application.
	.mpg	Motion Pictures Experts Group (MPEG) video: any MPEG player [May require special hardware.]
Virtual reality	.wrl	Virtual Reality Modelling Language (VRML) 'worlds' file: VRML player or Web browser (with appropriate plug-in.)

* File suffixes indicating file compression formats are listed in Table 7, p46.

† See also Table 12, p159.

TABLE 7 File compression suffixes and example expansion programs

Suffix	Computer platform and expander program			
	PC	Mac	UNIX	Amiga
.arc	ARC	ArcMac	arc	ARC
.arj	ARJ	unArjMac	unarj	UNARJ
.cpt	EXTRACT	Compact Pro	macunpack	–
.dd	–	DD Expand	macunpack	–
.gz	GZIP	MacGzip	gzip	GZIP
.lha	LHA	MacLHA	lharc	LHA
.sea	–	Self-expanding	–	–
.sit	UNSTUFF	Stuffit Expander	macunpack	UNSIT
.Z	COMPRESS	Stuffit Expander*	compress	COMPRESS
.zip	WINZIP	UnZip	zip	ZIP

* Enhanced version.

Choosing a file-transfer protocol

When using certain client software, such as the FirstClass or CompuServe client, you don't need to worry about choosing a protocol for file transfers (see Table 5). Other services, however, may ask you to nominate a file-transfer protocol before a download or upload takes place. In this instance, your choice of protocol may be limited by the BBS software on the remote computer, or by the communications software you are running on your own machine. Given a choice on a BBS, Zmodem is the most reliable (error-correcting) and efficient (fast) binary file-transfer protocol. It can also begin receiving files automatically, and resume partially completed downloads if transmission is disturbed. On the Internet, file transfers take place in either ASCII (7-bit) or binary (8-bit) 'mode' (explained in Chapter Twenty One), and Zmodem is not used.

Computer viruses

Viruses are small segments of code that insert themselves into your software, often with malicious intent. An 'infected' file may cause annoyance or the loss of data. In theory, any program you download is a potential vector. Most online services screen for virus infection before making their files available for downloading. There are a number of commercial and shareware antiviral solutions available for every platform which you can obtain to run on your system as a further safeguard. These programs act like the body's immune system in that they are always on the lookout for 'foreign' material—in this case, foreign program code.

Upload areas

A BBS encourages its users to **upload** (send to it) files as well as download them, if these files are not already present on the BBS and are likely to be of use to callers. Some even operate a policy where the amount of downloading you are allowed is related to uploads you have made to the BBS. Sometimes there will be a designated area for uploads, which may or may not be made available to other users before the BBS administrator has approved them as suitable or cleared them of viruses (see above). It is a good idea to include a description of anything you upload, so the administrator will know where to file it and other users can choose whether to spend money downloading it.

Chat

Chat is a novel but expensive way to communicate in '**real-time** typing' with another person online. If a BBS has more than one modem line, you can type messages to another caller who will respond in kind; otherwise you can chat with the system administrator. This sort of facility is also available on the Internet (as 'Internet Relay Chat', p.229).

Bulletin-board networks

Some BBSs exchange mail and conference messages with each other on a regular basis, effectively creating a 'part-time network'. Examples are the FidoNet and OneNet networks.

FidoNet

FidoNet is the largest amateur network of bulletin boards. Aside from local messages, you can send mail to someone on another FidoNet BBS (referred to as 'NetMail'), or to a conference which can be read by many people through being 'echoed' by other FidoNet BBSs (referred to as 'EchoMail'). It is also possible to request specific files from other BBSs. FidoNet-style addresses are explained on p.157. FidoNet BBSs can use a 'UUCP gateway' (e-mail exchange with a network of UNIX computers) to enable e-mail access to the Internet.

Medical echoes include **GRAND_ROUNDS** (discussing of all medical topics), **MED_RAYS** (radiology), and various electronic support groups such as **ALZHEIMERS**, **LARYNGECTOMY**, **DIABETES**, **MENTAL_HEALTH**, **MULT_SCLEROSIS**, and **SPINAL_INJURY**. UK Healthlink (p.89) is an example of a FidoNet BBS.

OneNet

OneNet is a network of BBSs running FirstClass server software. OneNet conferences are based somewhere in the chain of FirstClass BBSs around the world. Any BBS which carries a particular conference mirrors its contents at all other sites. You can also send messages to anybody on another OneNet site simply by adding the server name after the person's name. In the UK, several conferences are typically carried by FirstClass BBSs:

- **Medical**: a general discussion/non-file area. Largely questions from lay people to doctors/fellow patients. International.
- **Medical Library**: informational text files and messages, notices of conferences and symposia. International.
- **Medical Software**: for discussion of medical software and posting of files. Mostly about medical accounts packages, but little actual software posted. International.
- **Medical UK**: covers topics such as doctors' hours, NHS management, conferences, and diagnosis requests. Local to UK.

Like FidoNet, some FirstClass BBSs operate gateways to the Internet.

CHAPTER SEVEN
Making contact

In preparation for dialling into an online service you must configure your communications software and modem. Whilst modem configuration is infrequently changed by many users, a change of software configuration is necessary for each new online service or bulletin board you wish to contact.

Configuring your software

To ensure that your modem and the host modem are, quite literally, speaking the same language, you need to configure your communications software (Fig. 7). The configuration required depends partly on your modem's attributes, and partly on the characteristics of the online service you intend to dial. Configuration involves specifying *connection settings* and *terminal settings*. Many of these settings need to be shared by both modems in the connection; if they differ, garbage may embellish your screen. The settings for each service are sometimes stored in a separate file.

Connection settings

Telephone number: Client software sometimes requires you to enter the phone number of the modem you intend to dial in advance. Alternatively, numbers may be selected from a phonebook (p.33), or typed in manually using Hayes AT commands (p.21).

Speed setting: This determines how fast data travel back and forth across the connection. A discrepancy between modem speed settings causes garbage to appear on screen. However, since today's modems feature 'automatic speed fallback' (i.e. they drop down to the highest common setting), it is reasonable to specify the highest speed your modem is realistically capable of.

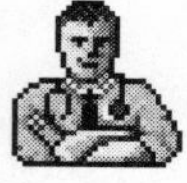

Setting a V.34 (28 800 bps) modem to 57 600 bps is normally reliable. This allows for any realistic speed gains brought about by data compression, yet acknowledges that driving a connection too fast can introduce errors as the computer's serial port struggles to keep up.

In practice, the speed savings brought about by data compression when downloading files are often not as stunning as modem manufacturers would have you believe, since most files stored online are already compressed.

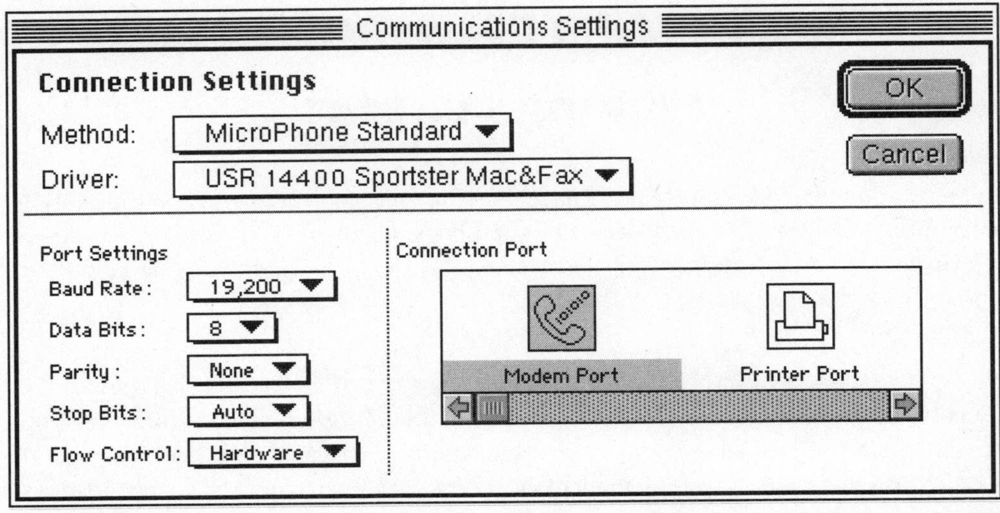

Fig. 7 Configuring communications software. On the Mac and PC running Microsoft Windows, this can be a simple matter of choosing options from pull-down menus.

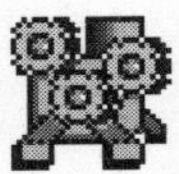

Remember that bits per second is not technically equivalent to baud rate (p.22), although the terms are often used synonymously. High-speed modems typically transmit data (in bits per second) well in excess of the baud rate.

Data bits: **Data bits** refers to the number of bits that make up a character, thus the synonym 'character bits'. A character is a sequence of bits that forms a meaningful unit of information (a letter, number, or symbol—p.29). Usually set to 8 (for binary-protocol file transfers), or alternatively to 7 (for ASCII-protocol file transfers). File-transfer protocols were discussed on p.31.

Stop bits: **Stop bits** are extra bits positioned at the end of a sequence of character bits. They are usually set to 1. This means that for every 8-bit character, 10 bits are actually transmitted (a 'start' bit is assumed).

Parity: Now a rarely used technique for error detection, **parity** is most often set to 'None'. If used, it is set to 'Even' or 'Odd' in reflection of the even or odd number made by the sum of bits in a character.

A feature used in 7-bit ASCII file-transfer protocol, the parity-correcting bit has been incorporated into the 8-bit characters used in binary file-transfer protocols.

Handshake: A way of regulating data flow between computers and modems (see p.23). If you set your software to use hardware handshaking, your modem must be likewise configured. XON/XOFF (software) handshaking is more frequently used by bulletin boards offering slow connection speeds.

Communications port: Specifying which serial-communications port you are using is necessary. This will be a COM port on the PC, or the Modem or Printer port on the Macintosh.

Terminal settings

Communications programs tend to vary in their handling of terminal settings, which define the characteristics of the type of terminal to be emulated. Some 'high-powered' packages can make things quite complicated. Your manual should be useful here. The more common settings follow:

Terminal type: Although TTY (the simplest type of terminal emulation) can be used for most connections, if the service being called is run on a PC then ANSI is likely to be supported. Larger online services based on UNIX machines typically expect VT100 emulation. See also Table 4, p.28.

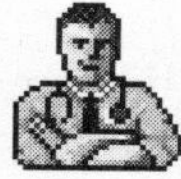

It is often a good idea to make an initial connection to a service you have not tried before using TTY or VT100. If ANSI or other terminal types are supported, the service will let you know. Reconnect to the service after changing your software configuration to make the most of its features.

Line feeds: When an online service sends a carriage return (**CR**) to your terminal software, the cursor on your screen is moved back to the left margin. Usually the carriage return is combined with a **line feed** (**LF**)—a signal to begin a new line. On screen, the text will then move up one line, displaying the next line of information. Since most PC-based services automatically send **CR**/**LF** as a pair, *automatic* line feeds can be left *off*. A few systems send only the **CR** control character and not **LF**, in which case automatic line feeds may have to be enabled (or new lines of text will be written on top of existing text).

Duplex: **Duplex** refers to the direction of data transmission across a communications link. In a *full* duplex link, data can be sent and received at the same time. In a *half* duplex link, one modem is the sending modem and the other is receiving. Full duplex is common, and means that on some services (and on the Internet) you can upload a file whilst downloading your mail (for example).

Local echo: **Local echo** means that your typing at the keyboard is 'echoed' or sent to your own *local* screen as well as being sent via the modem to an online service. If this did not happen, you would not see what you were sending. Since most online services automatically echo your commands or words, local echo does not normally have to be turned on. If it is, all you type will appear twice (as in '**ttwwiiccee**'). You will need to turn local echo on if the computer being called does not echo your typing (for example, if you are sending a file direct to a colleague's computer).

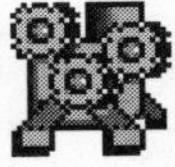

'Full duplex' and 'local echo off' are often mistaken to mean the same thing. This is because full duplex services (which send data in both directions) typically *do* echo what you have transmitted back to your screen, once it has been received by the remote host computer. Since this is a *remote* echo, there is no need for a *local* echo (from your own modem) as well. If a full-duplex service provided no remote echo, you would have to switch local echo on. Thus although they are most often set together, 'full duplex' and 'local echo off' do mean different things.

Other settings

Sometimes it is necessary to specify whether you are using tone (the usual digital exchange) or pulse dial (older phones). You may have to add a dialling prefix, such as a '9' followed by a comma, to get an outside line. If you have call waiting, incoming calls cause the modem to drop the line; it can be temporarily disabled for the duration of your modem calls (in which case, contact your telephone company who will know how to do this). Further settings include how the modem should be 'reset' after a call, modem speaker volume, how long to wait before re-dialling an engaged number, and whether to use a modem 'driver' (a file containing instructions for operating a particular make of modem). Your manual should be of assistance here.

Occasionally experts talk about 'mode', referring to 'asynchronous' and 'synchronous' communications. It is sufficient to know that communications involving personal computers are asynchronous.

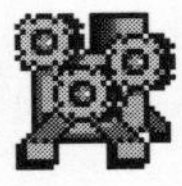

Asynchronous serial-communications protocols use start and stop bits to mark the beginning and end of a transmitted character. A special circuit (the 'Universal Asynchronous Receiver/Transmitter') in your PC transmits and receives these characters at a variable rate through the serial-communications port, so that start bits do not occur at a fixed interval. 'Asynchronous' in this context therefore means 'lack of fixed timing'. The alternative is synchronous communications where characters are processed at a timed interval. Consequently, start and stop bits become redundant.

Configuring your modem

The initialization string

Having configured your software, the modem is prepared to carry out the instructions given to it. This process is called **initialization**, ensuring that modem settings match software settings and that certain modem functions (like data compression and error control) are enabled. Initialization is achieved via the Hayes AT command set (p.21), or other similar proprietary commands.

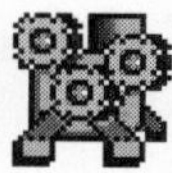

A number of commands can be joined together in a string, beginning with **AT** (from 'attention') and implemented using **Enter** or **Return**. As an example, **ATS0=0V1E1** means 'Attention modem: don't auto-answer the phone; send **CONNECT** to the screen when establishing link; and turn off local echo'. Typing '**AT&F**' will restore the default settings stored within the modem.

Although there are some instances where you may wish to alter the default settings, generally they enable all the 'good' features your modem can use. The modem's manual will detail how to change these features. Note that some software uses modem 'scripts' (initialization instructions) optimized for a particular modem and/or online service.

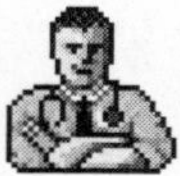

To send a file direct to a colleague's computer (rather than via an online service) telephone first to ensure his or her modem will be on and initialized to auto-answer the phone. Hang up and have your software call the number.

Testing the modem

Having now configured both software and modem, you can run a simple test to confirm that computer and modem are talking to each other. With both devices switched on, load your terminal emulator and type '**AT**'. If the modem responds with '**OK**', then the modem is listening and awaiting your instructions. If there is no response, check again that the modem is connected to the serial port specified in your communications software. If you have an external modem and its lights (if present) do not flicker, there may be a fault with the cable or with the modem itself.

Before dialling anyone the modem must be plugged into a telephone socket. Few people have an extra telephone line dedicated to their modem. You can purchase an inexpensive socket adapter from many hardware and electronics stores which allows the telephone, modem, and even answering machine to share the same wall jack. You can't, however, use the modem while someone is on the telephone, and incoming calls can disrupt your modem sessions.

Making contact

Dialling a bulletin board

Once you have initialized the modem and tested it successfully, you can dial a bulletin board, either using a number stored in a phonebook (if your software supports one), or by sending it to the modem manually using the **ATDT** command. After the dial tone and one or two rings, you will hear screeching noises when the two modems negotiate agreed modulation, handshaking, data compression, and error-correction protocols. The following example indicates the type of dialogue that may appear on your screen as you dial:

```
AT
OK
ATE1Q0V1X4B0&A3&B1&H1&I0&K1&M4&N0&R2&D0
OK
ATDT9,01614390617
CONNECT 14400/ARQ/V32/LAPM/V42BIS
Press RETURN twice to connect
You have connected to a FirstClass System. Please login...
UserID:
```

In this example, the software has sent **AT** to the modem to make sure it is listening, followed by a customized initialization string. **ATDT** attains the dial tone, inserting a 9 before the BBS number to get an outside line. A **CONNECT** message then appears, stating the agreed protocols resulting from negotiation. Here, the BBS software expects callers to hit the **Return (Enter)** key twice to connect and begin the log-on sequence.

If the number dialled is engaged the modem will return a message like '**BUSY**'. Some software can automatically re-dial busy numbers. If the number continues to ring, but no modem answers, the service may be offline through maintenance or mishap.

The log on procedure

Online services require that new and frequent users 'log on' to the system. For new users, this often involves supplying a user name, password, address, telephone number, and perhaps a 'terminal-preferences questionnaire' or other form of survey. You may be asked whether you agree to abide by the terms of membership. Once this has been done, the next time you log on you will be asked only for a user name and password, although should any other personal information (such as an address) change, it can usually be altered from one of the service's menus. Recording this information allows the sysop to monitor use of the service, set 'user privileges' (whether you have unlimited access to the service or not, how much time you can have per call, etc.), and capture billing information.

To prevent unauthorized use of your account, it may be wise to have a different password on each service that you call and to change it from time to time (although in practice the difficulty of remembering multiple passwords may outstrip its benefits). Once logged on you may be taken to the main menu by default, or alternatively the BBS will present you with unread mail or updated bulletins. It should be easy to identify the commands used in the message, file, and chat areas (as discussed in Chapter Six).

Logging off

If you have called a colleague directly, the connection can be closed simply by typing **ATH**, the hang-up command. All bulletin boards and commercial services, however, have some sort of procedure for logging off. Logging off in the correct way avoids the risk of being charged for extra time on a commercial service, and reduces the chances of the sysop having to reset the service's modems. Before you do log off, the BBS software may ask if you would care to send a note to the sysop.

More communications jargon

Settings shorthand

An informal shorthand is often adopted to describe communications settings succinctly. You may be given, as an example, '8-N-1 to 14 400 bps'. Your action in this case should be to set 8 data bits, no parity, 1 stop bit, and a port speed of 14 400 bits per second (or higher).

Set your software to 8-N-1, the most common configuration for PC-based bulletin boards, unless you know that the settings are different. Seven data bits, even parity, and 1 stop bit (i.e. 7-E-1) is more common for UNIX-based services.

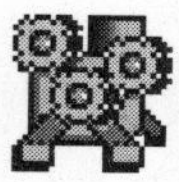

CompuServe is an example of a 7-E-1 service. Since 7-bit communications links use the 7-bit ASCII codes, one might wonder how it could be possible to transfer 8-bit binary files (p.30). CompuServe gets around this by on-the-fly switching to 8-bit communications using its proprietary CompuServe B+ protocol, thus enabling file-downloads. Aside from the actual file transfer, the user interacts with the service over a 7-E-1 link. If you wish to use a more conventional 8-bit binary protocol like Xmodem or Ymodem, you must reconfigure your CompuServe account to 8-N-1. The Kermit protocol gets around the problem of transferring binary files over 7-bit links by slicing the 8-bit bytes into 7-bit sequences. These sequences can therefore be transmitted as ASCII codes and reassembled into 8-bit extended characters on the receiving computer.

Characters per second

Characters per second (cps) is a better measure of the speed of data transfer than bits per second (bps). This is estimated from the bps rate and the length of the transmitted character.

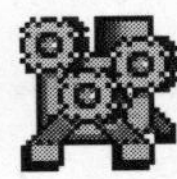

Whether you are using 8-N-1 or 7-E-1, 10 bits are typically transmitted per character. This is because 8-N-1 implies 8 data bits, no parity bit, 1 start bit, and 1 stop bit (i.e. 10); 7-E-1 implies 7 data bits, 1 parity bit, 1 start bit, and 1 stop bit (again, 10 bits). As an example, if a modem is set to 14 400 bps and is handling 10-bit characters, then 14 400 bps divided by 10 bits per character would transmit 1440 cps. However, this calculation is theoretical as a number of factors influence the final cps. Factors like data compression can increase the cps. The cps falls off when retrieving a file from an Internet computer, depending on how many other users are sharing that computer's resources.

CHAPTER EIGHT
Online ethics

Netiquette

Usenet, the discussion area of the Internet (p.171), has adopted several principles of etiquette in relation to the posting of electronic mail messages. Known widely as **netiquette**, these principles are equally applicable to postings on bulletin boards, commercial online services, and to mailing lists (p.165). The following points are of relevance to postings in the medical newsgroups (p.173) and conferences.

- Respect others as you would have them respect you. Your message may have an international audience with greatly varied backgrounds, experience, and ages. Consider using 'emoticons' or 'smileys', such as **:-)** to indicate something said in jest (this gives your message context).
- Post concise messages. The inclusion of acronyms such as IMHO (in my humble opinion...) is a common practice, but by no means essential.
- Pay attention to formatting. DON'T TYPE IN CAPITALS—it is harder to read. Avoid special symbols (e.g. use UKP instead of £). Limit line length to 80 characters (the width of a standard terminal window). Note that the **Tab** key can have different results on different machines. Lay out your message using a 'monospaced' font (where all the characters are the same width) when trying to align characters (as in creating a table).
- Think about the subject header: it can determine whether people take the time to read your message. For example, 'Lupus info needed' is preferable to 'Read this please!!! Help urgently needed!!!'. If a **thread** (a sequence of related messages) wanders off the topic, don't continue with it but post on a new subject.
- Before posting be sure you have the appropriate newsgroup/conference. It is a good idea to 'lurk', or just read rather than post, until you know the focus of a particular group. Lamenting the decline of the NHS is better done in a local forum than an international one. Giving notice of major symposia is another matter. Don't 'cross-post' to several groups at a time if posting to one will get a response (this causes annoyance).
- Follow-up postings should be by e-mail whenever possible, unless the group as a whole will benefit from your reply. For example, request a copy of a file from the author, not by posting 'Send it to me too!'. Summarize very briefly what you are replying to; don't quote entire messages. If appropriate, post a summary of replies made to a question which you have had answered.

- Keep signatures short and relevant. You might include your qualifications, position, and contact details, etc., but not artworks drawn from text characters (called 'ASCII art').
- Before posting a new user question, read the relevant FAQ (frequently-asked questions) file. FAQs are discussed in Chapter Eighteen.
- Don't infringe copyright; cite relevant references; and do not start or take part in flame wars. These issues are discussed separately below.

Medical ethics online

Giving medical advice in online forums

Many online medical conferences are characterized by numerous requests for diagnosis. Some conferences and mailing lists (p.165) intended for health-care professionals specifically discourage the posting of such questions, although this rule is not infrequently violated. Many doctors, it seems, do not enjoy reading these messages. This is not necessarily a reflection of an unwillingness to be helpful, but, at least in some cases, uncertainty over the appropriateness of giving advice to an unseen patient. Indeed, the giving and receiving of advice online can be fraught with risks for both patient and doctor.

Some doctors fear that misinformed advice from other 'doctors' may promote unnecessary invasive procedures, or cause morbidity or even mortality, making it essential to verify the status of the person giving the advice (Sharma 1995). There is presently no easy way to do this on the Internet.

Likewise, patients cannot be sure whether the person replying to their questions—who may be recommending a particular treatment or other course of action—is professionally qualified. Because electronic mail messages are usually brief, important details may be omitted by the poster. In contrast to a traditional face-to-face consultation, online dialogue imposes a severe limitation on the development of a doctor–patient relationship; it also does not permit further questioning and examination of the patient and his or her records. Consultation over live video links (p.126) remains experimental but may overcome some of these concerns.

Currently a number of doctors have taken to appending disclaimers to their electronic signatures to lessen the risk of legal action resulting from erroneous advice given online. It is uncertain, however, whether the giving of advice with altruistic intent would in any case constitute a professional contract of care between the 'patient' and doctor. An alternative approach is not to reply directly to questions, but rather to recommend an information source (such as a cancer society or, of course, the patient's general practitioner). If there is to be an on-going dialogue, it is advisable to use private e-mail messages, rather than continuing to post to a public forum. When replying to a posting by another health professional, it may be good practice to cite references which can be used to verify an opinion or obtain further information. Discretion rests with the individual as to whether and how they should respond to these requests.

Electronic communication with patients

This author is aware of several instances where doctors and patients are using e-mail as a basis for on-going dialogue (for various reasons). It is highly probable that, with the upward trend in rates of Internet connectivity, such unusual instances will become commonplace occurrences. However, using e-mail as a routine (or even occasional) tool in clinical practice raises a number of complex issues. These are discussed separately in the following chapter by Beverley Kane.

Sharing personal health information between professionals

Some bulletin boards offer closed forums where doctors can discuss medical matters without fear of misinforming (or frightening) the public. Validation of professional status is commonly far from stringent (if required at all). In this setting, is it ethical for doctors to disclose personal health information within such a forum in the interests of sharing experience or seeking clinical help? This question will become even more topical as health-service networks experiment with electronic forums and professional communications (and with the transfer of electronic medical records). The opportunity to bring together geographically dispersed health professionals afforded by online conferencing promises multi-disciplinary cooperation as never before. But what about the confidentiality of personal health information?

There is no ethical debate that we, as doctors, are duty-bound to preserve the confidentiality of such information. The General Medical Council states, as a principle of confidentiality, that doctors '...must make sure that patients are informed whenever information about them is likely to be disclosed to others involved in their health care, and that they have the opportunity to withhold permission' (GMC 1995).

There are, however, circumstances in which it would seem reasonable to share information pertaining to individuals with other health professionals—when the patient stands to benefit from shared knowledge and experience. This is how we learn. Some may argue that the patient's consent to such discussion is implied at the outset of consultation. It is widely recognized that a patient's explicit and informed consent is a prerequisite to the use of identifiable health information for teaching purposes. In *Duties of a doctor,* the GMC (1995) states that 'Patient's consent to disclosure of information for teaching and audit must be obtained unless the data have been effectively anonymised.'

The Department of Health has published guidance for the NHS on *The protection and use of patient information* (DoH 1996). This guidance emphasizes the desirability of using anonymized information wherever possible, and also stresses the need to inform patients how their information will be used. However, the Office of the Data Protection Registrar (see below) is not convinced that the guidance sufficiently emphasizes the need to inform patients of the extent of their right to prevent their information being passed on to others, and continues to call for statutory guidelines (DPR 1996).

These principles should hold true for the electronic sharing of personal health information between professionals. If identifiable personal health information is to be shared in an e-mail message to a colleague or online forum, the patient's express and informed consent must first be sought. If the data are not identifiable, the patient's express consent is not a prerequisite (although a duty of confidence remains).

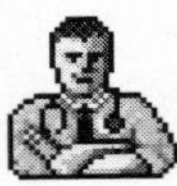

Confidentiality is enhanced online as elsewhere by removing any references within a message that could lead to the identification of the individual being discussed, and by encrypting sensitive information.

It may be good practice if discussions of case management, for example, are not undertaken online without the express and informed consent of the patient—even where identifiable personal health information is not disclosed. In the UK, the Data Protection Act may impact on the appearance and storage of personal health information in online forums (and other computer files such as surgical logs, case presentations, etc.). The Act of 1984 offers protection to individuals where data relating to them may be held in electronic form (DPR 1994). Those holding identifiable personal health information may be required to register with the Data Protection Office as data users and therefore to comply with the Data Protection Principles.

Many issues remain unresolved, and extend in scope far beyond those briefly considered here. With the adoption of statutory or 'common law' guidelines, the question becomes one of ensuring the integrity of e-mail messages and that only qualified health professionals are admitted to closed online forums. These, however, are security issues, not ethical ones.

Security issues in brief

Doctors using the same computer system for storing personal health information and connecting to the Internet (or other networks and dial-up services) may be placing their patient's trust in jeopardy if they have not fully considered the security risks this may pose.

Although the risks may seem small, we are told that 'systematic and automated probing of new Internet connections is being carried out by a shady cast of characters that includes hackers-for-hire, information brokers, and foreign governments' (Cobb 1995).

Whether the threat is exaggerated or not, there is no question that all confidential medical information must be protected from misuse. At the same time, data security must provide access to the protected information for those who require it. There a several efforts in progress to establish a standard way of protecting commercial information (such as credit card details—p.110) as it travels over various networks, and these same standards may find applications in a health-care setting. In the interim, public-key cryptography and firewalls are the mainstay of protection.

Public-key cryptography has been advocated as a means to provide the secure transmission of confidential medical information on insecure networks (Andreae 1996). In essence, the sender uses his or her 'private key' to uniquely 'sign' a file. The file is then encrypted or locked using a mathematical algorithm prescribed by the intended recipients 'public key' (which is advertised). Once transmitted, the recipient can unlock the file using his or her private key (which is secret), and confirm the origin of the file by checking the signature against the sender's public key. If the message were to be intercepted and altered, decryption would fail—so providing further security. See also Chapter Nine, p.76.

Firewalls are commonly employed by network administrators to prevent unauthorized access to an internal network by outsiders. A firewall is a hardware and/or software gateway through which all in-bound and out-bound network traffic can be forced to pass. Only certain kinds of traffic may be allowed (or not—Telnet connections, for example).

Readers interested in the security aspects of clinical information systems and the risks inherent in their connection to outside systems such as the Internet may wish to read the paper (1996) and editorial (1995) by Anderson on this topic.

Flaming doctors

A **flame** is an inflammatory criticism directed at someone posting a message to one of the Internet's Usenet newsgroups (p.171). So-called 'flame wars' erupt when other users flame those doing the criticizing. From time to time (in the newsgroup **sci.med** in particular), doctors are the object of these flames. Some have been the recipients of vicious attacks on their personal character and professional reputations and accused of malpractice by people who are hostile for no apparent reason. This public defamation does little to encourage confidence in the medical profession. The experience of being flamed can discourage medical involvement in Usenet, leaving questions unanswered and advice withheld.

Although the nature of the Internet means that it is easier to publish one's opinions than ever before, the flamers themselves could be libelled for defamation in some cases. There may not always be the right of reply to an accusation where a newsgroup moderator decides 'enough is enough' and demands an end to discussion of the topic. Although such experiences are not common, there does seem to be a reluctance on the part of some doctors to identify themselves online. A few choose to make anonymous replies to medical questions.

Copyright and citation of online sources

The principles of electronic copyright

Under the Copyright Designs and Patents Act of 1988, copyright is automatically attached to any original work created by a qualifying author (or published in a qualifying country). Not everything can be protected by copyright, however, notable exceptions being facts and ideas themselves—although the selection of facts and the context in which these ideas are expressed will be protected in the UK. Copyright, giving the owner (subject to limited statutory exceptions) the sole right to copy, publish, modify, or publicly display a work (or to authorize another to do so), commences as soon as the work is recorded in writing or otherwise. These rights generally last for the period of life of the author plus seventy years.

Because no organization has authority over the entire Internet, some material is available without the consent of the copyright owner. The use of this material is a violation of the copyright attached to it. Even if the text files, software, or graphics you find online do not originate in the UK, international copyright conventions make use of them without the owner's consent unlawful within the UK.

A common online and (providing all conditions are met) legal method of obtaining software is the 'shareware' concept. With such software, one is usually allowed to make a copy for personal evaluation, and pass it on to others. If the author asks for payment, the users are obliged to forward it within a specified time frame if they continue to use the software. If they do not continue to use the software, then no payment is necessary, but the evaluation copy must be deleted or passed on. Shareware authors permit their software to be held on bulletin boards and Internet sites because this aids distribution. Some shareware authors follow the tradition of commercial software and include licence agreements that describe terms of use. There are many medical shareware programs on the Internet (see Chapter Twenty One).

Authors of 'freeware' software retain copyright on their work but do not request any money for you to use their programs for as long as you like. Rarely, an author puts material into the 'public domain', for example the Center for Disease Control's *Morbidity and Mortality Weekly Report* (MMWR). In this case, the author does not wish to exercise copyright over the material and no special acknowledgement is necessary for its use. This does not necessarily mean that the author waives the right of integrity (that is, the right not to have the work subjected to derogatory treatment by modification).

Often a notice will accompany literary copyright material setting out the uses which the author permits and those which would constitute a breach of copyright. For example, this notice may specify that copying in part or *in toto* is permitted providing the source is acknowledged; that it cannot be altered without permission; that it is freely distributable on non-commercial services only; or that commercial distribution requires express permission. Sometimes the author will request that those wishing to use the material include a specific copyright notice, or detail how the material should be cited.

The Copyright Designs and Patents Act provides for certain permitted acts in relation to copyright works including 'fair use' for the purposes of criticism and review, reporting current events, research and private study, as well as copying for educational purposes and by librarians. What uses are considered 'fair' depends on such things as the nature of the use, what proportion is to be copied, and whether doing so damages the commercial potential of the original work.

If one wishes to include part of an e-mail message in an article, it is a precondition to its lawful use to contact the author and obtain consent. The issues of electronic copyright are very complex: a stimulating treatise on the subject in several parts by Terry Carroll can be found on the Internet at:

<URL:ftp://rtfm.mit.edu/pub/usenet/news.answers/law/Copyright-FAQ/>

See *Universal resource locators* in Chapter Twelve (p.102) for an explanation of this Internet address.

Citing online sources

All academic journals have an established style for referencing printed sources, but guidance in dealing with current variations in online sources is lacking. In the future, health professionals may wish to cite references in the form of e-mail messages, mailing lists or other periodicals, online databases, or files held on Internet archives, Gopher, and World-Wide Web sites. The ability to cite electronic sources accurately will be essential as more health professionals become regular users of the Internet. Electronic citation is an issue critical to the development of the Internet as a viable tool for scientific (as opposed to casual) medical communications.

The Harvard system for the citing of references within books is preferred by Oxford University Press. According to this system, references are cited in the text like this: (McKenzie 1995). The list of references then follows the general form:

> *Periodicals*: Author/s (Year). Title. Journal, **Volume**, (Issue), Page numbers.
>
> *Books*: Author/s (Year). Title, Volume, (Edition), Page numbers. Publisher, City.

The Vancouver style (ICMJE 1991) is popular where references are to be cited in journal articles. According to this system, references are numbered consecutively in the order in which they are first mentioned within the paper. The list of references then follows the general form:

> *Periodicals:* (No.) Author/s. Title [Type of article]. *Journal* Year. Month; Volume (Issue): Page numbers.
>
> *Books*: (No.) Author/s. Title. Edition. City: Publisher, Year: Page numbers.

In citing a reference, one generally wishes to acknowledge the author, give a date to indicate currency, give a title, indicate a particular version or edition, and enable others to locate the cited work. Electronic sources can be accommodated within this scheme by relatively minor changes to both the Harvard and Vancouver systems. The importance of retaining location descriptions 'generic' to particular information sources, and of specifying the type of medium (e.g. printed book or journal as opposed to online or CD-ROM) has been identified (Li and Crane 1993).

In the case of Internet resources, the 'generic' location description is the 'universal resource locator', or URL. Aside from being an Internet standard, the URL system has inbuilt potential to accommodate future (as yet undefined) Internet services. If you are unfamiliar with URLs, read *Universal resource locators* (p.102) before continuing. The following suggestions serve as a guide only: there are no established standards. For online sources, references are cited in the text as already described; the list of references then follows the general form:

> *Harvard*: Author/s (Year, Date). Title, (Version) [Medium]. Location. Publisher, City.
>
> *Vancouver*: (No.) Author/s. Title [Medium]. *Journal* Year Date;Version. Location. City: Publisher.

There are several points to note:

- Adding *Date* to the scheme opens up the problem of transient or dynamically updated sources that typify the Internet. Not everybody follows the 'dd/mm/yy' date convention; it is better to use, for example, Jun 10 (as opposed to 10/06/95, which could be interpreted as October 6). *However*, World-Wide Web pages in particular undergo a process of constant revision. It remains to be seen whether the scientific community will accept the validity of a non-permanent document as a legitimate reference source. The ability to consult references exactly as cited is paramount to the process of peer review. Thus, only archived, retrievable versions may be regarded as valid.
- The *Title* element may be the name of an occasional article (taken from the subject heading), a file name, or the name of an article and the periodical carrying it (with a full stop separating the titles).
- *Version* is the online equivalent of *edition*. Version or revision numbers are particularly common in files held in Internet archives. The *Date* may be optional if a particular version number is identified (although it would indicate currency).
- [*Medium*] will be replaced by [Online] in the case of sources referenced over a telecommunications link. Alternatives might be [CD-ROM], [Laserdisk], [Videodisk], [Disk], etc.
- *Page* numbers are not usually a feature of electronic documents, as pages will change depending on the viewing method.
- *Location* refers to the URL as specified in *RFC 1738* in the case of Internet-accessible resources. In the case of disk-based sources, the Location element could be 'Disk, obtainable from: *postal address*', instead of a URL or generic online location.
- The Internet enables anyone to be a publisher, and *Publisher* may be omitted where the author has self-published. However, electronic publishing online is becoming an industry in itself, and the position of publisher in the scheme needs to be retained. The *City*, if known, is useful to identify the geographic relevance of the work.

Example electronic citations

The following examples illustrate the practical applications of this scheme. As this book concerns itself with online resources, these form the focus of the examples. You are best advised to return to this section after having familiarized yourself with the concept of URLs.

Private e-mail:

Example: (McKenzie, personal communication).

Note: E-mail can be cited as a personal communication, without being mentioned in the reference list. This system works equally well for e-mail messages received on bulletin boards or over the Internet.

Periodic mailing/online journal:

Example (Harvard style): Lee, T.H. (1995, Feb 10). Support for the prognostic value of PSA. Journal Watch, [Online]. <URL:news:sci.med>. Massachusetts Medical Society.

Example (Vancouver style): (1) Lee TH. Support for the prognostic value of PSA [Online]. *Journal Watch* 1995 Feb 10. <URL:mailto:jwatch@world.std.com>. Massachusetts Medical Society.

Note: In this case the article was available to readers of Usenet's **sci.med** newsgroup, or subscribers to the *Journal Watch* mailing list. Mailing lists are more likely to have retrievable archives than Usenet items, so the subscription address may be preferred.

Occasional article:

Example (Harvard style): Parsons, D.F. (1994, Aug 22). Telemedicine in New York State, (ver. 1.01.) [Online]. <URL:mailto:LISTSERV@albnydh2.bitnet> Send: get NYS SUMMARY.

Note: This article is under 'dynamic review' (updated as an ongoing process), exemplifying the value of date and/or version information. The *Location* element contains further information necessary to retrieve the article (i.e. what should be in the body of the e-mail message) in addition to the URL e-mail address. This is because the message is sent to a machine (the *LISTSERV*). If more than one command is to be given, these can be separated by a semicolon (e.g. **Send: get file; quit**). Where the message is variable (i.e. addressed to a person), brackets in the format **Send: (personal message)** can be used.

Example (Vancouver style): (1) McKenzie BC. Re: Is chemotherapy good for people? [Online]. 1995 Apr 13. <URL:news:sci.med.diseases.cancer>.

Note: 'Conference'-type messages typically identify an author, date, subject/topic, and conference name. In some cases postings (such as those on CompuServe) can be identified precisely by a message identification number. Individual Usenet articles can be identified uniquely by a URL with the syntax **news:<message-id>**, where **<message-id>** is taken from the 'Message-ID' in the article header. Unfortunately, this is of no more help in locating an old message. It is debatably more meaningful to refer to the newsgroup in which the article was posted, as above. In any case, the transience of articles in these conferences currently invalidates them as means of recording academic communications.

Online database:

Example (Harvard style): Anon. (1995) Chest Tap (Thoracocentesis). HealthNet Reference Library, [Online]. CIS:HRF-2987. CompuServe Incorporated, Columbus.

Note: This example retains the generic location information for CompuServe: users can retrieve this database article by typing **GO HRF-2987**.

FTP server:

Example (Harvard style): Gaffin, A. (1995). EFF's guide to the Internet, (ver. 3.1) [Online]. <URL:ftp://ftp.eff.org/pub/Net_info/EFF_Net_Guide/netguide_3.1.txt>. Electronic Frontier Foundation, Washington.

Example (Vancouver style): (1) Gaffin A. EFF's guide to the Internet [Online]. 1995;3.1. <URL:ftp://ftp.eff.org/pub/Net_info/EFF_Net_Guide/netguide_3.1.txt>. Washington: Electronic Frontier Foundation.

Note: If retrieving files using a mail server, it is sometimes the subject line in the message that is important, rather than the body. In this case, use the format:

<URL:mailto:faq-server@rtfm.mit.edu> Subject: help; Send: (empty)

Gopher server:

Example (Harvard style): Advisory Committee for the Co-ordination of Information Systems. (1994). The Internet: An introductory guide for United Nations organisations, [Online]. <URL:gopher://gopher://nesirs01.iaea.or.at:70/11/unintgd/inetasc>. United Nations, Geneva.

Example (Vancouver style): (1) Advisory Committee for the Co-ordination of Information Systems. The Internet: An introductory guide for United Nations organisations [Online]. 1994. <URL:gopher://gopher://nesirs01.iaea.or.at:70/11/unintgd/inetasc>. Geneva: United Nations.

WWW server:

Example (Harvard style): McKenzie, B.C. (1995, Oct 13). Medicine and the Internet, [Online]. <URL:http://www.oup.co.uk/scimed/medint>. OUP, Oxford.

Example (Vancouver style): (1) McKenzie BC. Medicine and the Internet [Online]. 1995 Oct 13. <URL:http://www.oup.co.uk/scimed/medint>. Oxford: OUP.

Note: Many WWW pages are now including 'Page last updated on ...' statements, making it easier to cite the version that was consulted.

Telnet:

Telnet is an interactive service requiring the user to navigate a series of menus leading to resources held on another Internet Service. The syntax for Telnet URLs does not provide for the description of these menu choices (McCahill, personal communication). In order to acknowledge sources located via Telnet, it is therefore necessary to specify a non-Telnet URL (such as Gopher, FTP, WWW etc.). Unfortunately, this information is not always obvious from Telnet menus.

Bibliography

Anderson, R. (1996). Clinical system security: interim guidelines. *BMJ*, 312, 109–11.

Anderson, R. (1995). NHS-wide networking and patient confidentiality: Britain seems headed for a poor solution. *BMJ*, 311, 5–6.

Andreae, M. (1996). Confidentiality in medical telecommunications. *Lancet*, 347, 487–8.

Berners-Lee, T., Masinter, L., and McCahill, M. (ed.) (1994, Dec). *Uniform resource locators*, (RFC 1738) [Online]. <URL:ftp://ds.internic.net/rfc/rfc1738.txt>. Internet Engineering Task Force.

Cobb, S. (1995). Internet firewalls. *Byte*, October issue, 179.

Data Protection Registrar. (1994). *The Data Protection Act 1984: the guidelines* (3rd series). Booklet, obtainable from: Office of the Data Protection Registrar, Wycliffe House, Water Lane, Wilmslow, Cheshire SK9 5AF.

Data Protection Registrar. (1996). *DoH guidance for the NHS on 'The protection and use of patient information': comments from the Registrar*. Document, obtainable from: Office of the Data Protection Registrar, Wycliffe House, Water Lane, Wilmslow, Cheshire SK9 5AF.

Department of Health. (1996). *The protection and use of patient information: guidance from the Department of Health*. Booklet, obtainable from: Publications Unit, Department of Health, PO Box 410, Wetherby LS23 7LN.

General Medical Council. (1995). *Duties of a doctor: confidentiality*. Booklet, obtainable from: GMC, 178-2002 Great Portland St., London W1N 6JE.

International Committee of Medical Journal Editors (1991). Uniform requirements for manuscripts submitted to biomedical journals, (4th edn). *BMJ*, **302**, 338–41.

Li, X. and Crane, N.B. (1993). *Electronic style: a guide to citing electronic information*. Meckler, Westport.

Moraes, M. and von Rospach, C. (1995, Jul 12). *A primer on how to work with the usenet community*, [Online]. <URL:ftp://rtfm.mit.edu/pub/usenet-by group/news.answers/usenet/primer/part1>.

Oxford University Press. *Notes for authors: preparing references and bibliographies*. Booklet, obtainable from: Science and Medical Division, OUP, Walton Street, Oxford OX2 6DP.

Sharma, P. (1995). Popular medical information on the Internet. *Lancet*, 346, 250. [Letter.]

CHAPTER NINE
Electronic communication with patients

by Beverley Kane

This Chapter addresses the lack of established guidelines concerning the use of electronic communications between doctors and their patients. The advantages and disadvantages of the medium are first discussed. Suggested guidelines follow, many of which are equally applicable to casual discussions about health issues in online forums, and to the electronic sharing of personal health information between professionals (p.58). This Chapter forms the basis of a White Paper for the Internet Working Group of the American Medical Informatics Association, and your ongoing contributions are encouraged (see the Contributors page for the author's contact details).

Technically minded health-care consumers have accelerated the demand for fax and electronic mail (e-mail) access to their health-care providers (Fridsma *et al.* 1994). In contrast to unauthenticated online medical exchanges between anonymous parties (see below), electronic communication has a more obvious role in the established doctor–patient (or more broadly, clinic–consumer) relationship. In many locales, consumer-driven demand is forcing health-care providers, both as individuals and on an institutional basis, to establish guidelines for such exchanges.

Guidelines for using e-mail in a clinical setting address two inter-related aspects: interpersonal dynamics between the doctor and patient, and the observance of medicolegal prudence. Since many malpractice claims can be traced to faulty communication, good communication equals good insurance. Medicolegal restrictions, however, should not be allowed to disable open communication as the basis for a healthy provider–patient relationship.

From a sociological standpoint, e-mail is a hybrid between letter-writing and the spoken word. From a technical standpoint, unencrypted electronic messages (p.77) provide less privacy than postal mail or telephone calls. In practice, e-mail replaces and is used more like the telephone—but with less urgency. Due to its necessarily asynchronous (back and forth over hours or days) nature, e-mail is personal in function but impersonal in form.

Initially, clinic-to-patient e-mail traffic will be limited by the number of patients who routinely have access to e-mail accounts. In one study at a University-based health centre, a majority of the the patients in the internal medicine clinic had e-mail accounts (Fridsma *et al*. 1994). However, most Internet services were supplied, and to some extent monitored, by the patient's employers. Thus, many patients were reluctant to use these accounts to convey medical information.

A consideration of the advantages and disadvantages of electronic mail will help you decide whether it is appropriate to provide patients with your Internet address.

Advantages of e-mail in doctor–patient communications

E-mail may offer several advantages over existing communications channels between health-care providers and their patients.

- E-mail messages are less intrusive than phone calls. Half or more of all phone calls to clinics are non-urgent, and patients might naturally gravitate to e-mail for routine enquiries. E-mail messages can thus be batch-processed at the convenience of the recipient.
- Responding electronically to patient enquiries creates a written record that removes any doubt as to what was said during the patient's appointment. Often patients under duress forget to ask important questions. Self-care instructions might not be fully understood or retained. E-mail follow-up allows retention and clarification of information provided in clinic.
- E-mail is especially useful for information the patient would have to commit to writing anyway. Examples include addresses and phone numbers of other facilities to which the patient is referred; test results, interpretation, and subsequent instructions; instructions on how to take medications or apply dressings; and pre- and post-operative instructions. Some of these details lend themselves to a permanent position on a health-care provider's home page (p.202) on the World-Wide Web. If the patient has Web-browsing capabilities, an e-mail response can include the appropriate Web address (URL—p.102).
- E-mail messages are less likely to fall through the cracks of a busy practice. Phone messages are often lost or ignored. Voice mail systems are plagued with irksome branching menus, lapses on hold, and the threat of telephone 'tag'—many callers opt to just hang up. With or without annoying automated systems, telephone messaging often relies on a physical chain of human transmissions from front desk, to nurse, to doctor—with many 'While you were out...' slips getting lost.
- E-mail messages can be more detailed than those left in voice mailboxes (especially systems with a 60-second limit) or taken down by amanuensis. However, e-mail

tends to constrain the conversation to a single focus and avoids the rambling, multi-agenda phone call whose polite termination is difficult to manoeuvre.

- From an administrative standpoint, when e-mail has been established as the patient's preferred route of communication, appointment reminders, insurance questions, and routine follow-up enquiries lend themselves well to that medium.

Disadvantages of e-mail in doctor–patient communications

Like any communication medium, e-mail can be abused and misused.

- Many practitioners are concerned that answering e-mail will further burden their over-taxed schedules, without the prospect of reimbursement for time spent online. In the early stages of adoption, providers might be responsible for their own e-mail. Administrative support might be weak or non-existent.
- Some patients, fascinated by the novelty of the medium and the prospect of direct access to their physician, will become long-winded and frequent correspondents.
- When the volume of e-mail reaches critical mass, it might be necessary to retrain existing personnel, or hire additional support to handle the load.
- Most e-mail systems over the Internet do not provide confirmation that the message was delivered, although most do notify the sender if a message could not be delivered to the recipient's mailbox. Even software that returns notification of receipt cannot assure that the message was actually read and understood.
- For novices, uncertainty exists around netiquette (p.57) and other subtleties of correct usage. Some clinic–patient relationships will not tolerate a trial-and-error approach to the electronic persona.
- The medicolegal standing of e-mail-based communications has not yet been established clearly (see below, under 'Administrative and medicolegal guidelines').
- The electronic medium poses many issues relating to data security (see below, under *Data security*).

Communications guidelines

In these times of increasingly impersonal, truncated, and regulated care, clinic time with patients is often compromised. Presenting a business card with your e-mail address to the patient at the conclusion of the clinic visit invites an ongoing caring relationship. If you anticipate a need to re-contact the patient with regard to test results or other near-term follow-up, you should always enquire about the patient's communication preferences. Informally, you can ascertain preference for e-mail, voice mail, or postal exchange at the time of visit and document this in the chart. A more formal arrangement entails the documentation of informed consent (discussed below). Keep in mind that patients may elect telephone, e-mail, or the postal route at different times for different purposes. You should confirm on a visit-by-visit basis which route to take. At that time you should:

- Ascertain how often both parties retrieve e-mail and establish a maximal turn-around time for patient-initiated messages. In some messaging cultures, natural selection has evolved a one-business-day turn-around for non-urgent phone calls and a 2–3 business-day turn-around for e-mail. Often, the context of the patient's message will indicate the expected turn-around time. A patient who enquires about the results of a routine cervical smear will tolerate a longer messaging interval than one who is experiencing even mild side effects from a medication.
- Inform patients about whether your account is private or screened by ancillary staff. Will the office staff or nursing staff triage messages, or will mail addressed to your private account be read exclusively by you?
- Establish whether the patient may send you e-mail with express instructions to omit certain parts from the chart. If the patient is allowed to censor messages from his permanent record, is it advisable for you to keep an unexpurgated copy in your private files?
- Especially if other clinic staff will be processing e-mail from your patients, establish the extent of action you will permit over e-mail—prescription refills, medical advice, test results.
- E-mail exchanges constitute a form of progress note. Until a fully integrated electronic medical record affords automatic storage, back-up, and retrieval of data, e-mail should be printed in full and a copy placed in the patient's chart. The following steps result in efficient archiving:

    1. Include the full text of the patient's query in your e-mail reply.
    2. Copy the reply to yourself.

  When the Internet delivers your copy, which now includes both the original message and your reply, you should print it and file it in the chart. Be sure the printout arrives in an area which is accessible only to staff and not to other patients.
- For messages containing important medical advice, and in absence of software with built-in notification features, instruct the patient to acknowledge messages by sending a brief reply. When such acknowledgment is expected, the printed copy should await this final volley.
- Never assume that the patient has received important instructions. When in doubt, as when acknowledgment of receipt is not forthcoming, you must escalate communication to telephone contact.
- Include a footer (signature file) that invites the patient to escalate communication to a phone call or surgery visit, should they feel e-mail to be insufficient, and

give the appropriate contact information. You may need to wield a firm hand in discouraging the use of e-mail as a substitute for clinical examination.

- Use automated out-of-the-office replies on any e-mail account which will not be serviced by staff or covering doctors during an absence which exceeds your established e-mail response time. Such messages should include your estimated date of return and instructions for whom to contact for immediate assistance.
- Maintain a list of patients who communicate with you electronically in the address book feature of your e-mail software (p.155). If it becomes necessary to notify correspondents of an impending shutdown for network maintenance, recent mail blackouts, new clinic services, or change of address, you will have a ready-made mailing list (p.165). However, never use group-addressing, where those in the group see each other's names, to send mail to patients. The fact that a person sees a particular health-care provider is confidential information. Additionally, patients have become indignant over inclusion on lists such as the age-revealing list of 'women who are due for mammograms'.
- Keep in mind that the impersonal nature and ambiguity of e-mail often results in a real or imagined exaggeration of animosity toward the recipient. Sick, anxious, or angry patients might indeed express stronger sentiments than in a face-to-face encounter or in a voice message.
- Be prepared to encounter patients who are sophisticated Internet users, aware of its privacy limitations, who nevertheless initiate unencrypted e-mail discussions of a surprisingly intimate medical nature.

Administrative and medicolegal guidelines

Aspects of electronic messaging of particular interest to risk management and legal departments concern data security and liability for advice. The most wary approach dictates that patients be asked to sign printed guidelines—a sort of informed consent—at the time an electronic relationship is established. In addition to the points in the above communications guidelines, electronic messaging agreements should include:

- an explanation of the general nature of the network and its level of security. Are you using an intranet (p.113) with a firewall (p.61)? Are you or the institution directly connected to the Internet or do you use an Internet service provider who conceivably monitors transmission? Are you using encryption software (see below, and p.61)?
- the facility for a patient to specifically 'opt out' of the use of encryption if he or she does not wish to comply with the extra processing required;
- a clause to limit liability for network infractions beyond the control of the health-care providers.

Additionally, you should:

- avoid leaving open e-mail on your computer screen. If your computer is in the same room as other patients, be sure to use a password-activated screen saver so that patient files are not visible to other patients, especially if you are called out of the room;
- never forward the patient's message or patient-identifiable information to a third party without the express permission of the patient;
- never use a patient's e-mail address in clinic marketing schemes nor supply such addresses to third parties for advertising or any other use;
- as with other parts of the medical record, do not take patient-identifiable e-mail out of the office or surgery. If you answer e-mail from home you must take special precautions to prevent other household members from intercepting messages from patients. Do not share e-mail accounts or passwords with friends, family, or non-medical coworkers. If you communicate with patients, you should have your own account for professional use. You must see to it that e-mail processed off-site on home systems or via personal digital assistants (PDAs—p.17), for example, is subsequently printed in the office and included in the medical record;
- as soon as practicable, establish a means of secure communication using the data encryption methods described below.

Data security

In order for electronic transactions to be trustworthy, users must have authenticated identities; data must be transmitted accurately; and sensitive information must be protected from interception or malicious hacking. Maximum patient privacy requires that all e-mail exchanges be encrypted. From the standpoint of data security, unencrypted e-mail is like sending a postcard or talking over a wireless phone. As wireless access to the Internet becomes more common, data encryption of medical information will probably become an absolute requirement.

Terms used in talking about data security include:

Authenticity:

Authenticity refers to validation of the message-sender's identity, often by means of a 'digital signature'.

Confidentiality:

The degree to which the message is impervious to interception by eavesdroppers. A **confidential** message is one whose contents are seen only by those so authorized.

Data integrity:

Data integrity is a measure of system robustness which indicates that the data have been unaltered in transfer either deliberately by malicious intent or inadvertently through network failures.

Digital signature:

A **digital signature** is a means of authentication. In 'public-key' encryption schemes, the sender encodes their document or document header with a private key. If the document can be decoded with the sender's public key, the sender's identity is confirmed.

Encryption:

Transforming information by means of a mathematical code so that it is unintelligible (see *Security issues in brief*, p.60). Encrypting messages with a prearranged code ensures confidentiality. Encrypting a signature authenticates the sender.

Note that both parties to e-mail must have compatible encryption–decryption software on their computers. PGP (Pretty Good Privacy) is a freely available encryption package that runs on most platforms and uses the popular RSA (Rivest, Shamir, and Adleman) algorithm. It can be downloaded by anonymous FTP (p.179) from many places including:

<URL:ftp://ftp.ox.ac.uk/pub/crypto/pgp/>

This addressing scheme is explained in Chapter Twelve. Alternatively, public-key encryption capabilities are available as a feature of some e-mail and Web applications (such as Netscape Navigator, p.200), and from companies specializing in encryption software. An institutional licensing fee may be required.

Spoofing (an e-mail message):

Sending a message purporting to come from someone else.

Other issues

Mistakes due to poor interface design and lack of fail-safe mechanisms are particularly troublesome in medical communications. There is litigation pending in the US courts (as of this writing) involving a physician who allegedly inadvertently posted his patient's diagnosis of breast cancer to the public area of a major commercial online service. As the doctor and patient had had prior e-mail exchanges, the mistake was almost certainly an interface problem with the client software. Until fool-proof software is available, and unless communication uses public-key encryption systems, it is advisable to make a habit of checking the 'To:' box in your message prior to sending.

Institutional considerations for e-mail communication

There is growing evidence to suggest that electronic resources, both e-mail and Web-based self-help documents, will result in substantial cost savings to clinics (Gareiss 1994). Savings of time spent on the telephone will result from a reduction in telephone 'tag' and in repetitious instructions. Many clinics, especially those with 'capitated plans' (allocation of funds on a per-head basis), anticipate replacing inappropriate office visits with online support, including teleconferencing (Gareiss 1994).

Institutional policies will need to be developed to address communication and medicolegal guidelines. Questions that must be answered include the following.

- Who will triage e-mail and what is to be the response time?
- Who will print messages and place them in patient's charts?
- Will each provider have his or her own account or will there be categorical accounts for all billing questions, medical questions, and scheduling questions?
- Should all patients be given the provider's e-mail address or can the provider give it out on a selective basis?
- How is e-mail cleared from the server? Does it stay on your local machine and/or on your mail server (p.141)? How are both repositories archived and cleared?
- Will the patient be given a choice as to what appears from his or her e-mail message in the chart? Do you wish to give the option for 'private' sections of the message that may not be placed in the chart? If you opt not to put all parts into the chart, do you wish to establish a secure repository, either electronic or paper-based, to recall the text of the original message for your own purposes? Or do you want the transaction to be more like a phone call where the conversation is relegated to second-hand progress notes?
- Will encryption systems be required? If so, what kind? Will patients be given the encryption software by the clinic?
- Should clinics provide patients with e-mail accounts on the institutional server?

Eventually e-mail storage and retrieval must be integrated with a comprehensive electronic medical record (EMR). World-Wide Web-based EMRs (p.113) over secure internal Internet sites (called 'intranets', p.113) are a likely model for the future.

E-mail is not a substitute for face-to-face clinical evaluation. When in doubt, encourage the patient to make a personal appearance.

References

Fridsma, D.B., Ford, P., and Altman, R. (1994). A survey of patient access to electronic mail: attitudes, barriers, and opportunities. In *Proceedings of the Eighteenth Annual Symposium on Computer Applications in Medical Care*, pp.15–19. American Medical Informatics Association, Bethesda.

Gareiss, R. (1994). Electronic triage. *American Medical News*, 25 April, 23–7.

CHAPTER TEN
Example online services

In this Chapter we take a brief look at a selection of five online services offering medical content. The examples given here include a large commercial online service (CompuServe), commercial databases (DataStar and DIALOG), a not-for-profit network (HealthNet), a service provided through the UK's National Health Service (NHS Viewdata Information Services), and a small 'hobbyist' bulletin board (UK Healthlink). The examples illustrate the variety and potential usage of online medical information resources.

Other non-profit bulletin boards of interest to UK doctors include the Andy's Clinic BBS (8-N-1, VT100, 0161 439 9429), Primary Health Care Specialist Group BBS (8-N-1, ANSI, 0191 5192 542), and Pry Marie Care BBS (8-N-1, ANSI, 0126 0299 782). The UK Healthlink BBS maintains a listing of British BBSs with a health focus (p.89).

Physicians' Online, a commerical American service, offers a range of databases (including MEDLINE) free to US physicians. Access is through a local call in most instances, although the custom PC and Mac client can also connect across an IP (Internet Protocol, p.100) link. More information is available by telephoning 1(800) 332-0009, e-mailing the Member Services Department at **general@po.com**, or using the following Internet address (URL—p.102). Physicians' Online have announced plans to extend into Europe:

<URL:http://www.po.com/>

The Black Bag Medical BBS List, maintained by Edward Del Grosso, covers North American bulletin boards with medical and paramedical themes. To retrieve ths list, send e-mail to **list@blackbag.com**.

Medicine on CompuServe

CompuServe can be accessed through local numbers in many countries. Content on CompuServe is divided into forums and databases. Each forum contains a message board, library, and conference area. Both the message and library areas are subdivided into topic areas. Conference 'rooms' allow private online chat, and participation in planned medical conferences (in real-time typing). Some databases are only available at extra cost ('premium services'), and these are indicated below by the '($)' sign, as in Physicians' Data Query ($).

Health services can be reached by navigating menus using the CompuServe Information Manager (CIM, a graphical interface), or by typing in 'GO words' (quick reference words).

Getting a complete picture of the available services using menus in the CIM or broad GO words (such as HEALTH and MEDICAL) is difficult owing to extensive cross-referencing. It is easier to 'GO' for a specific service (see Table 8). Note that the following list of services is not comprehensive; it is intended only to illustrate the diversity in services available.

TABLE 8 Overview of CompuServe health services

Forums	**GO words**
AMIA Medical Forum	GO MEDSIG
Attention Deficit Disorder Forum	GO ADD
Cancer Forum	GO CANCER
Diabetes Forum	GO DIABETES
Disabilities Forum	GO DISABILITIES
Health and Fitness Forum	GO GOODHEALTH
Natural Medicine Forum	GO NATMED
Human Sexuality	GO HUMAN
Information USA (Health section)	GO INFOUSA
Muscular Dystrophy Association Forum	GO MDA
Retirement Living Forum (Health and Medicine section)	GO RETIRE
Time Warner Lifestyles Forum (Health and Fitness section)	GO TWLIFE
UK Professionals Forum	GO UKPROF
Databases	**GO words**
Comprehensive Core Medical Library ($)	GO CCML
Consumer Reports Complete Drug Reference	GO DRUGS
Handicapped User's Database	GO HUD
Health Database Plus ($)	GO HLTDB
HealthNet	GO HNT
IQuest Medical InfoCenter ($)	GO IQMEDICINE
NORD Services/ Rare Disease Database	GO NORD
PaperChase (MEDLINE) ($)	GO PAPERCHASE
Physicans Data Query ($)	GO PDQ
PsycINFO- Psychological Abstracts ($)	GO PSYCINFO
Other health-related services	**GO words**
AIDS News Clips	GO AIDSNEWS
Business Database Plus	GO BUSDB
Government Publications	GO GPO
Syndicated Columns (The Medical Advisor)	GO SYN-30
Sports Medicine	GO INFOUSA

($) Incurs additional charges aside from connect-time.

Health services: Forums

Natural Medicine Forum: Message/library areas on topics including holistic medicine; herbs and plants; homeopathy and Bach flowers; chiropractice; healing and the mind; women's health; health education, and rethinking AIDS.

Information USA (Health section): Message/library areas on topics including AIDS and cancer information; pregnancy and contraception information; health-care letters; cigarette smoking and tobacco use; stress and mental illness; and health-related questions and answers. US Government health information.

Retirement Living Forum (Health and Medicine section): Contains information from the National Institutes of Health, the National Heart, Lung, and Blood Institute, and others relating to the treatment and prevention of heart diseases and cancer.

Time Warner Lifestyles Forum (Health/Fitness section): General lifestyle discussion; exercise; dieting; stress management, etc.

Disabilities Forum: Covers developmental disabilities; emotional disturbance; deaf/hard of hearing; learning disabilities; visual impairment; mobility impairment; epilepsy and multiple sclerosis—among other topics.

Attention Deficit Disorder Forum: Diagnosis; treatment; family and social issues; parenting; sources of further information, etc.

Muscular Dystrophy Association Forum: Research; support; resources; insurance, etc.

Human Sexuality: Includes a dictionary; family planning information; questions and answers; homosexuality issues, and men's and women's health information.

AMIA Medical Forum: Supported by the American Medical Informatics Association, a place to meet American health professionals. Topics under discussion include research; informatics; pharmacology; computers in medicine; CME; subspeciality practice; nursing, and more. Frequent conferences on a variety of topics.

Cancer Forum: Includes a support library; hospice issues; research, and information on various forms of cancer.

Diabetes Forum: Hypoglycaemia; insulins; complications; diet and exercise; travel; blood sugar monitoring, etc.

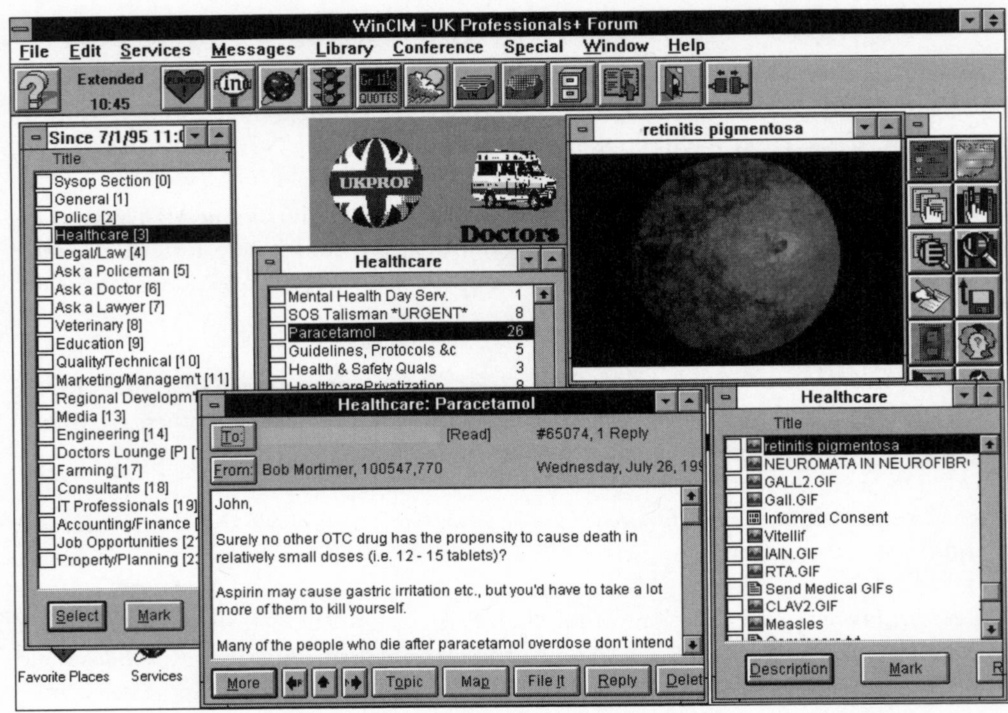

Fig. 8 CompuServe's UKPROF Healthcare section provides a forum for health professionals to join real-time nationwide discussions, exchange messages, and download UK-focused health information. [Screen capture: Dr. I. Kewley.]

Health & Fitness Forum: Mental health; family health; exercise and fitness; addiction and recovery; women's health; CFS/ME, etc.

UK Professionals Forum: There are three forum areas of interest: *Healthcare* includes UK meetings and symposia; NHS information and computing; medical GIF images; pharmacology; ethics; health service privatization; inter-professional discussions; medical shareware programs, etc. *Ask a Doctor* covers UK credentials; medical records; long-term care; all health problems, etc. *Doctor's Lounge*—a private section for doctors only—includes journal club; clinical cases; medico-political discussion; sports medicine; peer support, etc. A closed conference for doctors is held on the third Sunday of each month at 9.00 pm. The application form to gain access to the Doctors Lounge can be downloaded as **SEC15.TXT**, from within the Healthcare library. See Fig. 8.

Health services: Databases

Comprehensive Core Medical Library: A database of medical literature abstracts from the general journals and major medical references. Searchable by subject, author, title, publication, article type, and publication date.

Consumer Reports Complete Drug Reference: Compiled by the *US Pharmacopeia*, you can enter a generic or (US) brand name to obtain information on drug use, dosage forms, cautions and contraindications, storage instructions, side effects, etc. In consumer-oriented language.

HealthNet: A menu-driven library with articles covering sports medicine; disorders and diseases; symptoms; drugs; surgeries/tests/procedures; home care and first aid; obstetrics/ reproductive medicine; and ophthalmology/eye care.

Health Database Plus ($): Although oriented to non-professionals, this database contains abstracts from several sources of interest to health professionals including the *Morbidity and Mortality Weekly Report*, *Journal of the American Medical Association*, *The Lancet*, and the *New England Journal of Medicine*. Instructions for using the service via the CIM or by terminal emulation are online. Offers two levels of searching, QuickSearch (subjects only) and PowerSearch (by subject, author, date, journal, article title, keyword, and combined searches). Searches can use **wild cards** (e.g. gyna*cology) and **Boolean operators** (and, or, not). Marked articles can be downloaded for offline viewing.

PaperChase ($): An interface to MEDLINE. See Chapter Twenty Nine.

NORD Services/Rare Disease Database: From the National Organization for Rare Diseases (NORD), a database for lay people searchable by illness name, symptoms, cause, and type (e.g. neurological). The resulting list of diseases can be examined to gain information about synonyms, symptoms, causes, affected population, related disorders, therapies, and resources.

IQuest Medical InfoCenter ($): A menu-based collection of databases including citations, abstracts, and full-text articles (no graphics). Can search a single database, or across several at a time. Permits wild cards and Boolean operators. Charge for unsuccessful searches.

Physicians' Data Query ($): Contains the Consumer Cancer Information File (treatment options, staging, and prognoses by cancer name—for lay people); the Professional Cancer Information File (treatment options, staging, prognoses, and bibliographies by cancer name—for health professionals); the Directory File (listing National Cancer Institute designated cancer centres or other career-approved programmes, directory of specialist physicians), and the Protocol File (protocols by cancer name and stage, treatment type, or medication).

PsycINFO-Psychological Abstracts ($): From the American Psychological Association, contains abstracts from psychology and behavioural sciences literature. Can be searched by subject, author, language, or publication year.

For further information, contact CompuServe Information Services Ltd, 1 Redcliff Street, PO Box 676, Bristol BS99 1YN, telephone Sales on 0800 289 378, or e-mail **70006.101@compuserve.com**.

DataStar and DIALOG

Another type of online service is the searchable database from commercial providers. Examples are DataStar and DIALOG, two large collections of databases offerred in the UK by Knight-Ridder Information Ltd. The cost of using services such as these can be prohibitive to the individual, but they exist to fill a particular market niche. Users of these services tend to work within commercial organizations or undertake extensive research. Whether this type of specialist service represents value-for-money for any given user is dependent on a number of factors. Information presented in this way is currently more accessible, comprehensive, and better organized than Internet-based resources. MEDLINE and full-text medical journals are also available on CompuServe, for example, and offer an attractive alternative for occasional use.

Both DataStar and DIALOG can be accessed in the same way as other online services, using an ordinary personal computer and modem transmitting at up to 9600 bps. Both collections include bibliographic databases such as EMBASE (formerly Excerpta Medica), CANCERLIT (cancer literature), MEDLINE, CINAHL (Nursing and Allied Health), and combinations of full-text and bibliographic data such as the Health Periodicals database. DIALOG also includes MEDTEXT, a full-text database of articles from the *New England Journal of Medicine*, the *Journal of the American Medical Association*, and other AMA speciality journals. DataStar includes several UK-oriented databases, such as the *The Lancet* and General Practitioner (full-text of the periodicals *General Practitioner*, *Mims Magazine*, *Medeconomics*, and *Fundholding*).

Aside from normal telephone charges, the cost of accessing this service comprises annual service fees, network charges (BT or SprintNet), a fee for each document output, and a connect-time fee. Training, usage documentation, and DialogLink software (Mac or Windows) are optional extras. Charges are calculated from Swiss francs (DataStar) or US dollars (DIALOG). As of writing, a 3-month introductory offer was available at a fixed price of SFr 1500 for DataStar and $US 1500 for DIALOG.

The service is also available over the Internet. Further information is available from Knight-Ridder Information, Haymarket House, 1 Oxendon Street, London SW1Y 4EE. Telephone 0171 930 5503 or fax 0171 930 2581.

HealthNet

HealthNet (HealthLink in South Africa) is a unique online network that sprang from the realization that the developing world was under-served by the revolution in medical information technology. A project of the Boston-based not-for-profit organization SatelLife, it provides both a telecommunications infrastructure and medical content at prices suited to health professionals in developing nations. Using existing telephone systems, radio, and its own low Earth-orbiting satellite and ground stations, HealthNet links doctors in the developing world with each other and with the medical databases most of us take for granted.

HealthNet in its present form is presented as an alternative to the relative expense of an Internet connection. Although its clients are able to exchange e-mail with Internet users and access Internet-based mailing lists, they also have their own e-mail and file-transfer tools. Together these tools enable physician collaborations, the collection of clinical data from remote sites, dissemination of medical alerts, transmission of referrals, and the scheduling of consultations. Using Grateful Med (p.244) and BITNIS, users can save search strategies as a text file which can be transmitted by e-mail and used to interrogate databases at the National Library of Medicine (and retrieve article abstracts).

HealthNet News is a publication distributed exclusively to HealthNet users and contains relevant full-text articles culled from major peer-reviewed journals. SatelLife also sponsor several moderated conferences (equivalent to Internet mailing lists, p.165) covering emerging diseases, AIDS, and essential drugs. These conferences are open to anyone with an e-mail account, whether or not they subscribe to HealthNet itself. To join a conference or view archives of the discussions, visit the SatelLife Web site.

SatelLife have announced plans to integrate optional full Internet access into their current service using a custom software interface. For further information contact SatelLife, 1360 Soldiers Field Road, Boston MA 02135, USA, e-mail **hnet@usa.healthnet.org**, or view the SatelLife Web site at:

<URL:http://www.healthnet.org>

NHS Viewdata Information Services

NHS Viewdata Information Services provide three online services targeted specifically at National Health Service users.

TOXBASE, from the National Poisons Information Service, is a clinical toxicology database. It includes sections on assessment and management of poisoning, with references to relevant literature. Aimed primarily at accident and emergency departments but useful to general practitioners, registration for access to this service is free within the NHS.

The TRAVAX information service is provided by the Scottish Centre for Infection and Environmental Health. The database is continually updated to provide advice on immunizations by country with vaccine details, malaria prophylaxis, and HIV risks, as well as information on other health risks travellers may encounter (such as food, water, and insect-borne infections). Special attention is given to recent outbreaks of disease and changes in vaccination and other prescription schedules. General Practitioners are not charged to use the service (charges do apply to some other groups).

VADIS is from the Scottish Pharmacy Practice Centre. It consists of a database covering the basic pharmacology, pharmacokinetics, usage and doses, contraindications and precautions, use in organ dysfunction, adverse effects, therapeutics, and interactions for drugs in clinical use in the UK. A subscription fee of £75 is applied to all users, with a surcharge for heavy usage.

Any PC running terminal-emulation software can be used to access the services. **Viewdata** emulation is preferable, providing colour.

The service can be called direct, or accessed via the AT&T Istel Infotrac network which allows most UK users to make a local call. A demonstration database is available for those with Viewdata emulation. Set your terminal software to 7 data bits; 1 stop bit; even parity; and a speed of 1200/75 bps. Dial 0131 536 3333, type **DEMO** at the **Login ID** prompt, and press **RETURN**. Technical help is available on (voice) 0131 536 5050. For further information, contact the Viewdata Services Manager, The Old Residency, The Royal Infirmary NHS Trust, 1 Lauriston Place, Edinburgh EH3 9YW.

UK Healthlink

UK Healthlink is a FidoNet bulletin board located in Wigan (FidoNet node 2:250/232.0). It is a voluntary service linking those interested in the use of computers in the health services, and providing a forum for communication between health-care workers. To connect to the BBS, dial 01942 722 984 using the following settings in your terminal emulator software (p.49):

- Speed to 14 400 bps
- 8 data bits
- No parity
- 1 stop bit
- Hardware handshake
- Full duplex
- ANSI (or VT100 terminal type)
- Local echo off

Full access is available to registered members only, but visitors are allowed limited access. Registration is £10 per annum for individuals or £30 for groups of up to ten in Colleges of Education, plus usual telephone charges. Registration for overseas health workers is free. New users are requested to give their name and choose a password online. Health professionals also complete a brief questionnaire. Registration details are confirmed by post, indicating that full access has been granted. UK Healthlink is organized like many small non-profit bulletin boards; it is essentialy divided into message areas and file areas.

The message areas contain public conferences and the facilities for private messages, including the option to exchange e-mail with the Internet (an Internet e-mail address is automatic for registered users). Public message areas include news on NHS computing, several FidoNet echos (p.47), and nursing conferences. Through the International FidoNet Association, UK Healthlink communicates with up to thirty thousand similar BBSs worldwide.

File areas include health-related files, conference and course information, and nursing informatics files. A range of file-transfer protocols are supported for downloads and uploads, including Zmodem, Xmodem, Ymodem, Kermit, and ASCII (see p.31).

For more information, contact **sysop@healthlink.fido.zetnet.co.uk**, telephone 01942 712 385, or write to UK Healthlink, 164 Windsor Road, Ashton-in-Makerfield, Wigan WN4 9ES.

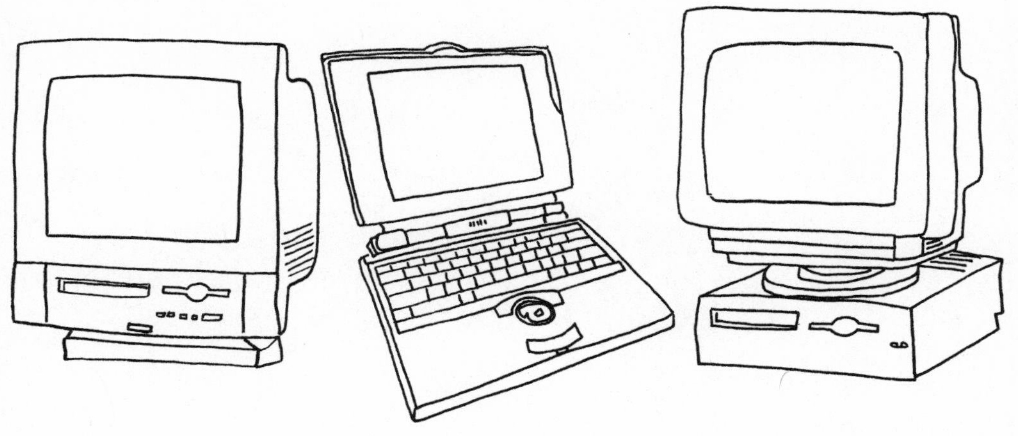

PART 3

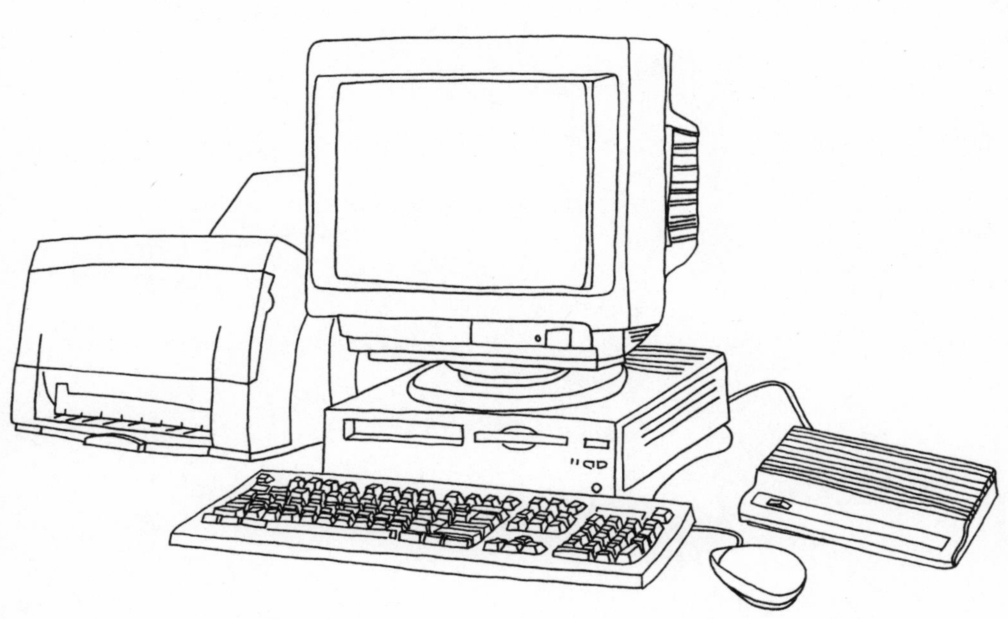

CHAPTER ELEVEN
Internet introduced

The Internet has the been subject of extraordinary publicity in recent times. For many it remains some ill-defined entity bordering on the mythological. How is it possible to talk to America without the cost of a transatlantic telephone call? Colourful terms such as 'surfing the Web', 'cyberspace', 'information superhighway', and 'e-mail' are becoming integrated into the lay vocabulary. But what exactly is the Internet? And more specifically, what is its place in the practice of medicine? How do you become involved? This Part provides answers to these questions.

The Internet is actually a simple concept. Imagine several computers in a Medical Physics Department linked together by a series of cables. These cables allow the connected computers to swap files and exchange all kinds of information, providing that they communicate with each other using the same 'language'. This arrangement is called a **local-area network** (LAN), because all the computers are directly connected to one another within a relatively small area. Some larger networks use telecommunications services in place of electrical cables to link together computers that may be many miles apart. This is known as a **wide-area network** (WAN). But the ability to link together computers doesn't end here.

Telecommunications links (such as the telephone system, satellites, and fibre optic cabling) can also join whole networks together, forming an even larger one. As before, if these INTER-connected NETworks speak a common language, information can be passed from one network to another. The Internet (with a capital I) refers to the worldwide internet of computer networks that speak a language called TCP/IP. This Part begins by expanding on our explanation of what the Internet is and how it works.

A network of networks

People are attracted to the Internet for a variety of reasons. Some simply enjoy the concept of using their PC to access a computer thousands of miles away by making a local telephone call. Others find its interactive nature more stimulating than television. Still others, however, hope to gain something useful from it. The Internet offers rapid communications with millions of users all over the globe, thousands of discussion groups covering all facets of life, vast storehouses of computer software, vendor support and product news, and free electronic libraries of text and pictures. These offerings are given an overview in this Part, with an emphasis on those that have applications in medicine.

Despite the criticism levelled at the Internet because of the unsavoury nature of some material accessible through it, it is not something that is inherently evil. It may provide access to a discussion of the most effective techniques for committing suicide, but there will always be those who exploit its capabilities or air objectionable views.

Virtually all online services offer some form of Internet access, and computer magazines often give away access packages from a plethora of new companies specializing in Internet access. We look at options for getting connected beginning on p.135.

The Internet versus the online service

America OnLine (AOL in Europe) is the world's largest commercial online service, followed closely by CompuServe, each with over 4 million subscribers. Internet users number somewhere in the tens of millions—a number growing every month. The Internet supports so many more users because it is a fundamentally different service. Superficially there may be similarities: you pay a connection fee; run communications software to log on over a modem connection, and upload or download messages and files. Underneath, the Internet is an extremely large but loose association of many individual networks, none of which owns or operates the service as a whole. It is run by mutual cooperation, not a profit-motivated Board of Directors.

Many bulletin boards and online services incorporate some part of the Internet in their offerings (see Chapter Fifteen). Each different online service based on proprietary software requires unique communications software settings and navigational skills, whereas directly accessed Internet resources can be tied together seamlessly by the World-Wide Web (p.197) in a uniform point-and-click interface.

Chapter Five considered the sometimes difficult distinction between a bulletin board and a commercial online service. But what is the difference between these two, and an Internet **service provider**?

Early 1996 saw many online services begin moving away from selling content via proprietary client software, gravitating toward the more 'open standards' of the Internet. In many instances, content once accessed through proprietary software on closed networks can now be accessed via the World-Wide Web (see Chapter Twenty six). Content on Web sites can be password-protected giving access to subscribers only, although some material may be available to non-subscribers. Some Internet service providers also publish content on their Web sites. Consequently, the distinction between an online service and Internet service provider is not so clear at first glance.

There remain, however, a few differences that are useful to bear in mind—if only for the fact that they have a bearing on how much you end up paying for Internet access.

- A service that relies solely on its own secure network to deliver content to subscribers, which cannot be accessed via an alternative access provider over the Internet, is clearly an online service.
- Online services sell access to unique content, and may also sell access to the Internet. Because this unique content is described as 'value-added', it usually justifies higher fees compared to an Internet-access only service.
- Online services usually charge on a 'pay-as-you-go' basis, whereas companies selling just Internet access typically charge a flat fee for unlimited use.
- The type of content on an online service versus content on the wider Internet differs, based on the premise that people expect to pay more for quality products that have commercial potential. Some online services offer a number of commercial medical databases that are unlikely to be made available 'free' on the Internet. Even so, the combined resources of the networks making up the Internet enable it to offer more in terms of scope and volume than any one online service could alone. Online services (and smaller bulletin boards) can exert far greater control over the content they choose to offer.
- Online services are generally better at providing all the software, manuals, and other paraphernalia needed to use the service compared with dial-up Internet service providers. Analogous to an all-inclusive package holiday, this approach can avoid the need to 'mix and match' the elements you need to explore the online world—at the expense of customization.

The rising popularity of the Internet does not necessarily herald the death of local bulletin boards and online services. A different heritage inherently suggests different strengths and weaknesses. Perhaps, most obviously, spreading expenditure across numerous network providers helps ensure the viability of the Internet with minimal charge to individual users. Commercial services seeking to provide expansive network access with high-quality products—and generate profit—can only do so at cost to subscribers. Local bulletin boards, on the other hand, are typically the least expensive way to get online.

In summary, a BBS or commercial online service offers unique content, possibly in addition to Internet access. An Internet access provider strictly provides just that, although the term is loosely applied to anyone—BBSs and online services included—who provides *any* form of Internet access.

When you've finished this Part you should:

in relation to the Internet,

- be able describe the Internet as the global interconnection of networks to a colleague
- know (in outline) the purpose of the main Internet services
- know what is meant by domain name and URL

in relation to online medicine,

- be aware of what the Internet offers today, and what it doesn't
- appreciate the potential of the Internet as a tool in health care—and also the potential problems
- have an idea how to find resources on the Internet

know what is involved

- in obtaining Internet access
- in setting up a dial-up TCP/IP Internet connection.

CHAPTER TWELVE

What is the Internet?

A 'network' is simply the linking together of any number of individual computers. The 'Internet' is the interconnection of many smaller networks to form a single network that is very vast indeed. It connects together governments, universities, businesses, online services, hospitals, professionals, and millions of people across the globe from all walks of life. The Internet began life in the US Army in 1969, and grew to include academic and government computers until, in the early 1990s, it became accessible to anyone who owned a computer, a modem, and an account with an Internet access provider.

When connected, one has access to all of the public resources stored on the computers that make up the many networks (see Fig. 9). These resources include informational text files, software, electronic magazines, journal articles, pictures, sounds, video clips, and animations, etc. On the Internet, distance is irrelevant. The computer on your desk effectively becomes a terminal for computers all over the planet. Surprisingly, it is possible to access these international resources for the cost of a local telephone call.

How does the Internet work?

The high-speed communications backbone of the Internet is today formed by a number of large commercial networks such as Sprintlink and MCInet. A great many smaller networks are linked to these commercial backbones. Each network is run independently and paid for by whichever academic, government, or private organization owns it. The Internet itself, however, has no central authority; it operates by mutual cooperation.

In essence, the Internet's computers talk to one another using a language known as **TCP/IP**. Computers that connect to the Internet via telephone lines need a kind of interpreter (called **SLIP** or **PPP**) to make TCP/IP understood over this type of connection.

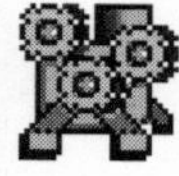

Internet-linked computers talk to each other using a communications protocol suite known as TCP/IP (Transmission Control Protocol/Internet Protocol). Firstly, your Internet software ensures its instructions or data are organized according to TCP/IP conventions. TCP breaks up the data into 'packets', adding an address, reassembly instructions, and error-correction controls. IP breaks TCP packets into even smaller units, each with an 'address header'.

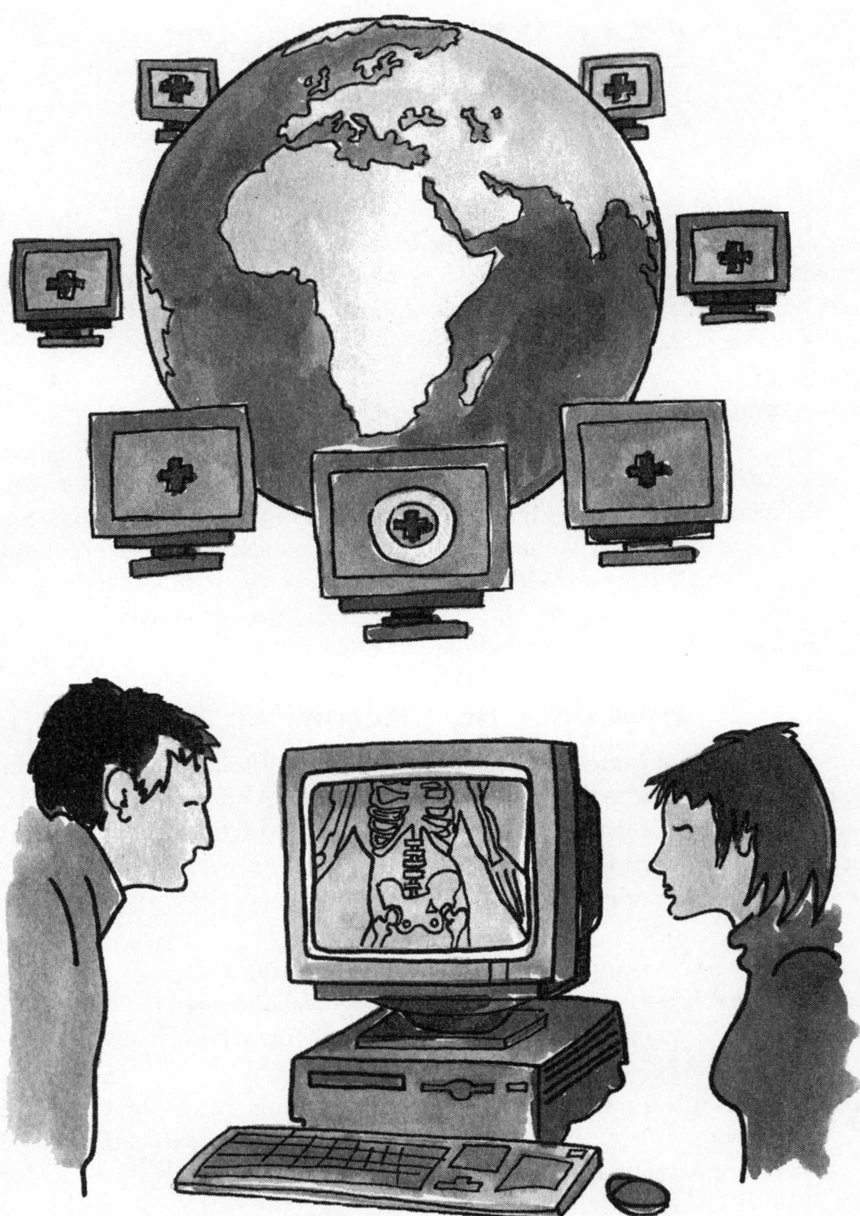

Fig. 9 What is the Internet? By connecting your home PC to the Internet through an Internet access provider, you become part of a network of networks spanning the globe. You can 'ride' one network to reach another, with instant access to the resources on that network for the cost of a local call.

These IP packets may be further modified by various network protocols, or by a protocol that allows them to be sent over telephone lines (Serial Line Internet Protocol or Point to Point Protocol). SLIP or PPP are actually network interfaces for dial-up links using modems, effectively making your machine a part of the networks you are using (although you continue working in a familiar operating system). In fact, you can simultaneously link to several networks at once. Using a news reader, file-retrieval software, and an information browser for example (see below), you might exchange data with three different computers in three different countries, each task utilizing a percentage of your modem's total capacity (or **bandwidth**).

The packets are sent as a 'stream' across any possible series of intermediary networks, via the shortest possible route (not necessarily the most direct), to the address specified in the header. In reflection of its military heritage, however, should part of this network be 'taken out', IP will automatically divert the data to its destination along an alternate path. At the remote computer, the packets are interpreted and reassembled into the original data, whether it be a command or a file of some description. This packet exchange is a two-way process.

Strictly speaking, only those networks which use TCP/IP are part of the Internet proper. However, many bulletin boards, networks using different protocols, and commercial online services have **gateways** to this IP traffic (machines that translate between different network protocols). Being a part of the Internet has *informally* come to mean that you have some sort of ability to communicate electronically with other Internet-connected people.

Internet services overview

Historically the three primary Internet applications are electronic mail, File Transfer Protocol, and Telnet. Electronic mail (**e-mail**) allows us to send messages from one computer to another either as a personal message, or to a group of people via a mailing list or newsgroup. **Mailing lists** discuss particular topics and messages relating to that topic are e-mailed to all the people who subscribe to that list. **Network news** (including **Usenet**) is not unlike a global bulletin board, but without a fixed home, where messages are organized into **newsgroups** to be passed around Internet sites, read, and added to. **File Transfer Protocol (FTP)** allows the user to upload or download files. **Telnet** lets us log in remotely to other computers and use them as if we were at a terminal in the same location. These primary applications appeared early in the course of the development of the Internet and are crucial to the workings of later Internet applications. Both primary (traditional) and secondary (later generation) applications are referred to collectively as **Internet services**.

Secondary applications have greatly modified the way people use the Internet, with facilities such as Internet Relay Chat (multi-user real-time conversations across the globe) and Multi-User Dimensions (MUDS—role-playing games) reflecting the Internet's newer role in entertainment. For readers of this book, however, the most important group of secondary applications are information retrieval tools.

Information retrieval tools share the characteristic of helping to locate information and/or files held on various Internet computers. The important tools are Archie, Gopher, Wide Area Information Servers, and the World-Wide Web—each unique in its capabilities to retrieve usable information. **Archie** is a searchable database of the location of files that are available for the public to download. **Gophers** organize information on different computers into a menu and, with the help of 'Veronica' (p.193), can lead you to relevant resources. **Wide Area Information Servers (WAIS)** go further than Archie and can search the contents of files looking for a match to your query. The graphical **World-Wide Web (WWW**, or simply 'the Web') has become so prominent that calling it a 'secondary' service is rather misleading. Gopher and the WWW link together assorted elements so seamlessly that their client applications are known as **browsers**, reflecting the casual nature of accessing resources through them. The important Internet services are summarized in Table 9, and each is discussed in greater detail in the next Part. With a little experimentation it will become clear which tools are best suited to a particular task.

Finding your way about

To access any of the Internet services, you need to understand how machines and resources on the Internet are uniquely identified. The three basic ingredients for Internet navigation are IP addresses, domain names, and uniform resource locators.

Internet Protocol addresses

Every machine directly connected to the Internet is uniquely identified by an Internet Protocol or **IP address**. This address takes the form of a grouping of four numbers separated by full stops, such as 158.152.64.237.

The Domain Name System

IP addresses aren't exactly memorable, and can in fact change occasionally. To overcome this the Domain Name System (DNS) uses a hierarchy of named 'domains' (subdivisions of computers) to make things more intuitive (sometimes). The broadest category is called the 'top domain', and in the US is a three-letter acronym such as **org** for organizations, **edu** for educational institutions, and **gov** for government computers. The rest of the world uses a two-letter acronym, such as **uk** for the United Kingdom and **nz** for New Zealand. A variable number of sub-domains then describes the name of the organization or institution, a particular department, or a certain machine. The combination of these elements is called a **domain name**. As an example, a computer called CyberTas might have Internet access via a commercial service provider called Demon Internet based in the UK. Its domain name is therefore:

cybertas.demon.co.uk

The **.nhs.uk** domain is provided for National Health Service organizations. Note that domain-name elements are also separated by full stops, and by convention are written in lower case. An alphanumeric name followed by the @ symbol can precede the domain name and is used to address a specific person or software robot on certain machines (such as **bruce@cybertas.demon.co.uk**. See also p.153). Dedicated computers called 'DNS name servers' invisibly map domain names to current IP addresses, although it is possible to access an Internet computer by typing in the IP address directly.

TABLE 9 Summary of useful Internet services

Primary Internet services	**Electronic mail** e-mail (general use) mailing lists (e-mail subscriptions) network news (discussion groups)
	File transfer File Transfer Protocol (FTP)
	Using other computers/remote control Telnet
Information retrieval tools	Archie Gopher and Veronica Wide Area Information Server (WAIS) World-Wide Web (WWW)
Other ways to communicate	Internet Relay Chat (IRC) MUD, object-oriented (MOO) Streaming audio Internet telephony and videoconferencing Web-based conferencing Internet fax

Uniform resource locators

Uniform resource locators (URLs) refer to a standardized syntax describing the location and method of accessing Internet resources. They are defined formally in *RFC 1738* (see below, *Learning more*), and are crucial to navigating the Internet. By entering a URL into a computer, you can find any specified resource without having to search manually, directory by directory. The basic format of URLs follows:

service://host[:port]/path

The **service** element is the type of Internet Service, as in:

mailto Electronic mail

ftp File Transfer Protocol server

news Network news

telnet Telnet remote access

gopher Gopher server

wais Wide Area Information Server

http HTTP (Hypertext Transfer Protocol), used by World-Wide Web

The **host** element is the domain name (see above) of the actual server hosting the service. The optional **port** element specifies a 'contact address' for the server application on the host. Some servers are addressed through a default **port number**, such as port **70** in the case of Gophers. The **path** element is used to specify the directory location (**path name**) and/or **file name** of a particular resource on the host service. The '**/**' symbol is used to separate out the different elements in the hierarchy. *RFC 1738* recommends that URLs be preceded by **URL:** and enclosed in angle brackets (**<** and **>**) to improve identification. Typing the whole string (without the angle brackets or **URL:** part) into a WWW browser, for example, will take the user to any given Internet resource. Study the following example URLs, which illustrate the more common variations (note that double forward-slashes are not normally included in mail or news URLs):

<URL:mailto:bmj@bmj.com>

<URL:ftp://ftp.eff.org/pub/Net_info/EFF_Net_Guide/netguide_3.1.txt>

<URL:news:sci.med>

<URL:telnet://bubl@bubl.bath.ac.uk>

<URL:gopher://gopher.internet.com:2100/11/>

<URL:wais://imsdd.meb.uni-bonn.de:210/CancerLit_MedLine>

<URL:http://www.oup.co.uk/scimed/medint/HOME.html>

E-mail, news, and Telnet URLs have no path element. URLs that end with the '/' symbol point to a specific directory, rather than a certain file. File name suffixes indicate the type of file, such as **.txt** for text files (see p.44).

Because some Telnet servers require you to log on with a certain **user name** and/or password, there is an option to precede the host name (**bubl.bath.ac.uk** in the above example) with this information. The syntax in this case will be **<URL:telnet://user:password@host[:port]>**. In the above example no password is required, so only the user name is shown (**bubl**). Because no port is specified, it can be assumed to be the default (**23** for Telnet). In the above example, the Gopher server is addressed through port **2100** rather than the default of **70**, so this time it must be included.

The example URL for the WAIS server indicates that the name of the database available for searching is 'CancerLit_MedLine'. If the port is omitted, it defaults to **210**. You might come across a WAIS URL that specifies a particular search on a given database. In this case, the syntax is **<URL:wais://host[:port]/database?search>**, where **search** is a word which occurs in the database, such as 'pain'.

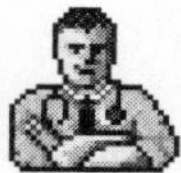

URLs must be spelled exactly; if a URL doesn't work, check the spelling. If a file name has changed, you may be able to find it by dropping the file name and ending the URL with the '/' symbol.

How do I locate usable material?

Most criticism of the Internet falls as a consequence of its anarchic nature (which has ironically permitted it to flourish). Specifically, it can be difficult to locate what you want, and only a small proportion of content is actually usable. The Internet is rather vast, and in its vastness there are a lot of 'data' (as opposed to information)—but while the relative proportion might not be large, the absolute proportion of real information is significant. The trick is to know where to look before you go looking.

Luckily, a number of efforts are in progress to catalogue medical Internet resources and improve our ability to locate specific information. Like all Internet resources, those targeted at consumers and providers of health care suffer alike from variable quality. This technology is still, in terms relative to the everyday practice of medicine, in its infancy, with burgeoning acceptance as a valid tool for 'ordinary' doctors. Perhaps in time the full potential of the Internet as a medical knowledge base will be realized.

It can be unproductive (and possibly expensive) to simply 'browse' the Internet using Gopher or the WWW. A good place to start is a document pointing to other specific resources (see below).

Much health information of use to the public is provided in the form of **frequently asked questions** files, or **FAQs** (see p.175). Aside from containing pointers to other electronic sources on the subject, many FAQs are well referenced, answering the questions most relevant to our patients. The World-Wide Web plays host to a large number of resource catalogues, pointing to sites of interest to both health-care consumers and professionals. Other tools such as e-mail, Archie, FTP, Gopher, Veronica, WAIS, and WWW search engines all have their place in locating and retrieving medical information. These tools are discussed in more detail in Part Four.

To help you locate the resources mentioned in this book, Oxford University Press has put up complementary Web pages (see p.301) that enable you to try out e-mail, newsgroups, Telnet, FTP, Gopher, WAIS, and the WWW:

<URL:http://www.oup.co.uk/scimed/medint/>

Learning more

Despite criticism that the Internet doesn't contain much 'information', information about the Internet itself is easily located in both paper and electronic formats.

Books and magazines

Visit your local bookstore. It is possible to buy separate titles covering the World-Wide Web, e-mail, the Internet for Macs, the Internet for PCs, the Internet for beginners, the Internet for advanced users, Internet directories, guides to online services, and more guides. The choice can be overwhelming and if this book has not satisfied your appetite, the *Unofficial Internet book list* may limit the alternatives. This list by Savetz reviews hundreds of Internet-related titles; you can get an abridged (but nevertheless large) version by sending e-mail to **booklist-request@northcoast.com** with the subject heading **archive**, and **send booklist** in the body of the message. Alternatively, the full searchable list is on the World-Wide Web at:

<URL:http://www.northcoast.com/savetz/booklist/>

Many new magazines devoted to the Internet have appeared, and at least one will be stocked by your local newsagent. Guides are also available on video for your VCR.

Medical journals

Interest in the potential role of the Internet in medical communications, education, and publishing has seen the appearance of a growing number of Internet-related articles in the medical journals. Major general journals have already published brief guides to the Internet (below), as have several specialty journals, concentrating on resources relevant to their own disciplines. In addition, many of these journals have migrated on to the Internet themselves (see p.115 and p.216). A MEDLINE search (Chapter Twenty nine) for Internet-related articles is a simple way to stay up-to-date with the topical issues—such as electronic peer review and patient confidentiality online.

Glowniak, J.V. (1995). Medical resources on the Internet. *Annals of Internal Medicine*, 123, 123–31.

Glowniak, J.V. and Bushway, M.K. (1994). Computer networks as a medical resource: accessing and using the Internet. *Journal of the American Medical Association*, 271, 1934–9.

Millman, A., Lee, N., and Kealy, K. (1995). ABC of medical computing: the Internet. *BMJ*, 311, 440–3.

Pallen, M. (1995). Guide to the Internet: introducing the Internet. *BMJ*, 311, 1422–4. [First article in a series.]

Electronic new user guides

Netskills, based at the University of Newcastle, was developed for the UK Higher Education community. Self-paced tutorials are available on disk and on the WWW (as TONIC: The Online Netskills Interactive Tutorial):

<URL:http://www.netskills.ac.uk/>

One of the best-known electronically available and free Internet guides is EFF's *Guide to the Internet* (formerly *The big dummy's guide to the Internet*), by Gaffin and the Electronic Frontier Foundation. It can be obtained from:

<URL:ftp://ftp.eff.org/pub/Net_info/EFF_Net_Guide/>

'Request for comments' documents

'Request for comments' or **RFC** documents are a record of evolving Internet protocols and standards. There are many such files discussing all aspects of the Internet, with a less technical subset of 'For your information' (FYI) titles. Particularly useful are:

- RFC 1206/FYI 4: *FYI on questions and answers: answers to commonly asked 'new Internet user' questions* (Feb. 1991)
- RFC 1392/FYI 18: *Internet users' glossary* (Jan. 1993)
- RFC 1462/FYI 20: *FYI on 'What is the Internet?'* (May 1993)
- RFC 1738: *Uniform resource locators (URL)* (Dec. 1994)

You can obtain these documents from many places, including the Imperial College archive at:

<URL:ftp://src.doc.ic.ac.uk/rfc/>

An easy alternative is to point your World-Wide Web browser at:

<http://www.cis.ohio-state.edu:80/hypertext/information/rfc.html>

Other electronic sources

A number of documents relating to the use of specific Internet services are mentioned throughout Part Four of this book as each service is discussed.

CHAPTER THIRTEEN

What use is the Internet in medicine?

Connecting the medical profession and health-care institutions to the Internet is an ongoing experiment. Various groups are developing medicine-related Internet resources that utilize e-mail, FTP, Gopher, WAIS, and the WWW to make online text, graphics, and multimedia content available. Paralleling this development are efforts to catalogue and peer review these resources. More and more doctors are realizing that the Internet is a tool—like the stethoscope or coat-pocket handbook. It extends our experience and complements our ability to learn and practice medicine.

This increasing realization spawned the European Society of the Internet in Medicine in September 1995, promoting the use of the Internet in the medical sciences. Indeed, during the writing of this edition in October 1996 the Society hosted MEDNET 96—the European Congress of the Internet in Medicine. For more information, use the following URLs:

<URL:http://www.mednet.org.uk/mednet/>

<URL:mailto:info@mednet.org.uk>

The Internet is primarily a tool for individuals, but it can also be a tool for health-care organizations, a means of disseminating electronic journals and of teaching medicine, a tool for research, and a means of delivering health care. As with any relatively new technology, the Internet faces a number of hurdles—only some of which are technological. Perhaps one of the biggest hurdles to its wider acceptance in medicine is ignorance. In this Chapter, we introduce some of the applications that the Internet has in the practice of medicine (see Fig. 10). The reader will be aware that not all the applications described below will apply to the individual with a home computer—the onus of this book—but there is benefit in gaining a slightly wider view.

A tool for the individual

A personal computer represents a considerable investment for most of us. Computers are at their best as productivity tools, but the machine can easily become an under-utilized resource. The Internet provides opportunities to enhance its value as a productivity tool in medicine. One can ask for recommendations on a suitable program for preparing slides; learn how to expand the computers memory, or make it run faster; download a reworked printer driver to improve the appearance of a *curriculum vitae*; find a shareware database to store case histories; or contact the vendors of the applications you are using, etc.

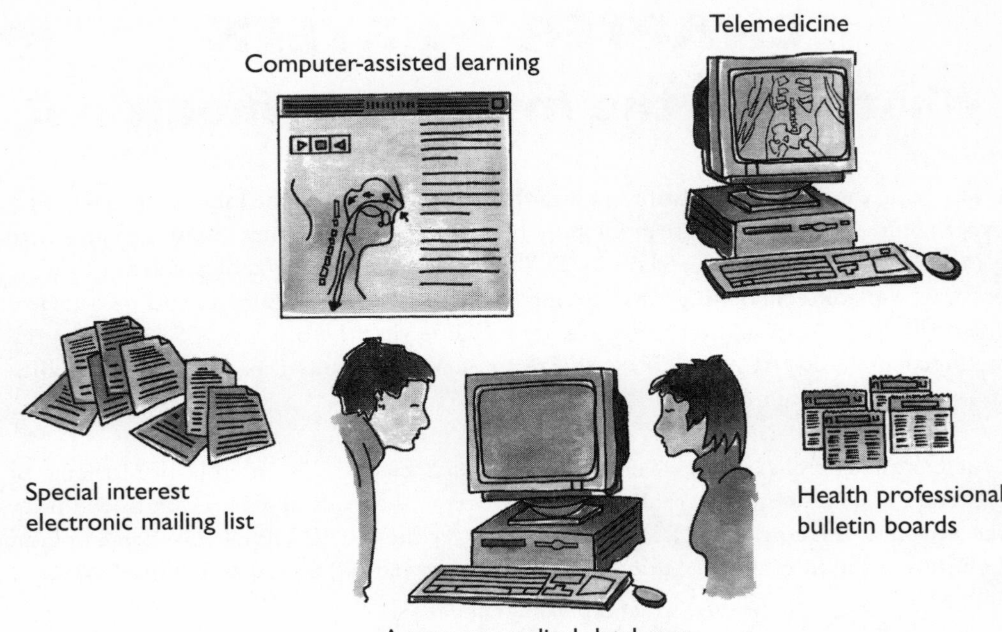

Fig. 10 What use is the Internet in medicine? With access to more people and more resources than could ever come together at one site, the Internet could be utilized to deliver computer-assisted learning, access to medical databases, telemedicine and videoconferencing, special-interest mailing lists, and health professional bulletin boards.

Professional and personal communication

The Internet provides an easy method of keeping in touch. Indeed, it is sometimes easier and faster to send e-mail than it is to find a pen, paper, envelope, stamp, and post box. Electronic mail is discussed in Chapter Eighteen.

Mailing lists foster contact between like-minded international colleagues. Typically rather informal affairs, contributions are actively encouraged from all subscribers. Some of these lists require subscribers to verify their professional status by supplying a registration number or photocopies of their qualifications. This goes some way to ensuring that list subscribers are a 'known quantity'. These lists allow subscribers to share experiences to their mutual benefit, and for those far from main centres this can limit what has become known as 'professional isolation'. Mailing lists are discussed in detail in Chapter Nineteen.

Enjoyment

One cannot deny that enjoyment is an additional reason to use the Internet. It can be very satisfying to find a mailbox full of international messages, or to utilize the resources of faraway institutions from one's home computer. Informality is the general rule, and the House Officer can correspond with the Professor without the usual inhibitions imposed by hierarchy.

Obtaining information

As Wyatt (1991) points out in an enlightening paper on sources of medical knowledge, journals are not normally available on the ward or clinic, and it can be difficult to find clinically relevant advice. He also notes that textbooks—aside from being dated—typically offer few references and superficial indexes. Furthermore, the standard textbooks are not usually available in all clinical areas where they might be called upon, but rather reside in a central or departmental library. Perhaps the future will see computers used routinely at the point of care to access keyword-searchable full-text electronic journals and 'classic' medical texts, via a MEDLINE-like WWW interface. See below, *Electronic journals*, and *MEDLINE by modem* (Chapter Twenty nine).

Perhaps one of the biggest advantages of electronic media over traditional paper-based publishing is currency. As a matter of course, the time scale of traditional publishing can mean that information within a textbook may be out of date before it appears on the shelves. On the Internet, information can be available almost from the moment it is written. Increasingly practice guidelines and management protocols are finding their way on to the Internet where they can readily be updated and available when needed—whether the doctor is at home, in the surgery, or at the departmental office.

While some books and journals boast usable indexes, the capacity to search the entire contents of many separate works simultaneously using 'intelligent' search tools has obvious benefits. Although this facility has not been fully realized in clinical medicine, one of the first such resources is a case in point. Cancernet, from the US National Cancer Institute, is a collection of documents relating to cancer diagnosis, management, and research, etc., and has been indexed on a WAIS server in cooperation with the University of Bonn Medical Center. The searcher can retrieve all documents containing a particular word or words, sorted by order of 'relevance':

<URL:http://imsdd.meb.uni-bonn.de/cancernet/>

WAIS, briefly discussed in Chapter Twenty five, is just one of many ways to find information. For example, if you are an anaesthetist all that is needed is a starting point, like a Gopher server (Chapter Twenty four), and a world of anaesthetic information becomes available:

<URL:gopher://gasnet.med.yale.edu/>

The public health physician can keep a finger on the pulse of social perceptions about HIV and AIDS, by dipping into Usenet's **sci.med.aids** newsgroup (Chapter Twenty). The pathologist can retrieve histological images from one of several online archives by FTP (Chapter Twenty one). We can all subscribe to informative mailing lists (Chapter Nineteen) and browse multimedia textbooks on the World-Wide Web (Chapter Twenty six).

Self-publishing

The individual doctor can become the author/editor of a newsletter or collection of Web pages with minimal investment; production and distribution costs are significantly diminished relative to paper-based equivalents. If necessary, a nominal subscription can still be charged. See also *Electronic journals*, below, and *Becoming an information provider* (Chapter Thirty).

Online purchasing

The future may see us making regular use of online purchasing facilities. For example, it is already possible to order medical texts direct from publishers such as Blackwell via the World-Wide Web:

<URL:http://www.blackwell.co.uk/bookshops/>

What constitutes a secure electronic financial transaction, however, is not clear as of this writing. Although the risk of credit card fraud online may even be less than with giving details by phone or to a shop assistant, public perception takes the opposite view. Encryption and 'digital signature' authentication (p.77) may offer reassurance, whether it is credit card details or a 'digital cash' transaction being transmitted. Although there are several potential standards vying for adoption, none has emerged favourite yet. In the interim most online retailers offer customers the option of giving out 'one-off' details by phone or fax; subsequent purchases can be made online using a user name and password.

Advertising medical products and services

The Internet is becoming ever more commercialized, providing many opportunities to doctors with entrepreneurial skills. Several sites provide for professional advertisement, such as MedSearch America:

<URL:http://www.medsearch.com>

Another example is the Cyberspace Telemedical Office from Digital Med Inc:

<URL:http://www.telemedical.com/~drcarr/>

From these Web pages, consumers and physicians can shop for health-care products including prescriptions; make use of 'telemedical' services (see below); consult fellow health professionals; order investigations after browsing preventive health information; request the services of an online librarian; employ a triage service for on-call physicians; link to continuing medical-education programmes; subscribe to a clinical trials information clearing-house, or order video monitoring and other home care services. They can also enter their medical records and obtain personalized disease, drug, and health-maintenance information.

Finding employment

A number of journals publish their Classified section on the WWW, enabling readers to look for a new position online. Examples are given in Chapter Twenty six.

A tool for health-care organizations

At an institutional level, the Internet provides passage to an extended information service without great expense—more resources than could ever be held by a single institution. Through telecommunication links even the smaller organizations can access resources such as bibliographic and other databases, and all forms of electronic medical information. The Internet can also help break down the barriers between primary and secondary health care by improving communications between workers in these sectors—providing security concerns can be resolved.

Health professional communications and development

The potential of the Internet as a means of disseminating communications to large groups of health professionals is enormous. Health services can use the Internet as a tool for professional development by providing access to resources for self-directed learning and by fostering professional contact on electronic bulletin boards. Without needing to conform to a regular schedule, doctors will find it easier to fit this type of activity into the working day. For general practitioners and the staff of smaller hospitals it can be a means of keeping up-to-date with current practice at centres of excellence. Working groups, both clinical and managerial, will be able to hold 'virtual conferences' (see Chapter Twenty eight). Precursors of such facilities can be viewed online today, such as the multimedia case histories at the Virtual Hospital in Iowa, and in the physician contact seen in newsgroups and mailing lists:

<URL:http://indy.radiology.uiowa.edu/VirtualHospital.html>

In the UK, rather than being simply a medium for transmitting medical records and laboratory results, etc., NHSnet provides the infrastructure necessary to achieve similar ambitions by allowing health service staff access to the Internet (p.137). Such an ambition is, however, fraught with difficulties in an era of diminishing financial flexibility in health services worldwide. Worthwhile services demand significant development and maintenance time—and therefore expense.

Health services on the World-Wide Web

The visual 'point-and-click' navigation afforded by browser tools and the World-Wide Web in particular has been welcomed enthusiastically as a salvation from archaic text-based interfaces. Perhaps, in the not too distant future, the health services will provide unique content and WWW pages pointing to the best of the Internet in a manner attractive even to computer-phobic users. With regard to developing content attractive to physicians, a WWW interface probably needs to support documents such as up-to-date treatment protocols, practice guidelines, employment databases, and moderated bulletin boards on practice issues (Malet, personal communication). Those who discuss this issue on the Internet are confident that such a service will need to be private in order to encourage health professional participation. That is, it should not be open to public requests for diagnostic help; a separate service might be dedicated as an online 'help page'.

Brighton Health Care NHS Trust became the first non-teaching hospital in the National Health Service to introduce a presence on the Web in December 1994 (although it has since moved from its original Web site):

<URL:http://www.rsch.org.uk/rsch/>

In a press release dated 20 December, the stated aims of the service included providing general practitioners with information about available diagnostic services, the clinical backgrounds of hospital doctors, and the Trust's performance in the 'national league tables' (comparing NHS hospitals on the basis of waiting times, etc.).

Further examples of health services on the WWW are given in Chapter Twenty six. A hypertext list of worldwide hospitals on the WWW is at:

<URL:http://neuro-www.mgh.harvard.edu/hospitalweb.nclk>

Increased use of telecommunications to disseminate information rapidly (via the Internet, NHSnet, or other services) may have avoided public and professional dissatisfaction with the Department of Health's handling of recent 'health scares' in the UK concerning oral contraceptive use and the safety of British beef. Although this author is not aware of any studies reporting the efficacy of electronic communications in such 'medical alert' situations, it has been shown to improve the speed of and satisfaction with communication in relation to laboratory and discharge reports sent from hospitals to general practitioners (Branger *et al*. 1992).

Electronic medical records and clinical information systems

A clinical information system developed by the University of Minnesota Hospital and Clinic, based on WWW protocols, was instigated at a fraction of development costs associated with custom clients (Willard *et al.* 1995). Laboratory results, order entry, and protocols for standardized patient care were made available on the hospital network where they could be accessed by any computer capable of running a WWW client (p.199). Freely available graphics utilities were used to produce graphics created dynamically from raw patient data. A small survey of clinicians using the clinical microbiology results reporting system (Fig. 11) suggested significant reductions in interpretation time and incidence of major errors.

Aside from result-reporting facilities, researchers have begun to evaluate the possibilities for Web-based access to entire electronic medical record systems. In addition to displaying searchable clinical case notes, such a system would be capable of incorporating various medical images (such as X-rays and electrocardiograms) and integration with other information sources (such as online 'look-ups' or databases and diagnostic decision-support systems). One major advantage in the 'dynamic collation' of a Web-based record from multiple elements distributed on a network is that there ever only need exist one up-to-date copy of each element. Thus, a radiology department (for example) is able to retain ownership of and control over all X-ray reports, ensuring any new reports are available simultaneously to all those browsing that patient's record; there need only be one source of patient demographics, etc.

The Department of Medical Informatics at Columbia University maintains a list of links to real or experimental electronic medical record systems on the WWW at:

<URL:http://www.cpmc.columbia.edu/edu/medinfoemrs.html>

Security issues

Professional isolation from diagnosis requests is not the only factor that may necessitate a separate 'closed system' for health professionals. Security and confidentiality are areas that need to be looked at in detail, particularly if health-service networks are directly linked to the Internet. A case in point is NHSnet; the British Medical Association warned that unless it was satisfied the network was secure (e.g. through encryption and a statutory 'code of confidentiality'), it might encourage doctors not to cooperate with it (*BMJ* 1995). These issues are complex and beyond the scope of a general introductory text such as this, although they were briefly touched upon in Chapter Eight.

If, for whatever reason, an institution or hospital did not wish to connect itself directly with the Internet, there is an alternative. An **intranet** is a private internal network based

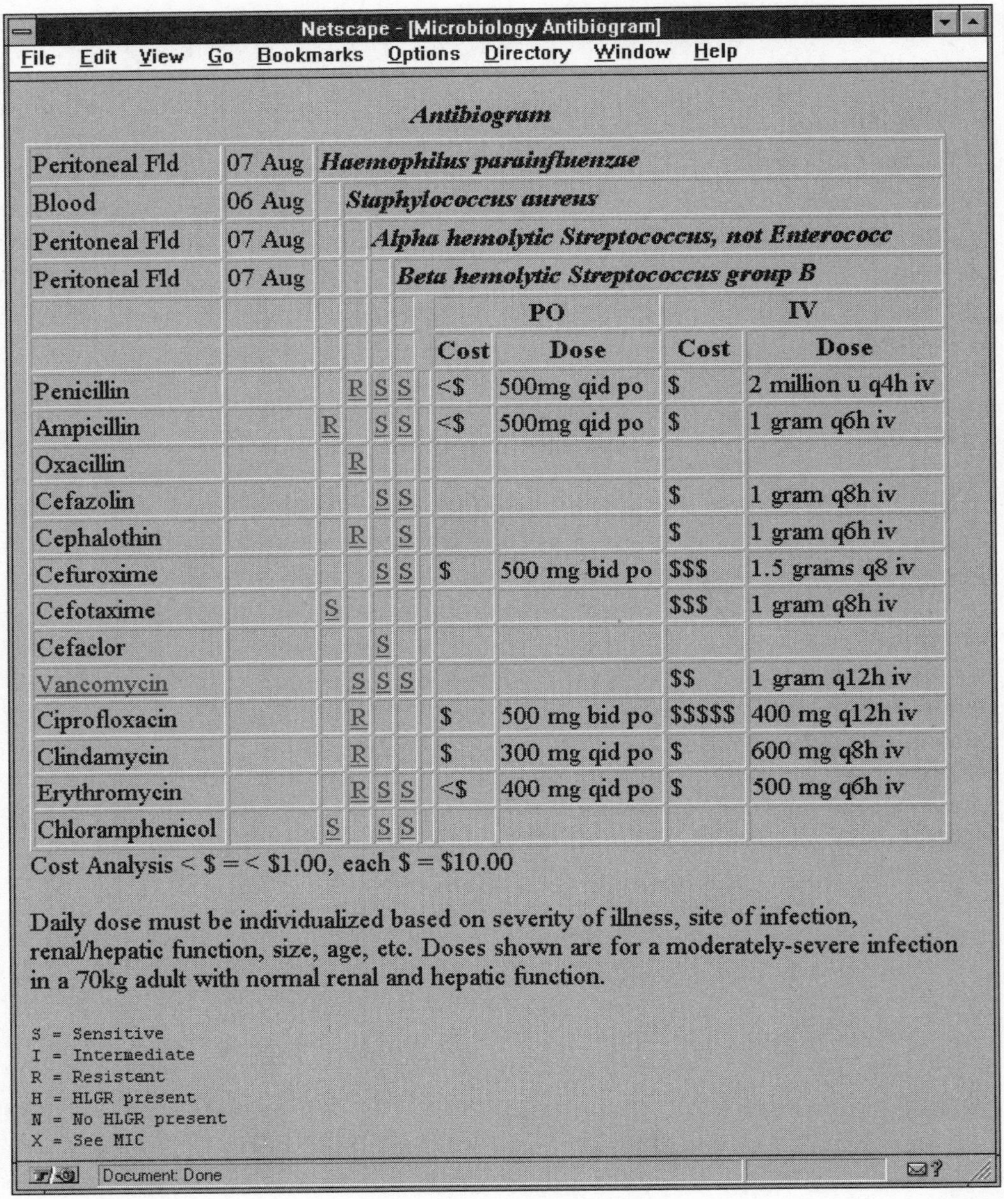

Netscape - [Microbiology Antibiogram]

File Edit View Go Bookmarks Options Directory Window Help

Antibiogram

Peritoneal Fld	07 Aug	***Haemophilus parainfluenzae***							
Blood	06 Aug		***Staphylococcus aureus***						
Peritoneal Fld	07 Aug			***Alpha hemolytic Streptococcus, not Enterococc***					
Peritoneal Fld	07 Aug				***Beta hemolytic Streptococcus group B***				
						PO		**IV**	
						Cost	**Dose**	**Cost**	**Dose**
Penicillin			R	S	S	<$	500mg qid po	$	2 million u q4h iv
Ampicillin		R		S	S	<$	500mg qid po	$	1 gram q6h iv
Oxacillin			R						
Cefazolin				S	S			$	1 gram q8h iv
Cephalothin			R		S			$	1 gram q6h iv
Cefuroxime				S	S	$	500 mg bid po	$$$	1.5 grams q8 iv
Cefotaxime		S						$$$	1 gram q8h iv
Cefaclor				S					
Vancomycin			S	S	S			$$	1 gram q12h iv
Ciprofloxacin			R			$	500 mg bid po	$$$$$	400 mg q12h iv
Clindamycin			R			$	300 mg qid po	$	600 mg q8h iv
Erythromycin			R	S	S	<$	400 mg qid po	$	500 mg q6h iv
Chloramphenicol		S		S	S				

Cost Analysis < $ =< $1.00, each $ = $10.00

Daily dose must be individualized based on severity of illness, site of infection, renal/hepatic function, size, age, etc. Doses shown are for a moderately-severe infection in a 70kg adult with normal renal and hepatic function.

S = Sensitive
I = Intermediate
R = Resistant
H = HLGR present
N = No HLGR present
X = See MIC

Document: Done

Fig. 11 An experimental WWW-based clinical information system at the University of Minnesota Hospital and Clinic. Here, an 'antibiogram' displays information about microbial sensitivities and prescribing information (patient details removed). As a 'restricted' drug in this institution, 'Vancomycin' is linked to further information from the hospital's Pharmacy and Therapeutic Committee. [Screen capture: Asst Prof. K.E. Willard.]

on the same protocols (i.e. TCP/IP) and applications (e.g. Web browsers) as the Internet. An intranet could host the same sort of information—searchable databases, informational WWW pages, e-mail, etc.—as on the Internet, but without all the risks of an 'outside' connection.

An intranet may, incidentally, be less subject to the 'traffic jams' that frequently bring the Internet to a virtual standstill during peak usage—not an ideal characteristic for a medical information system.

Electronic journals

The medical library of tomorrow may see clinicians making increasing use of electronic information, as recognized by the Follet Implementation Group on Information Technology, or FIGIT (1994). FIGIT (a subcommittee of the Joint Information Systems Committee, or JISC) sees libraries providing electronic document delivery (to reduce costs); electronic journals (via e-mail, hypertext, etc.); increased digitization (especially of little-used journals); 'on-demand' publishing (compiling and printing customized information); and access to network information resources (including training). The Internet is sure to play an important role in this vision. There are already many signs of the use of electronic communications in the production process and publication of journals.

Although it works well in the case of simple messages, e-mail has had mixed success as a means of conveying more complex information thus far. A few pioneering academic journals accept submissions in the form of e-mail, but the transition from paper-based manuscripts is not entirely without difficulty. Some mail 'gateways' slice long submissions into a number of segments, and all but the simplest of formatting is typically lost. If an author wishes to include digitized figures, the receiver must have the correct program to 'decode' them back into a readable form (see *Binary files by e-mail*, p.158), and the correct program to view them—there are no established standards. Despite these drawbacks, e-mail is a very efficient means of conducting ongoing dialogue between author, contributors, referees, and editor.

The amount of peer-reviewed medical knowledge finding its way on to the Internet is increasing, largely due to the relative simplicity and perceived advantages of WWW publishing (see Chapter Thirty). Journals such as the *BMJ* (Delamothe 1995), the *New England Journal of Medicine* (Campion 1996), and *The Lancet* (McConnell and Horton 1996) proudly announced their arrival on the World-Wide Web (see Fig. 12). However, full-text articles are few because of copyright concerns, restricted readership, anticipated loss of income (through a reduction in subscription and advertizing revenues), and a preference on the part of authors to publish on paper. The traditional journals have adopted a number of unique approaches to overcome these concerns. For instance, the *New England Journal of*

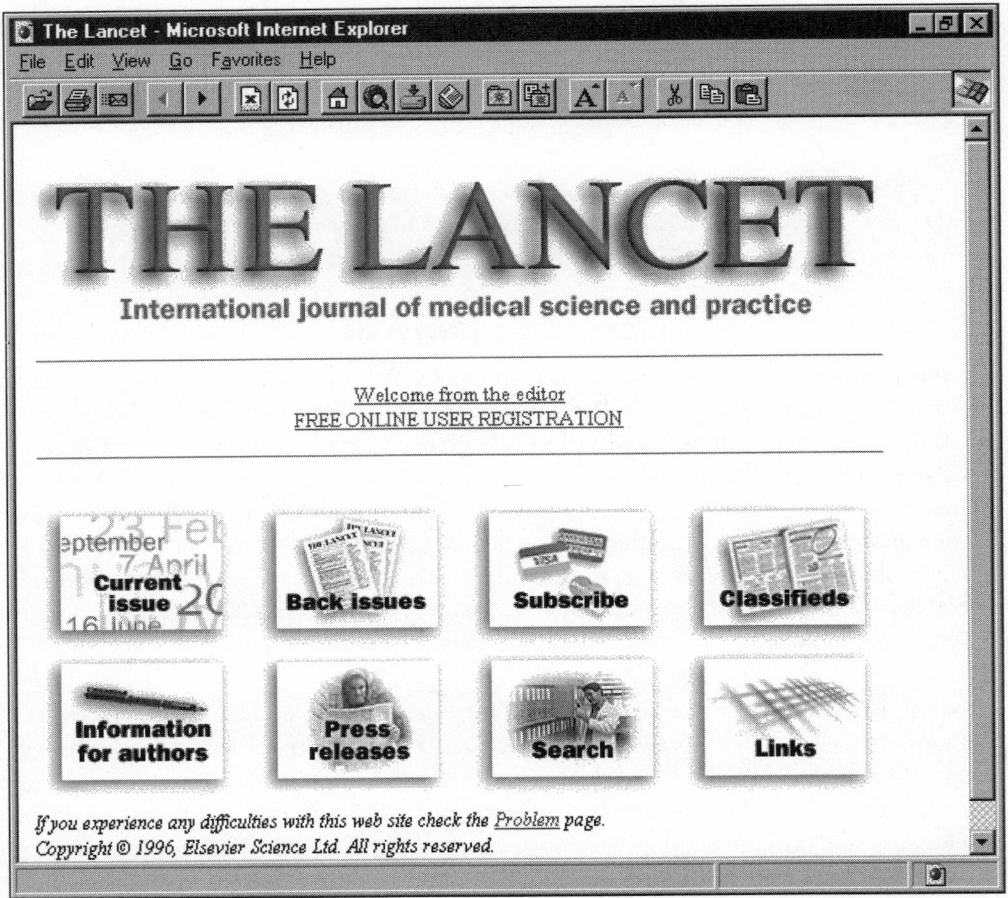

Fig. 12 Medical journals on the WWW. Journal publishers are looking to enhance their print publications with online material, yet face problems such as the protection of copyright, loss of revenue, a restricted readership, and the difficulties in reading on-screen editions. [Reproduced with permission.]

Medicine Web site offers abstracts for some of its articles, with a hypertext link to an order form whereby the researcher can obtain the full-text article for a fee. The URLs for journal sites are given in Chapter Twenty six.

Standards and peer review

There is concern that because any individual or organization can publish on the Internet, academic standards may fall. It is not clear that this will be the case, however, if the process of peer review is maintained. One of the prime reasons electronic journals have an edge is currency (as opposed to the familiar 'Received February 1995; comments to authors July 1995; accepted for publication November 1995, finally appears April 1996' scenario). This does not automatically imply the absence of peer review. The more rapid turnaround times afforded by electronic communication between author, editor, and reviewers can accelerate the traditional peer review process.

Traditional peer review involves a lengthy process whereby articles sent to the journal editor are referred to 'expert' reviewers, whose comments influence the editorial decision to publish the work (with the author incorporating the reviewer's suggestions) or not.

In a controversial article entitled *The death of biomedical journals*, La Porte and colleagues proposed an Internet-based 'global health information server' operating in association with an alternative 'democratic' system of peer review (La Porte *et al.* 1995). In this system, the 'quality' of a research communication is determined by reader-assigned ratings and comments; its 'impact' is determined by how many people have read it or created a hypertext link to it.

In the same article, La Porte and colleagues suggest that authors make ongoing changes to the communication in response to new analyses and comments. As Longmore (1995) muses, 'If the research communication I am referring to can be constantly changed and is perpetually provisional, what am I referring to?'. Needless to say, incomplete or frankly misleading information has the potential to do great harm. The issue of citing dynamic resources was raised in Chapter Eight.

La Porte's suggestions have been sharply rebuked by advocates of the traditional peer-review process. 'Direct electronic publishing of scientific studies threatens to undermine time-tested traditions that help to ensure the quality of the medical literature' (Kassirer and Angell 1995) was a typical response.

The University of Sydney Library and the Medical Journal of Australia have undertaken to examine an 'open' peer review process using the WWW to co-publish articles accepted for print publication (but not yet printed), together with the comments of peer reviewers (Bingham and Coleman 1996). Both article and comments can be viewed by Internet users and commented upon; any suggestions (after filtering) are passed on to the author/reviewer, providing for revision prior to print publication. Registered users can elect to be notified by e-mail when new articles are published within their nominated areas of interest. The results of this experiment are not available as of this writing.

<URL:http://www.library.usyd.edu.au/MJA/>

Many indices of medical resources offer peer review in the form of site annotations of variable quality and usefulness, depending on the objectives of the indexer (see p.223). Peer review in this context can, however, consider several facets beyond the purely academic standing of medical information. For instance, the AMIA Internet Working Group's Medical Matrix Project asks reviewers to consider a number of factors including currency, authenticity, use of references, use of media (sound, graphics, etc.), search capabilities, navigation tools, general interface, integration with 'back-end' databases, the reliability and speed of connection to the site, and a general impression of how important the resource is to the discipline (Malet, personal communication).

Journals by e-mail

The Internet is not set to displace paper (television has not made newspapers redundant). While the office desk may have more work space, it is not always practical or easy on the eyes to read articles on screen. A paper journal is more portable and it is easier to underline key points or to send a copy to someone without a computer!

Since people sometimes would rather read articles offline, electronic journals can be downloaded for printing instead. Certain cross-platform document formats, such as Adobe's Acrobat, enable high-quality output that maintains the layout of the original document and incorporates figures in their proper place (p.260).

Web-based journals

Publishing on the WWW offers a number of advantages (see Chapter Thirty). Many Web authoring tools make it possible to convert existing documents into WWW pages, containing the same text and graphics as the original paper pages. Such straight conversions do not offer anything new apart from using hypertext to link citations to original works. Even this, however, has the potential to be very effective if the practice becomes widespread. As Pignone (1995) points out, '... the ability to access directly an article's references (or the author himself or herself) would allow a more critical reading of the literature, complete with the opportunity for direct response.' The typical journal site today, however, usually serves to advertise the print publication with a table of contents, details of subscription rates, and limited useful content aside from token abstracts and sparse full-text articles.

Web-based journals can come into their own by delivering multimedia. As clinicians, our experience of patients is not one of still images and silence; we make diagnoses based on movement and sound. Electronic media can come closer to life than paper media by incorporating audiovisual content. Current WWW browsers feature the ability to play back animated sequences and video (see Chapter Twenty six). New developments will increase the reader's ability to interact with a Web page, perhaps 'picking up' a scalpel to reveal a deeper tissue plane, or adjusting the focus of a histological specimen on a 'virtual microscope'. True multimedia medical journals with real-time interaction are, however, unlikely to become available to the majority of potential readers until such time as the Internet's information-carrying capacity (bandwidth) is improved.

Currently most Web pages, including those aimed at doctors, are accessible to the general public. This raises two interesting ethical issues for journal publishers. Firstly, pharmaceutical companies are restricted by law (in the UK) to making certain product information available to prescribers but not the general public. Secondly, some journals contain images that are decidedly 'graphic' to the lay eye, such as forensic or trauma photographs, and it could be argued that the public should be protected from this material.

When journals are published on the Web, 'adjuvant mailing lists' could provide for follow-up discussions around key articles and the publication of all correspondence received by the journal but not published in print.

Learning medicine on the Internet

Undergraduate education

With Internet access from campus or home, medical students can partake in lessons without the confines of a strict timetable, the need to travel, or cope with double-booked rooms. Interactive tutorials on the WWW ensure that all students are presented with the same material, which can be explored at each individual's own pace. Although 'interactive' in one sense, most educational material does not provide the real-time one-to-one interaction between teacher and pupil often critical to memorable learning. Well-constructed tutorials can, however, come much closer to simulating real-life patient encounters than can be gained from the traditional textbook, although cannot be a substitute for face-to-face clinical encounters or practical sessions in the laboratory. Examples of Web-based teaching material are given in Chapter Twenty six.

CAL software

Computer-assisted learning (CAL) is both a popular and effective way of making education fun. A modest selection of medical-education shareware for the pre-clinical student (and general public) is accessible via the Internet. These programs can be just as interactive as current Web-based tutorials, but have the advantage of being utilized offline. Some examples of software archives are given in Chapter Twenty one.

Distance teaching

E-mail has been used as a means of communicating between students and tutors, and lessons have been delivered via the Internet as part of an MSc in general practice from the University of Derby (Sanfey 1996).

Many people believe that a widely accessible 'information superhighway' with the bandwidth to carry video is just around the corner. Currently, this type of facility is generally only available in medicine at a research level. An example is the Interactive Teaching Project in Surgery, an experiment led by University College London in cooperation with other universities. Using the high-bandwidth SuperJANET network (p.136), students have access to clinical teachers over two-way real-time video links between the classroom and operating theatre. Further information is available from:

<URL:http://www.ja.net/SuperJANET/SuperJANET/SJ-Applics-Menu.html>

Another practical application of **videoconferencing** is the teaching of students on peripheral hospital attachments, which can be carried out using direct ISDN (p.135) communications links. Video hardware is now readily available for PCs, and using compression and slow scan rates, it is possible to produce reasonable moving images for transmission over ISDN lines. This technology has been quickly absorbed by the business world as an economical alternative to travel—with apparent success. In their trial of a system in Scotland, Furnace *et al*. (1996) found that although ISDN videoconferencing has potential, there are a number of technical obstacles which need to be resolved before it will be useful as a teaching aid. This is especially true when applied to real-time audiovisual data transmissions via the Internet itself. See also Chapter Twenty eight, p.233.

Where medical students meet

The Usenet newsgroup **misc.education.medical** provides a forum for discussion of issues related to medical education. Here, medical students have the opportunity to exchange messages with their peers all over the world, contribute to useful discussion, and to publish themselves electronically by writing occasional articles or newsletters. There are several mailing lists for medical students, including:

MEDFORUM:

<URL:mailto:listserv@arizvm1.ccit.arizona.edu> Send: (personal message)

MEDSTU-L:

<URL:mailto:listserv@unmvm.edu> Send: Subscribe MEDSTU-L Medical student discussion list

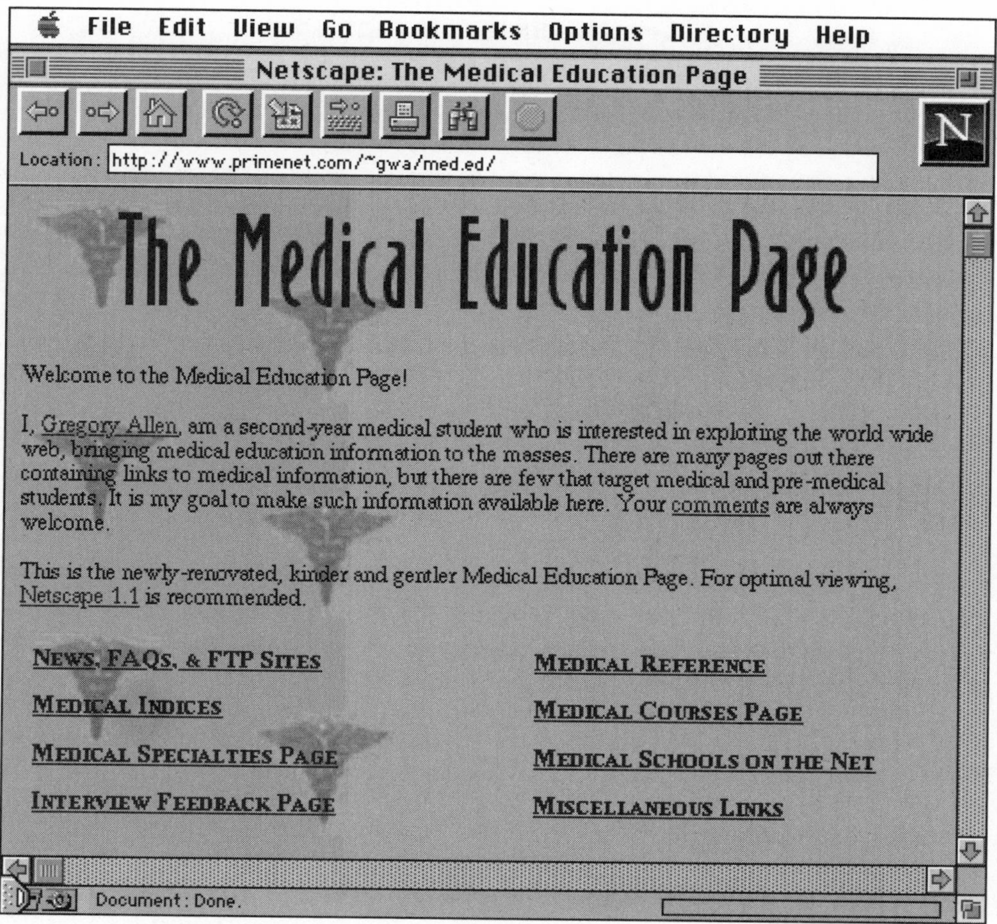

Fig. 13 Medical students on the Internet. Students from all over the world can share views on educational issues, explore the teaching resources of famous medical schools, and take a break from study. [Reproduced with permission.]

A number of resources specifically for medical students are available on the WWW (see Fig. 13), such as:

The Medical Education Page:

<URL:http://www.scomm.net/~greg/med-ed>

The Interactive Medical Student Lounge:

<URL:http://falcon.cc.ukans.edu:80/~nsween/>

A list of world-wide medical schools on the WWW is at:

<URL:http://www.anat.dote.hu/~tore/medfak/>

Postgraduate education

Even simple e-mail messages can be used to educate doctors. Using a basic but fundamentally interactive question-and-answer system , it has been shown that e-mail can be successfully utilized in helping resident doctors revise for examinations (Letterie *et al.* 1994). Aside from a growing number of special-interest mailing lists (Chapter Nineteen), an interesting American development is the ability to earn continuing medical education (CME) credits on the WWW. Contact URLs for these sites are given in Chapter Twenty six.

Formal continuing medical education is not yet mandatory in the UK, although strong pressures to engage in CME activities have been brought to bear by some Royal Colleges (Hayes 1995). Currently CME (or more broadly, continuing professional development) is measured primarily by attendance at courses and conferences—rather than by proof of learning. Didactic lectures do not permit active participation in learning or emphasize personal learning needs (Hotvedt 1996), and are not always convenient in time or place. Internet-based CME could help overcome these criticisms.

In the UK general practitioners can accumulate Postgraduate Educational Allowance (PGEA) hours through distance learning activities accredited by the Royal College of General Practitioners. As the title of the scheme suggests, these hours incur a financial reward. As of writing, only one Web site has PGEA approval:

> The management of dry eye in general practice (CIBAVision Ophthalmics):
>
> **<URL:http://www.cibavision.co.uk/pgea/dryeye/pgeadry.htm>**

Career-grade doctors in hospital-based specialties should likewise accumulate a certain number of CME hours, under the supervision of their respective Royal College. As of writing, no Web sites offer CME approval to UK specialists.

Quality issues

At present the authority or value of an educational resource is difficult to assess. One means of assessment is simply reliance on repeutation, or signs of obvious sponsorship from a trusted institution. More formal methods of assessing WWW-based medical education materials are however being developed. For example, the Leeds Interactive Medical Education (LIME) project seeks to create an up-to-date database of classified and peer-reviewed resources, all mapped to the local undergraduate cirriculum (Berry *et al.* 1996):

> **<URL:http://www.leeds.ac.uk/medicine/lime/>**

In the case of postgraduate resources, accreditation by professional organizations is a means of ensuring educational activities or materials are of a sufficiently high standard (see above and p.263). Another relevant initiative is the Code of Conduct from the Geneva-based

Health On the Net Foundation. Although not limited to educational resources, the code's self-governing Principles go some way toward promoting accountability on the part of information providers:

<URL:http://www.hon.ch/Conduct.html>

A tool for research

Online databases can obviate the need for further investment in hardware (such as CD-ROM drives), and the Internet may prove to be a cheaper means of accessing several databases rather than maintaining individual subscriptions to a number of CD-based collections. The researcher can browse medical library catalogues using Telnet (Chapter Twenty two), and conduct MEDLINE searches from the comfort of home (Chapter Twenty nine). There are at present some difficulties involved in citing electronic sources, particularly those which are transient; these were addressed in Chapter Eight.

It is increasingly possible for researchers to locate the manufacturers of biomedical instruments, sources of grants, and employment or collaborative opportunities with academic or commercial institutions through the WWW. Perhaps the online publication of one's research projects will constitute a new form of *curriculum vitae*? Alternatively, electronic publication of preliminary findings may encourage early and constructive feedback from *ad hoc* reviewers. PosterNet is an example Web site that offers a means to read feedback from readers and frequently asked questions with their answers from the authors of the 'poster':

<URL:http://pharminfo.com/poster/pnet_hp.html>

Authors should be wary that in publishing their work on the WWW, they may forgo subsequent publication in a paper-based journal (Kassirer and Angell 1995). In addition, placing previously published articles on the WWW without the permission of the journal in which it appeared may be an infringement of copyright.

The Web offers the opportunity for institutions to publish research results or disseminate evidence-based guidelines. The site administrator can score the number of visits to particular pages, providing feedback as to their effectiveness. With ready access to current research material, such as the online offerings from the National Institutes of Health, it is conceivable that research findings will be more quickly integrated into clinical practice (Ferguson 1996).

Another development of interest to researchers (and clinicians) is the e-mail alerting service. Such services enable users to create a personal profile which may be used to deliver tables of contents from selected journals, or to search for and notify users of new journal articles on specific topics. Example alerting services are:

Research Alert Direct (Institute for Scientific Information):

<URL:http://www.isinet.com/>

Reveal Service (The UnCover Company):

<URL:http://www.carl.org/reveal/>

The Internet has also been used as a promotional vehicle to recruit patients for clinical trials (Getz 1996), and to recruit trial centres and manage the submission of trial data (Kelly and Oldham 1996).

A means of delivering health care

Sometimes it seems health professionals have less and less time to involve themselves in the provision of health information. It is increasingly up to the patient to discover information in excess of what is offered in a brief medical consultation. The two principal benefits of the Internet for health-care consumers are health information (databases, mailing lists, and Web sites), and support newsgroups offering self-help advice or pointing to additional resources.

For health-care consumers who are immobile through illness or otherwise isolated (in rural areas, or with motor neurone disease, for instance), the Internet offers a potentially very accessible route to health information and support. Support forums in particular may contain a wealth of varied experiences and backgrounds. Rarely will a plea for information or advice go unanswered, and there is no intimidation, no face-to-face confrontation. Resources even seem to be more plentiful in those areas where, perhaps, there is the greatest need for support: AIDS, cancer, chronic debilitating neurologic conditions, physical disability, mental health, and nutrition. Indeed, annotated sites guides are now available to assist consumers in locating this material (for example, Lindon 1995).

A list of support newsgroups, Grohol's *Psychology and support groups newsgroup pointer*, is available from:

<URL:ftp://rtfm.mit.edu/pub/usenet/news.answers/finding-groups/psychology-and-support>

A similar document from the same author, the *Psychology and support mailing list pointer*, is at:

<URL:ftp://rtfm.mit.edu/pub/usenet/news.answers/medicine/support-mail-lists>

Improved access to information may, at least in theory, enable patients to participate more actively in the decision-making process with their doctors. Patients are equally likely to come across information about complementary therapies as they are information from conventional medical practice. Such a 'free market in information' (Coiera 1996) introduces a number of concerns aside from obvious issues such as ensuring the quality and authenticity of information, and the potential for breaches of confidentiality. The dangers of taking misinformed advice and issues of confidentiality were raised in Chapter Eight.

Although the publication of practice guidelines by respected medical organizations might counter some misinformation, Coiera (1996) asks whether ready access to knowledge of what is considered 'best practice' will see the resource-limited health service incapable of meeting heightened societal expectations of optimal care for all. While this may have unpleasant consequences for already litigation-prone clinicians, it is a sobering thought that our current system of health-care rationing is to some extent dependent on the ignorance of our patients. Of course, what is possible under one country's system of health care may not be feasible under that of another. Unfortunately (in some respects), information distributed via the Internet recognizes no such physical, financial, or cultural boundaries.

Kassirer (1995) has said that electronic 'communication between patients and medical databases and between patients and physicians promises to replace a substantial amount of care now delivered in person.' His vision is one of an increased role for physicians in the interpretation of information supplied electronically by patients who are more empowered in their own health care. Kassirer is not unaware of the many problems this would bring. Would quality and continuity of care suffer? What would become of the doctor–patient relationship? What types of problems can safely be handled remotely? How would the dangers of self-diagnosis and self-treatment be minimized? Would such a technological approach to health care further deprive those who cannot afford or are otherwise deprived of online access? Clearly, any transformation in health-care delivery will not be an overnight phenomenon, even if the necessary technologies were available to support an online health-care system.

Just how much of a problem these questions present depends on the extent of the 'revolution'. On one hand, 'electronic individualists' see physicians subordinate in health care; on the other, 'electronic institutionalists' are sceptical about the ability or desire of consumers to 'take control', and view access to information as an opportunity for more equal dialogue between all parties (*Lancet* 1995). Indeed, the 'art of medicine' lies in the skills doctors possess in the application of medical knowledge to individuals; it follows that replacing this with an impersonal 'vending service' would not equate to good medicine.

Perhaps some reassurance can be drawn from recent market research. Data from Find/SVP Emerging Technologies Research Group's *American Internet Users Survey* (Fig. 14) suggests that Americans who use the Internet regularly to locate health information would be most interested in accessing information directly from their own physician via the Internet (Brown 1996). For further information about the report, visit the following Web page:

<URL:http://etrg.findsvp.com/health/mktginfo.html>

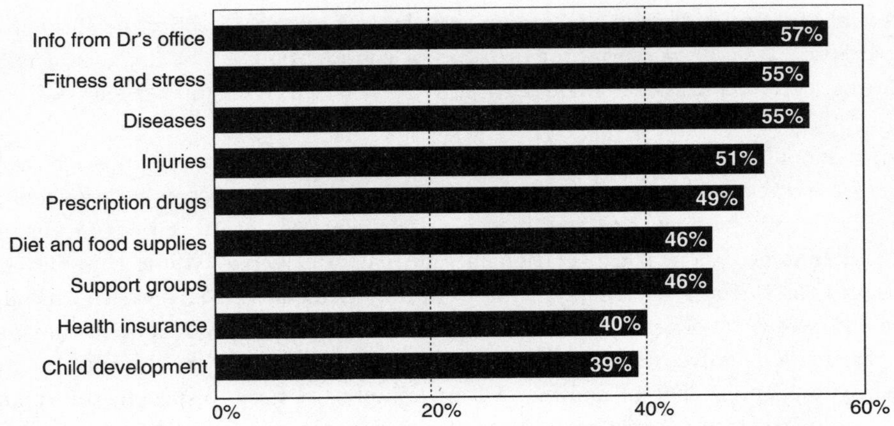

Fig. 14 Most of the 36.7 per cent of the American Internet-user population who regularly access health and medical information on the Internet would be interested in obtaining information directly from their own physician's office via the Internet. [Data from Find/SVP Emerging Technologies Research Group (see text) and used with permission.]

Another interesting suggestion is a personal password-protected Web page providing a travelling patient's clinical details in the event of emergency medical treatment (Doyle 1995). This would involve the patient wearing the equivalent of a Medic Alert bracelet stamped with the necessary access information (i.e. the URL and password). Doyle has even placed a demonstration version of such a page on the WWW:

<URL:http://www.inforamp.net/~djdoyle/pcwp.html>

Telemedicine

Telemedicine essentially involves using computers and telecommunication links to remove the factor of physical distance from medical interactions and information exchanges. Although an all-encompassing term, to many telemedicine equates solely to remote clinical consultation. This is perhaps because videoconferencing as a means of 'delivering' specialist care to patients in remote areas is the most visible and inspiring application of telemedicine. Many specialities are developing neologisms such as 'teledermatology' for the diagnosis of skin disease over real-time audiovisual links. In the US many radiologists based in larger centres can now report X-rays and other images made remotely in smaller facilities, speeding up the process and accuracy of diagnosis (known as 'teleradiology').

While telemedicine may promise to improve the availability and speed of access to specialist services—and at the same time reduce the cost of health-care delivery, no doubt some doctors and patients have reservations about taking such a 'hi-tech' approach. In addition there are a number of obstacles such as communications costs, data security, malpractice risk, and a lack of trials documenting effectiveness. However, these factors have not deterred academic and commercial experimentation.

One such experiment is the San Diego-based Cyberspace Telemedical Office (see above for the URL), offering an urgent primary-care telemedical service based on a WWW gateway (Carr, personal communication). Patients require access to a computer with a 14 400 bps or better link to the Internet, the ability to send scanned still images or video clips, and other devices such as a low-cost electronic stethoscope. Patients check in online, and whilst waiting to 'see the doctor' browse patient education material, enter their medical information, and perform computerized self-diagnostic evaluations. If clients meet certain criteria for a telemedical consultation they proceed by answering questions pertaining to their complaint, transmit their vital signs using home blood pressure devices, and provide details of their medical history (if this information is not already stored in the office's databases). If patients pass this 'triage' then they can conference directly with physicians via one of several techniques. This interaction may involve, in addition to keyboard and mouse input, real-time audio or video as necessary. Prescriptions or orders for tests can be sent via e-mail, fax, or phone directly to the patient's local pharmacy, radiologic facility, or laboratory.

Telemedicine on the Internet is discussed further in the following chapter by Richard Wootton.

Bibliography

Berry, E., Parker-Jones, C., Jones, R.G., Harkin, P.J.R., Horsfall, H.O., Nicholls, J.A., and Cook, N.J.A. (1996). In *A systematic methodology for assessing WWW medical education materials*, European Congress of the Internet in Medicine Programme and Abstracts, (ed. Arvanitis, T.N., Baldock, C., Lutkin, J., Vincent, R. and Watson, D.), pp.40–1. University of Sussex, Brighton.

Bingham, C. and Coleman, R. (1996). Enter the Web: an experiment in electronic research peer review. *Medical Journal of Australia*, **164**, 8–9. [Editorial.]

Branger, P.J., van der Wouden, J.C., Schudel, B.R., Verboog, E., Duisterhout, J.S., van der Lei, J., and Bemmel, J.H. (1992). Electronic communication between providers of primary and secondary care. *BMJ*, **305**, 1068–70.

BMJ (1995). The NHS network must be secure. *BMJ*, **310**, 1540. [News.]

Brown, M.S. (1996). *Consumer Health and Medical Information on the Internet: Supply and Demand*. Find/SVP Emerging Technologies Research Group, New York.

Campion, E.W. (1996). The *Journal's* presence on the Internet. *New England Journal of Medicine*, 334, 1129. [Editorial.]

Coiera, E. (1995). Medical informatics. *BMJ*, **310**, 1381–7.

Coiera, E. (1996). The Internet's challenge to health care provision. *BMJ*, **312**, 3–4. [Editorial.]

Delamothe, T. (1995). BMJ on the Internet. *BMJ*, **310**, 1343–4.

Doyle, D.J. (1995). Surfing the Internet for patient information: the personal clinical Web page. *Journal of the American Medical Association*, 274, 1586. [Letter.]

Ferguson, J.H. (1996). On-line medicine @nih.gov. *Journal of the American Medical Association*, 275, 94.

Follet Implementation Group on Information Technology. (1994, Aug 3) *Framework for progressing the initiative*, [Online]. <URL:http://ukoln.bath.ac.uk/elib/wk_papers/figit-4-94.html>. [JISC Circular 4/94.]

Furnace, J., Hamilton, N.M., Helms, P., and Duguid, K. (1996). Medical teaching at a peripheral site by videoconferencing. *Medical Education*, **30**, 215–20.

Getz, K.A. (1996). In *The Internet: a new patient recruitment resource*, European Congress of the Internet in Medicine Programme and Abstracts, (ed. Arvanitis, T.N., Baldock, C., Lutkin, J., Vincent, R., and Watson, D.), pp.59–60. University of Sussex, Brighton.

Hayes, T.M. (1995). Continuing medical education: a personal view. *BMJ*, **310**, 994–6.

Hotvedt, M.O. (1996). Continuing medical education: actually learning rather than simply listening. *Journal of the American Medical Association*, 275, 1637. [Letter.]

Kassirer, J.P. (1995). The next transformation in the delivery of health care. *New England Journal of Medicine*, 332, 52–3. [Editorial.]

Kassirer, J.P., and Angell, M. (1995). The Internet and the *Journal*. *New England Journal of Medicine*, **332**, 1709–10. [Editorial.]

Kelly, M.A. and Oldham, J. (1996). In *The Internet and randomised controlled trials*, European Congress of the Internet in Medicine Programme and Abstracts, (ed. Arvanitis, T.N., Baldock, C., Lutkin, J., Vincent, R., and Watson, D.), pp.40–1. University of Sussex, Brighton.

Kriz, H.M. (1995, Jun 26). *Teaching and publishing in the World Wide Web*, [Online]. <URL:http://learning.lib.vt.edu/webserv/webserv.html>.

Lancet. (1995). Leap of faith over the data tap. *The Lancet*, **345**, 1449–51. [Editorial.]

La Porte, R.E., Akazawa, S., Hellmonds, P., Boostrom, E., Gamboa, C., Gooch, T., *et al.* (1994). Global public health and the information superhighway. *BMJ*, **308**, 1651–2.

La Porte, R.E., Marler, E., Akazawa, S., Sauer, F., Gamboa, C., Shenton, C., *et al.* (1995). The death of biomedical journals. *BMJ*, **310**, 1387–90.

Letterie, G.S., Morgenstern, L.L., and Johnson, L. (1994). The role of an electronic mail system in the educational strategies of a residency in obstetrics and gynecology. *Obstetrics and Gynecology*, **84**, 137–9.

Lindon, T. and Kienholz, M.L. (1995). *Dr. Tom Lindon's guide to online medicine*. McGraw-Hill, New York.

Longmore, M. (1995). Permanence of paper puts authors on best behaviour. *BMJ*, **311**, 507. [Letter.]

McConnell, J. and Horton, R. (1996). The message, the medium, and *The Lancet*. *The Lancet*, **348**, 74.

Pignone, M. (1995). The Internet and the *Journal*. *The New England Journal of Medicine*, **333**, 1079. [Letter.]

Sanfey, J. (1996). MSc in general practice can be done over the Internet. *BMJ*, **312**, 978. [Letter.]

Willard, K.E., Hallgren, B.S., Sielaff, B., and Connelly, D.P. (1995). The deployment of a World Wide Web (W3) based medical information system. In *Proceedings of the Nineteenth Annual Symposium on Computer Applications in Medical Care*, pp.771–5. American Medical Informatics Association, Bethesda.

Wyatt, J. (1991). Use and sources of medical knowledge. *The Lancet*, **338**, 1368–73.

CHAPTER FOURTEEN
Telemedicine and the Internet

by Richard Wootton

Telemedicine can be defined as 'any medical activity practised at a distance'. As such it includes the processes of diagnosis and treatment, as well as all aspects of medical education. Clearly there are various ways in which the Internet can be used for telemedicine.

Teaching

Teaching on the Internet can consist of access to previously stored material, or may take place in real time (where both teacher and students have to be present simultaneously). There are many examples of the former, although much of the material is unstructured and not part of any formal syllabus. The quality of much of the teaching material accessible via the Internet is rather variable and the phrase *caveat emptor* springs to mind. Examples of teaching material are given in Chapter Twenty six. Examples of structured teaching material include:

> The Internet Dermatology Society's global lecture series:
>
> **<URL:http://telemedicine.org/lectures.htm>**
>
> A national project in teaching undergraduate surgery at University College London:
>
> **<URL:http://av.avc.ucl.ac.uk/tltp/insurrect.html>**

There are relatively few examples of live medical teaching on the Internet, although video of live surgery was recently transmitted from Germany by Health Online Services:

> **<URL:http://www.hos.de/>**

Diagnosis

For reasons explained below, most of the diagnostic work which has been conducted using the Internet has been experimental, rather than routine (operational). Examples include:

Store-and-forward telepathology:

> Pathologists in different locations have exchanged case material, including histological images, using multimedia electronic mail and the Internet. A formal evaluation of diagnostic agreement has been conducted. At image compression ratios between 6:1 and 40:1, satisfactory agreement was obtained in the majority of cases (Della Mea *et al.* 1996).

E-mail consulting in the developing world:

The HealthNet project (p.87) uses both satellites and the Internet to provide communications for doctors in areas of the developing world where the communications infrastructure is poor. There are stations in over a dozen countries, with eight in Africa (Fig. 15).

Intercontinental fetal surgery consulting:

Fetal surgery is not available in many countries, including the UK. Ultrasound images of a fetus in London were transmitted using FTP (p.179) to the Fetal Treatment Program in San Francisco for a surgical opinion. Surgeons and radiologists from the team in San Francisco reviewed the images and telephoned within the hour to speak to the referring physicians and the patient. Although the lesion was suitable for excision, they felt that the associated placentomegaly indicated a high risk of the mother developing other problems. The mother was thus spared the expense and anxiety of an unnecessary transatlantic trip (Fisk *et al*. 1993).

Treatment

At the time of writing, there are no known examples of the use of the Internet to deliver treatment in real time.

Communication

Another major use of the Internet for telemedicine, besides those listed above, concerns the general communication of medical information. Examples include:

The TIE database:

The TIE (Telemedicine Information Exchange) is an online information service comprising a number of linked databases dealing with various aspects of telemedicine. The bibliographic database, for example, contains over 2000 references on telemedicine, many with abstracts.

<URL:http://tie.telemed.org/>

Network news:

The newsgroup **sci.med.telemedicine** is for persons interested in telemedicine, not for persons seeking assistance with particular medical problems. See Chapter Eighteen.

The Journal of Telemedicine and Telecare:

The journal is the first academic journal intended specifically for publication of peer-reviewed papers on all aspects of telemedicine and telecare. The latter covers the emerging area of distance nursing and community support. Although the Journal is published by conventional means, up-to-date tables of contents and

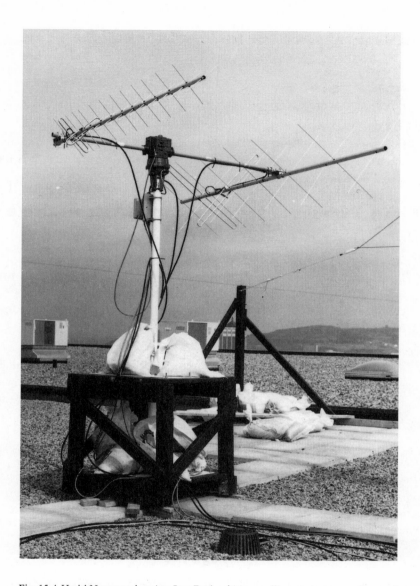

Fig. 15 A HealthNet ground station. Low Earth-orbiting satellites passing over such ground stations upload out-going e-mail and download incoming e-mail to remote locations. [Photo: Prof. A.M. House, Memorial University of Newfoundland.]

details about how to subscribe are maintained on the Web.

<URL:http://www.qub.ac.uk/telemed/jtt/>

Advantages of the Internet for telemedicine

The advantages of the Internet for telemedicine include:

Its low cost:
People can connect to the Internet via the telephone network using a modem.

It is (almost) ubiquitous:
Because of its connection to the telephone network it follows that access to the Internet is global. Even in areas without a telephone network, such as Antarctica, access is possible via a satellite link.

Disadvantages of the Internet for telemedicine

The disadvantages of the Internet for telemedicine include:

Lack of control:
By its nature, no single organization is responsible for the Internet. This makes it impossible to provide guarantees of service. It also makes the protection of confidential information transmitted on the Internet difficult, if not impossible (see p.60).

Low bandwidth:
Although new technologies such as high-speed fibre optic links are available, for reasons of cost they are more likely to be used by small or local-area networks rather than by wide-area networks (p.93). This is likely to mean that intercontinental data transmission will continue to be relatively slow.

Conclusion

The Internet certainly has something to offer telemedicine. However, because of the problems of its control, it is difficult to envisage clinical work being done on the Internet to a significant extent. It appears more likely that, with the possible exception of teaching, the majority of telemedicine work will take place on private networks in future.

References

Della Mea, V., Forti, S., Puglisi, F., Bellutta, P., Finato, N., Dalla Palma, P., Mauri, F., and Beltrami, C.A. (1996). Telepathology using Internet multimedia electronic mail: remote consultation on gastrointestinal pathology. *Journal of Telemedicine and Telecare*, 2, 28–34.

Fisk, N., Vaughan, J.I., Wootton, R., and Harrison, M.R. (1993). Intercontinental fetal surgical consultation with image transmission via Internet. *The Lancet*, 341, 1601–2.

CHAPTER FIFTEEN

How do I get on the Internet?

What are my options?

Network access via a LAN or WAN

Many universities run their own computer networks on campus, called local-area networks (LANs). If you have access to a network such as this, you may be able to sit at a terminal or PC where the central computer (often a UNIX workstation) has a direct link to the Internet. The Joint Academic Network, or JANET, interconnects UK campus-wide networks and is part of the global Internet. If you are a medical student or member of the academic staff at a teaching hospital in the UK, the chances are that you will have access to JANET (see below, p.136). Within the NHS, access may be possible via NHSnet (see below, p.137).

Dial-up modem access

If you don't have access to a LAN or WAN of some description, there are a number of 'dial-up' access options for modem users. These include terminal-based access, access via an online service gateway, or access using SLIP or PPP. The latter two are more popular, and are discussed below. It is also possible to dial a host computer (typically a UNIX machine) which is on the Internet using terminal-emulation software. Although not directly connected to the Internet yourself, you can use tools on the host to access virtually all Internet services through a command-line interface (p.16). Thus any files that you request will be sent to the host, from where they can be downloaded using a file transfer protocol such as Zmodem. The tools at your disposal will of course be limited to those provided by the administrator of the host computer.

Leased lines and dial-up ISDN

Many Internet access providers and telecommunications companies offer **leased lines**, providing a personal, direct, and constant connection to an Internet access point. The speed of the connection depends on the type of leased line available, ranging from standard telephone lines, through ISDN (see below), to super-fast digital lines (with names like 'T1'). Installation and running costs typically place this option beyond the reach of individuals.

An increasingly common alternative, although still expensive (in the UK), is an Integrated Services Digital Network, or **ISDN** connection. Operating like dial-up modem connections but using a dedicated high-speed digital telephone line and special hardware, data can be transmitted at 64 000 to 128 000 bps (depending on whether you are sending data down one or two 'channels'—and faster, if the data are compressed). These rates are achieved by transmitting a stream of digital bits, rather than performing the modulation/demodulation used by modems over an analogue telephone line. In addition to providing much faster access to the Internet than is possible using a modem, ISDN may be used for videoconferencing and distance learning (p.120). Note that you cannot use ISDN to access the Internet unless your Internet access provider offers an ISDN line to connect to.

Emerging access technologies

Cable access to the Internet (using television networks) has been tried experimentally, although is not yet offered on a wide scale. Although theoretically capable of receiving data at speeds much greater than conventional modems or even ISDN, it seems likely that in practice performance will be subject to bandwidth limitations (both within the Internet itself and those inherent to cable network technology).

Further competition for the existing telephone system and cable-based services may come from radio networks. Requiring a receiving dish, these radio-telephones are expected to allow videoconferencing as well as high-speed Internet access.

Conventional modems and copper-based telephone systems may yet deliver significantly more than 33 600 bps if ways to compress data into ever-smaller forms can be found. Personal fibre-optic Internet connections remain elusive due to cost.

JANET

The Joint Academic NETwork (**JANET**) was created in 1984. This network ties together all UK Higher Education Funding Council-supported universities, colleges, and research council establishments, and is itself directly linked to other networks on the Continent and in the United States. At its inception JANET was based on existing networks already using the **X.25** protocol (TCP/IP was not a contender). A variety of X.25-based standards permit file transfer, electronic mail, remote control of other computers, etc., as do similar standards on TCP/IP networks.

In 1989 the DES Computer Board, then responsible for funding JANET, endorsed plans to improve vastly the bandwidth (capacity) of the network using fibre-optic cables. This project was termed **SuperJANET**, and has made the transmission of real-time video and multimedia across the network possible. One of the earliest SuperJANET links was between Imperial College and Hammersmith Hospital in London.

In 1991 the JANET IP Service (JIPS) came into being, allowing TCP/IP and X.25 traffic to share the same bandwidth. JANET has essentially become a TCP/IP service, allowing medical students and academics full Internet access using, in theory, the same client software as is provided to dial-up users (see below). In practice the choice of client software will, however, be determined by each system administrator, partly because of the need to avoid abuse of the system. X.25-based services (like X.400 for mail and X.29 for terminal access) are being phased out as the original JANET infrastructure is dismantled.

For information on obtaining Internet access via JANET, contact the Computing Service at your university or institution. Guidelines for the use of JANET by NHS staff are documented in *Network News 43*, November 1994, which is available from the JANET WWW server at:

<URL:http://www.ja.net/>

The JANET Liaison Desk is at UKERNA, Atlas Centre, Chilton, Didcot, Oxfordshire OX11 0QS, tel. 01235 822212, e-mail JANET-Liaison-Desk@ukerna.ac.uk. A national dial-up service is also available in association with U-NET (e-mail janetdu@u-net.net for details).

NHSnet

The UK National Health Service (NHS) Executive, as part of its Information Management and Technology Initiative, instigated an NHS-wide Networking Project in 1992. The wide-area network (WAN), known as **NHSnet**, is run over the existing UK telecommunications infrastructure. NHSnet went 'live' in October 1995, despite unresolved security concerns (p.113). In addition to supporting an X.400-based message-handling service (MHS), NHSnet uses TCP/IP protocols, permitting Internet-style applications. High-bandwidth communications links (using leased lines and/or ISDN—see below) permit telemedical applications (Chapter Fourteen) in addition to high-speed access to NHS-specific WWW pages, etc. Using a secure *one-way* ('out-bound') gateway to the wider Internet, Health Service personnel can 'dial out' without unauthorized people having access to NHSnet itself (although e-mail is two-way). Individual NHS Trusts must subscribe to the TCP/IP service, and provide the necessary hardware and software for hospital-based doctors to utilize it. Access authorization for individual users is at a local level, although each Trust will be bound by an agreed 'code of connection'. General practitioners will be able to dial into a local access point, and through the WAN connect to their selected end-point—such as the Internet. This facility operates on a 'pay-as-you-go' basis. Further information is available by calling the NHS-wide Network Info Line on 0121 625 3838.

Online service Internet gateways

Online services differ greatly in the solutions they provide for access to Internet Services. Smaller bulletin boards commonly use a gateway to the **UUCP** (UNIX-to-UNIX CoPy) network, a cost-effective system linking together UNIX computers. Like most types of gateway access, this allows users to send and receive e-mail, read and post to Usenet newsgroups, and download binary files indirectly by e-mail. It does not allow the use of interactive services like Telnet or the use of a WWW browser. The next step up combines this sort of gateway with terminal-based access, as described above. Some services, such as CompuServe, offer the flexibility to access Internet Services via a gateway interface or a TCP/IP interface using SLIP or PPP (see below).

Commercial online services sometimes charge for the use of their gateway on a 'pay-as-you-go' basis, perhaps including connect-time charges on top of this. Although such an interface may have certain merits for some Internet services, such as the provision of a simplified means of accessing newsgroups, it may be a barrier to the full utilization of others. The user may feel restricted by the interface the online service has chosen to provide. They may also be forced to complete one task at a time (such as reading e-mail or downloading files), rather than undertaking several tasks simultaneously (as is possible with a direct Internet connection).

Dial-up modem access (SLIP and PPP)

Full access to the Internet means that you have an IP address for you own machine (p.100), and have a permanent connection to the Internet or dial-up link using SLIP or PPP. SLIP and PPP were introduced in Chapter Twelve. This type of access is being demanded by more and more Internet users. If you have a SLIP or PPP account with a service provider, the client applications on your computer directly interact with server applications on the Internet, typically by means of a 'user friendly' graphical interface.

Will any modem do?

Chapter Three recommended that you buy the fastest modem you can afford. This is of particular relevance on the Internet, where 14 400 bps is considered low bandwidth. At this speed some graphics-intensive WWW pages take so long to display that it is easier to turn off the display of graphics by your WWW browser. While this to some extent defeats the point of the WWW, it does dramatically speed up page-display times. It is still possible, however, to access the Internet at 2400 bps—although this is not recommended.

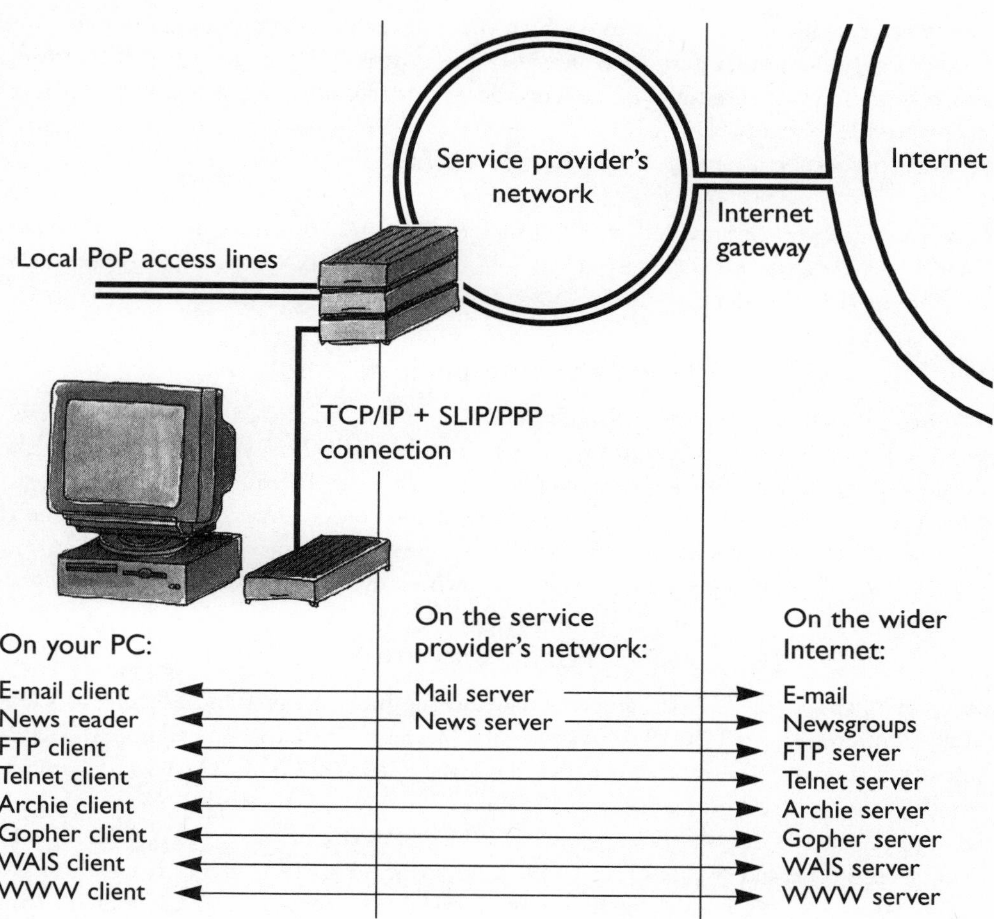

Fig. 16 The role of a SLIP or PPP Internet service provider. In addition to supplying modem access through 'Points of Presence', it operates the mail and news-servers required to transfer electronic mail, and to read or post to newsgroups. Other clients merely use the service provider's network as a gateway to interact directly with servers on the wider Internet.

What is a service provider?

A service provider is a company from which you rent the resources necessary to make your home/surgery computer a part of the Internet (intermittently, if using SLIP or PPP). **Points of Presence**, or PoPs, are banks of modems that provide local access to the service provider's high-speed IP network which is itself part of the wider Internet (see Fig. 16). Usually a monthly service fee is payable on top of the cost of telephone calls to the PoP.

So what does a service provider actually provide? To answer this question, we will look at each element of an access package individually. See Chapter Sixteen for help in choosing an Internet service provider.

A domain name and IP address

The first element of an access package is a domain name and IP address. Different service providers handle this in different ways. Some providers will allow you to specify a unique, personal domain name if they issue you with a static/fixed IP address. In this case, each time you connect to a PoP your machine is registered on the Internet with the same IP address. Other providers have a bank of IP addresses that are randomly assigned to your machine as you connect to the PoP (this is known as 'dynamic assignment').

TCP/IP software

In order to speak the TCP/IP language used on the Internet, PCs and Macintoshes (and other computers) need TCP/IP software. In the Microsoft Windows environment, TCP/IP software forms part of a 'stack' which includes a file called **WINSOCK.DLL**. This file provides compatibility with Windows socket-compliant IP software, a standard for Windows TCP/IP applications. Windows 95 comes with a TCP/IP stack (as does OS/2, Windows for Workgroups 3.11, and Windows NT), and shareware or commercial alternatives are available for Windows 3.1 users such as Trumpet Winsock (shareware) and Chameleon from NetManage.

Trumpet Winsock :

<URL:ftp://ftp.trumpet.com.au/winsock/>

Macintosh computers require either the MacTCP control panel (for earlier systems, obtainable from Apple separately or as part of System 7.5), or the TCP/IP control panel (a standard part of Open Transport system software).

Your Internet-access provider may provide pre-configured TCP/IP software (usually in the form of a settings file), or will provide instructions taking you though the setup process for their particular service.

PPP or SLIP

Point-to-Point Protocol (PPP) or Serial Line Internet Protocol (SLIP) drivers are necessary only for dial-up connections to the Internet (p.97). These protocols allow your computer to become a host on the Internet for the time that it is connected. PPP is more recent than SLIP and could be considered the current standard. Your service provider may offer one or the other, or both. Windows 95 provides PPP, and the popular shareware Trumpet Winsock stack has built-in PPP and SLIP functionality for Windows 3.1 (and Windows 95) users.

Some access providers (and Windows 95) offer a customized '**Internet dialer**' to PC users, replacing shareware alternatives. This is an application that may be used to manage PPP or SLIP configuration, other dial-up settings, connection/disconnection, and sometimes provides menu access to a range of Internet clients. On the Macintosh, PPP and SLIP are present as Extensions, and are configured via a corresponding Control Panel or application, which also serves as a dialer. Mac users can opt for a freeware solution for both PPP and SLIP software—FreePPP or InterSLIP, available from:

<URL:ftp://src.doc.ic.ac.uk/packages/mac-sumex/_Communication/_MacTCP/>

Your Internet service provider can assist in configuring the PPP/SLIP or dialer software for use with their particular service. They will also need to supply you with a UserID and password, and telephone numbers to access their network.

Mail-server address

The sending and receiving of Internet e-mail via a dial-up PPP/SLIP connection requires the use of a computer operated by the service provider known as a **mail server**. Because you are not continuously connected to the Internet you could not receive e-mail unless it was stored somewhere (i.e. on a mail server), waiting for your next call. Mail servers on the Internet use one of two protocols to send messages between the server and the e-mail client software on your computer: Simple Mail Transport Protocol (**SMTP**), or Post Office Protocol (**POP**). Your service provider will let you know the address of the SMTP server or the name of your POP account.

News-server address

In order to use a news-reader program on your computer, your service provider needs to run a **news server**. News servers receive all the articles posted to newsgroups that the provider carries. Using a protocol called Network News Transfer Protocol (**NNTP**) you can retrieve interesting-looking articles from the full list of subjects sent to you by the news server. The address of your news server will be something like **news.elsewhere.co.uk**.

Internet client software

Clients are the tools on your computer that communicate (using TCP/IP) with the corresponding server on the Internet. For example, to access a Telnet server, you need a Telnet client. The client–server relationship was explained in Chapter Four. This book does not attempt to take you through the installation of client software. Virtually all client software comes with at least a **README.TXT** file explaining how to use its features and giving installation instructions. Your service provider will be able to advise you on appropriate clients, and probably supplies a basic set of tools to get you started. New computers commonly ship with Internet clients pre-loaded (integrated into the operating system, or bundled separately).

Popular shareware clients are mentioned under the corresponding chapter in Part Three of the book, should you wish to replace a client provided to you as part of an access software kit. The best way to obtain the latest versions is to use an FTP client (p.179) to retrieve them from the Internet itself. If you cannot find a particular client by name in an FTP archive where you expect to find it, try an Archie search (p.187). Alternatively, download your clients from the file libraries of an online service or bulletin board, or look for a CD-ROM on the cover of an Internet or computing magazine.

One potential problem arising from the use of a diverse collection of shareware clients is that they all have to be configured separately. Commercial packages available for both Macs and PCs attempt to overcome this by providing an 'all-in-one' application (sometimes including TCP/IP and PPP/SLIP). Such packages may not be as flexible or feature-laden as the individual specialized clients, but are worthy of consideration (and may be the most cost-effective solution). Arguably, the World-Wide Web browser Netscape falls into this category.

Your Internet-access provider should be able to assist you in configuring client software for use with their particular service.

CHAPTER SIXTEEN

Choosing an access provider

Companies offering Internet access can be classified broadly into those that are historically online information services (such as AOL and CompuServe) and those that simply provide Internet access. However, as mentioned in Chapter Eleven, this distinction is becoming somewhat irrelevant. On another level, they can be divided into international, national, and local access providers.

Considerations in your choice of provider

There are a number of considerations that may help you decide with whom to open an account if you are looking for a dial-up Internet access provider.

Type of access

Perhaps you are interested in a simple e-mail account only? If you want to use a WWW browser like Netscape or Microsoft Internet Explorer (most people do) then a TCP/IP connection is required. For dial-up users, this entails a SLIP or PPP service (p.140). Alternatively, a BBS gateway may suffice. Many access providers offer a range of accounts to suit different requirements, including leased lines (p.135).

Local-call access numbers

Most access providers offer accounts to users on a national basis; some have less extensive networks and appeal to local users only (a particular city, for example). 'Local access' means a service is accessible at local call telephone rates (where applicable) to residents of the named area. Local access to high-speed modems (see below) will cut the cost of calling the service. This is even more advantageous in countries where local calls are free.

Find out how extensive the network of a potential access provider is. Junior hospital doctors, for example, often change posts every six months or so and if this involves a change of address, the greater the range of local access numbers, the better.

There are several large online services/Internet service providers that operate internationally. An account held with such a provider may be particularly useful to those who travel a lot, whether on overseas medical electives, voluntary work abroad, or to symposia. International services include America OnLine (AOL in Europe); CompuServe; IBM Global Network; MSN; TheOnRamp; and UUNET PIPEX.

TABLE 10 Example Internet access providers in the UK

Name	Telephone	E-mail and Web site
AOL	0800 279 1234	queryuk@aol.com http://www.aol.co.uk
CompuServe	0800 289 378	70006.101@compuserve.com http://www.compuserve.com
Demon Internet	0181 371 1234	sales@demon.net http://www.demon.co.uk
MSN	0800 750 800	MSNMembercommunications4@msn.com http://www.msn.com
UK Online	0645 00 00 11	sales@ukonline.co.uk http://www.ukonline.co.uk
UUNET PIPEX	0500 474 739	sales@dial.pipex.com http://www.uunet.pipex.com/

Some example providers operating in the UK are shown in Table 10 (note that inclusion in the table does not constitute an endorsement of any kind).

Speed of access

For modem-based connections to the Internet 28 800 bps is 'standard', and most providers offer this at their PoPs (p.139). It makes sense to verify that high-speed access will be available at the particular PoP you will be calling, as some providers offer high-speed access only in major towns, with slower modems manning the less urban PoPs. Companies offering dial-up ISDN access (p.135) may appeal to those with ISDN facilities.

Individual access providers also differ in the speed at which their own network operates, and in the speed at which they connect to the rest of the Internet; this ultimately influences the speed at which dial-up users can access remote resources via their provider's network.

Initial costs

Is there an initial 'start-up' fee to cover the setting-up of your account and/or the access software? What do you get for this fee? For example, how many e-mail addresses can you have?

On-going costs and type of charge

The cost of using a particular provider depends, quite logically, on how much use you will make of the service. Providers charge either on a 'pay-as-you-go' basis (usually online services), or allow unlimited access for a fixed monthly/annual fee. A 'pay-as-you-go' arrangement may be more suitable for occasional users, and unlimited connect-time for a fixed fee suited to heavy users. Some providers use a combination of both types of charging; you get a free allowance of connect-time per month, and when this allowance is exceeded, you pay per hour thereafter. Remember that aside from the access provider, your telephone company may be billing you for time online, so dial-up 'off-peak' whenever possible. Also, 'pay-as-you-go' is more expensive for users of slow modems.

Support facilities

The most important consideration in relation to support is whether or not the provider understands the workings of your particular computer type. For example, Mac users may risk strife by signing on to a 'Windows only' service provider. Is there telephone support available when you will be using the service (e.g. evenings and weekends)? Try dialing the support number; are you put on hold for a long time, or progressively routed elsewhere by an automated system? Are there online new-user forums where you can ask for help? Are printed instructions or a manual provided?

Software

Most companies supply a set of software programs to access and use with their accounts. This may be a collection of shareware (which you must then register at your cost), pre-registered or licensed software, or even a custom connection kit. Software supplied as part of a package generally works well together, but you might enquire about the potential to 'mix and match' should you have preferences for a certain client. Customized software usually has the distinct advantage of being pre-configured for use with the supplier's services, which can save a significant amount of time and frustration relative to configuring everything manually. Ask whether any supplied software includes setup instructions or a manual. Can you use an offline message reader (which will again cut the cost of connect-time to the service)? See also *Internet client software*, p.141.

'Real-world availability'

An advertisement for 100 per cent nationwide access at local call rates doesn't mean a first-time connection 100 per cent of the time, as bandwidth and modems are shared among callers. Popular services, by virtue of their popularity, often have engaged lines at critical times (like 7 pm, when everyone is trying to collect their e-mail or 'surf' the Web). This is where it can be particularly advantageous to take up the free trial offers that many companies promote. If you load the trial software and repeatedly have trouble connecting, consider an alternative provider. Sometimes people talk about 'modem-to-user ratio' which describes the statistical probability of a certain-sized group of users making a connection to a given modem at the same time.

Choice of e-mail address or domain name?

Do you have the option to specify at least the first part of your e-mail address, or will it be decided for you? Some providers also let you choose a unique domain name (p.100).

Range of services

Does a prospective provider offer value-added content such as news, online reference databases, forums, etc? Is that important? Some providers operate mailing lists, FTP archives, and IRC or Web servers (for example) for the use of their customers.

Personal Web space?

Many providers offer free Web space to individual customers, ranging from a single page to several megabytes of space. Make sure the provider supports the uploading of these pages and page creation software for your type of computer. Sometimes Web space is let to commercial concerns for a relatively small subscription.

How do I find out who sells access?

The easiest way to get an up-to-date list of providers in your area is to buy an Internet magazine that contains such a listing. Having worked out what considerations are important to you personally, it may be a good idea to ring around several companies to find out which comes closest to your requirements.

If you or a colleague already have some form of Internet access, British and Australasian readers may find the following useful:

List of Internet access providers in the UK, by Paola Kathuria:

<URL:http://www.limitless.co.uk/inetuk/>

Network access in Australia FAQ, by Zik Saleeba:

<URL:ftp://rtfm.mit.edu/pub/usenet/news.answers/internet-access/australia>

Internet access in New Zealand FAQ, by Simon Lyall:

<URL:ftp://rtfm.mit.edu/pub/usenet/news.answers/internet-access/new-zealand>

Another resource giving contact details for Internet access providers throughout Europe and worldwide is Mecklermedia's *The List*:

<URL:http://thelist.iworld.com/>

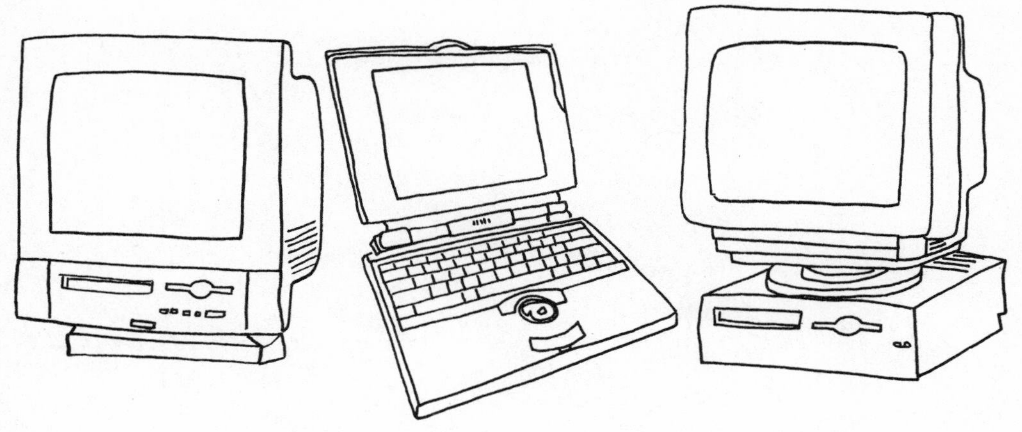

PART 4

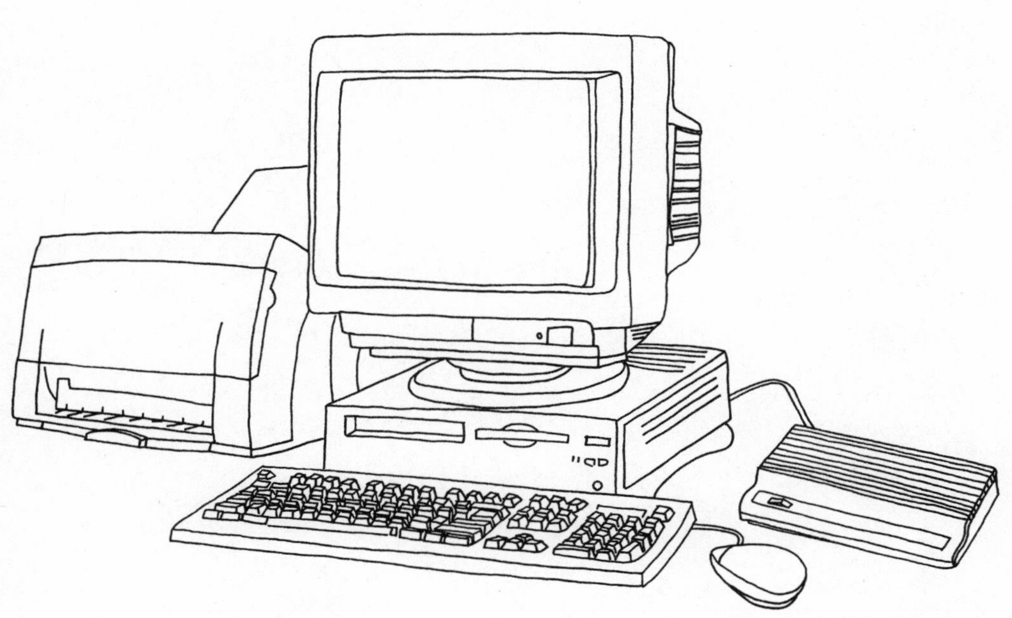

CHAPTER SEVENTEEN
Utilizing the Internet

Having introduced the Internet, in this Part we will take a closer look at each of the more common Internet services. Each service is examined with the assumption that the reader is using a personal computer with a graphical interface—a PC running Microsoft Windows or a Macintosh. Mention of UNIX commands is avoided; those using a command-line UNIX interface are likely to have on-site help. Further, the author will not provide installation instructions for client software, as these should accompany any software you intend to use. Nor will I attempt to mimic online catalogues and list every known medical resource on the Internet. Instead, we will look at a small number of examples.

Even with the right computer, modem, communications software, and guide book, it is not always easy to utilize the Internet. Given that you manage to find a free modem connection on your service provider's network, sessions can slow to a crawl as the available bandwidth is shared among callers. This waiting can get expensive in the UK, where local telephone calls are not free, unlike in many States in the US. 'This server is too busy to accept any more connections' messages are seen more frequently as one tries to connect to popular sites. Resources come and go. People come and go. Debate rages over commercialization and 'appropriate use' of the Internet, freedom of speech, 'crackers' (people who try to break into other people's computer systems), and encryption of commercial or sensitive data. This is because the Internet is all about people cooperating, not about technology. These considerations aside, utilization for most people falls under the headings of electronic messaging, file transfer, using other computers, information retrieval, and other ways to communicate.

Electronic messages

For most people electronic messaging implies e-mail between individuals. Many of the Internet services described in this Part can be utilized via electronic messages (see Table 11, p.150). Not with the same ease, granted, as is afforded by client software, but nevertheless making much of the Internet accessible to those who only have an e-mail account. In relevant chapters we briefly describe how to access various services by e-mail. The reader may also like to retrieve Rankin's *Accessing the Internet by e-mail* at:

<URL:mailto:mailbase@mailbase.ac.uk> Send: send lis-iis e-access-inet.txt

The basic use of e-mail is covered in Chapter Eighteen. Mailing lists, another common use, are discussed in Chapter Nineteen. The other major use of e-mail is bulletin boarding. The Internet is part of the distribution system for Usenet newsgroups (although Usenet as a

TABLE 11 Utilizing common Internet Services

E-mail	E-mail can be sent via	mail reader client software WWW client software
	You can use e-mail to	send and receive private messages send and receive messages to and from mailing lists send and receive messages to and from newsgroups retrieve files from FTP sites search Archie databases use Gophers and Veronica search WAIS databases retrieve WWW pages
Newsgroups	Send and receive news using	news reader client software e-mail Gopher client software (read only) WWW client software
File transfers	Access FTP sites using	FTP client software e-mail Gopher client software some Archie client software WWW client software
Telnet	Use Telnet via	Telnet client software WWW client software
	Using Telnet gives access to	other computer systems Archie Gophers and Veronica WAIS the WWW
Archie searches	You can use Archie via	Archie client software e-mail Telnet Gopher
	You can use Archie to	locate files you can download send FTP files to your computer (not all clients)
Gophers	Use Gophers and Veronica via	Gopher client software e-mail Telnet WWW client software
	You can use Gopher to	locate information send FTP files to your computer
WAIS	You can search WAIS via	WAIS client software e-mail Telnet Gopher WWW client software
	You can use WAIS to	locate information
WWW	You can read WWW pages via	WWW client software e-mail Telnet
	Using a WWW client access	multimedia information e-mail (send and receive) FTP Newsgroups Telnet Archie Gopher and Veronica WAIS

e-mail: Electronic mail WAIS: Wide Area Information Servers
FTP: File Transfer Protocol WWW: World-Wide Web

whole doesn't rely on Internet protocols). Usenet and other newsgroups provide a forum for Internet users—and those on other networks—to exchange points of view, ask for and give help, etc. See Chapter Twenty.

File transfer

In Chapter Twenty one we consider FTP, the Internet's workhorse for moving files from one computer to another. You might use an FTP client to download medical software, illustrations, and other files.

Using other computers

The Telnet protocol is essential to the working of client software, facilitating its interaction with the server. Telnet can also be used as an Internet service, with a client that allows you to log on to another computer and control the information which it sends you. Telnet is considered in Chapter Twenty two.

Information retrieval tools

If you know where to find a particular file on the Internet then an FTP client will take you to it. If you know the name of the file—but not where to find it—then Archie may be of service. See Chapter Twenty three.

A Gopher client presents the user with a series of menus linked to other menus, documents, or even other Internet services. Especially when combined with Veronica (p.193), a Gopher server can locate distributed information (i.e. information located in more than one place) on many medical subjects. See Chapter Twenty four.

Searching a WAIS database will result in a menu of documents being returned, ranked according to 'relevance' as determined by WAIS. See Chapter Twenty five.

The WWW is covered in somewhat more depth (Chapter Twenty six). The WWW has become *the* interface to the Internet, with current WWW clients integrating other services. Some clients (browsers) let you handle e-mail, subscribe to mailing lists, access FTP sites, perform Archie searches, read newsgroups, Telnet to other computers, visit Gopher sites, and of course explore WWW pages—all from within the familiarity of your WWW browser. Chapter Twenty seven follows with an introduction to searching for medical information on the Web.

Other ways to communicate

Internet Relay Chat, MOOs, streaming audio, telephony, videoconferencing, and faxing via the Internet are covered in Chapter Twenty eight.

Keeping up with new resources

This author highly recommends the American Medical Informatics Association's Internet Working Group MMatrix-L mailing list as a means of keeping up-to-date with new international resources. Focusing on clinical medical resources, the list encourages discussion relating to medical use of the Internet, and periodically sends out updates ('What's New') to the corresponding Medical Matrix WWW site (p.224), grading new resources on a scale of usefulness. Further details about the list are given in Chapter Nineteen. The 'What's New' postings can also be viewed and collectively searched on the WWW, courtesy of the University of Occupational and Environmental Health in Fukuoka, Japan:

<URL:http://www.uoeh-u.ac.jp/MML/MMS-e.html>

New health and medicine resources as indexed by Yahoo, a large general catalogue, are listed by the Hardin Meta Directory (University of Iowa) at:

<URL:http://www.arcade.uiowa.edu/hardin-www/mednew.html>

When you've finished this Part you should:

in relation to electronic messages,

- recognize the versatility of e-mail alone in accessing other Internet services
- know how to subscribe to a medical mailing list
- be aware of the health-related newsgroups, and the concept of FAQs

in relation to File Transfer Protocol,

- understand the use and value of FTP clients

in relation to using other computers,

- understand the use and value of Telnet clients

in relation to information retrieval tools,

- know how to find a file using Archie
- understand the use and value of Gopher clients
- understand the use and value of WAIS
- appreciate the significance of the WWW in popularizing the Internet, and its potential medical applications
- become familiar with ways to search for medical information

in relation to other ways to communicate,

- understand what the Internet may offer

have considered whether the Internet is simply a technology looking for a use, or a tool that could enrich your personal experience of medicine.

CHAPTER EIGHTEEN
Electronic mail

Electronic mail, or e-mail, is one of the most versatile Internet services (see Table 11, p.150). While not as quick as a service like Telnet or a facsimile, it is probably unrivalled in terms of convenience and cost-effectiveness. There is no need for stationary, stamps, or postmen. E-mail can be sent to another time zone without waking the recipient—and their computer does not need to be on at the time the message is sent. Compared to most handwriting it is highly readable, and can easily be edited and incorporated into other documents such as word-processor files. Current e-mail programs make it very easy to attach non-text files (e.g. illustrations) to an e-mail message, avoiding the sometimes messy exchange of floppy disks. Because electronic data is so reproducible, it is a simple matter to copy parts of a message into a reply, or forward a message to other recipients (electronically or printed). Furthermore it is the service least demanding on your computer, modem, or method of Internet access.

Exactly how long a message takes to get from person A to person B depends on several factors such as whether person A's Internet access is direct or indirect, how much traffic is on the Internet, how many networks are involved in handling the message, and how often person B checks his or her mailbox. If your message can't be delivered, the system will normally send a 'failed delivery' notice to the author of the message. Hopefully this will give a clue as to why delivery was impossible (e.g. you might have misspelled the address, or the person may no longer have an account on that machine).

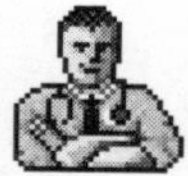

Anybody (with appropriate privileges) on any machine through which your message passes will be able to read it. There have been (very infrequent) reports of e-mail being routed to the wrong address. Bear this in mind if sending confidential clinical details. Potentially sensitive e-mail could be encrypted (converted into an indecipherable code).

For dial-up accounts, e-mail waits in your mailbox on another computer until you pick it up; your computer need not occupy the telephone line all day. When you receive an e-mail message, you will notice that it contains a lot more than just the message itself.

The structure of e-mail messages

Everyone on the Internet has a unique e-mail address, and like a telephone number it must be entered *exactly* in order to make a connection. Each address is made up of the person's name (or number), then an '@' symbol, followed by the domain name (as explained in

Chapter Twelve). This information appears in the **To:** line in the example below. This and several other lines form what is known as the 'message header'. Study the example below and note the following:

- The **Received:** lines give routing information. At each stage in the journey of a message from network to network, each gateway adds its own 'postmark' indicating the time when the message was received at each point.
- The **Date:** line records when the message was sent, not received.
- Sometimes there will be a **Cc:** line as well, indicating that someone else was sent a copy of the message.
- The **From:** line indicates the real name and e-mail address of the person sending the message.
- The **Organization:** line can be used to specify an affiliation.
- **Reply-To:** provides for systems where any reply should be made to a different address than the one specified in the **From:** line.
- The **Subject:** line typically contains a brief description of what the message is about, although is not compulsory.
- **Message-Id:** is a unique message identification number.
- **Mime-Version:** and **Content-Type:** are explained on p.160.

Below the header is the 'body' of the message. Included in the body are the message itself and (usually) the signature of the sender.

Received: from relay-2.mail.demon.net (disperse.demon.co.uk [158.152.1.77]) by dub-img-2.compuserve.com (8.6.10/5.950515)
    id UAA05101; Mon, 15 Jul 1996 20:55:30 -0400
Received: from post.demon.co.uk ([158.152.1.72]) by relay-2.mail.demon.net
    id ck21686; 16 Jul 96 1:54 +0100
Received: from cybertas.demon.co.uk ([158.152.64.237]) by relay-3.mail.demon.net
    id aa27576; 14 Jul 96 21:53 +0100
Date: Sun, 14 Jul 1996 21:53:51 +0000
To: 75337.2274@compuserve.com
From: Bruce C McKenzie <bruce-m@cybertas.demon.co.uk>
Organization: None
Reply-To: bruce-m@cybertas.demon.co.uk
Subject: Updates article by Gupta
Message-Id: <v01530500ae0f1c503201@[158.152.64.237]>
Mime-Version: 1.0
Content-Type: text/plain; charset="us-ascii"

Here is the URL for the Updates article by Gupta on sexual issues in family planning:
http://www.dundee.ac.uk/meded/webupdate/sexual/spgupta.htm

Cheers, Bruce

Using an e-mail client

To use e-mail, one needs access to a computer capable of exchanging mail with the Internet, an account on that computer, appropriate client software, and a personal unique e-mail address.

A good e-mail client will offer features such as direct replies to received messages (often quoting the original text using an angle bracket, **>**), mail forwarding, and the ability to send multiple copies to other individuals. There should be a menu option to attach a file stored on disk to your message; a good client will automatically encode the file (see below) and likewise decode it at the receiving end. An address book allows you to enter a person's name and e-mail address once, and subsequently address messages to them simply by choosing their name from a pull-down menu or clickable list (or equivalent). Ideally you should be able to use 'nicknames' rather than sometimes cryptic e-mail addresses (so you can type 'Bruce' in the **To:** field, instead of **75337.2274@compuserve.com**, for example). Examples of popular e-mail clients are Pegasus Mail and Eudora (Fig. 17):

Pegasus Mail (for the PC):

<URL:ftp://risc.ua.edu/pub/network/pegasus/>

Eudora (for the Mac):

<URL:ftp://ftp.qualcomm.com/quest/mac/eudora/>

Mail clients exchange e-mail with either a POP or SMTP mail server (p.141). Depending on your Internet service provider you may require separate programs to handle the sending and receiving of e-mail. Be aware that some service providers will automatically 'purge' your mailbox after a specified message expiry date. It would be wise to find out how frequently (if at all) this occurs.

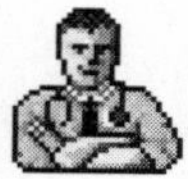

Whenever possible compose new messages offline, before initiating a communications link.

Contacting users on other networks

You can use Internet e-mail to contact doctors on other networks such as CompuServe and America Online. It is, of course, necessary to know their address on the system they are on. Given this, you may have to format the address in a particular way to meet the requirements of the gateway linking that service to the Internet. For a list of formats, see Yanoff's *Inter-network mail guide* at:

<URL:ftp://rtfm.mit.edu/pub/usenet/news.answers/mail/inter-network-guide>

The examples that follow illustrate the principles of contacting users via a few common gateways.

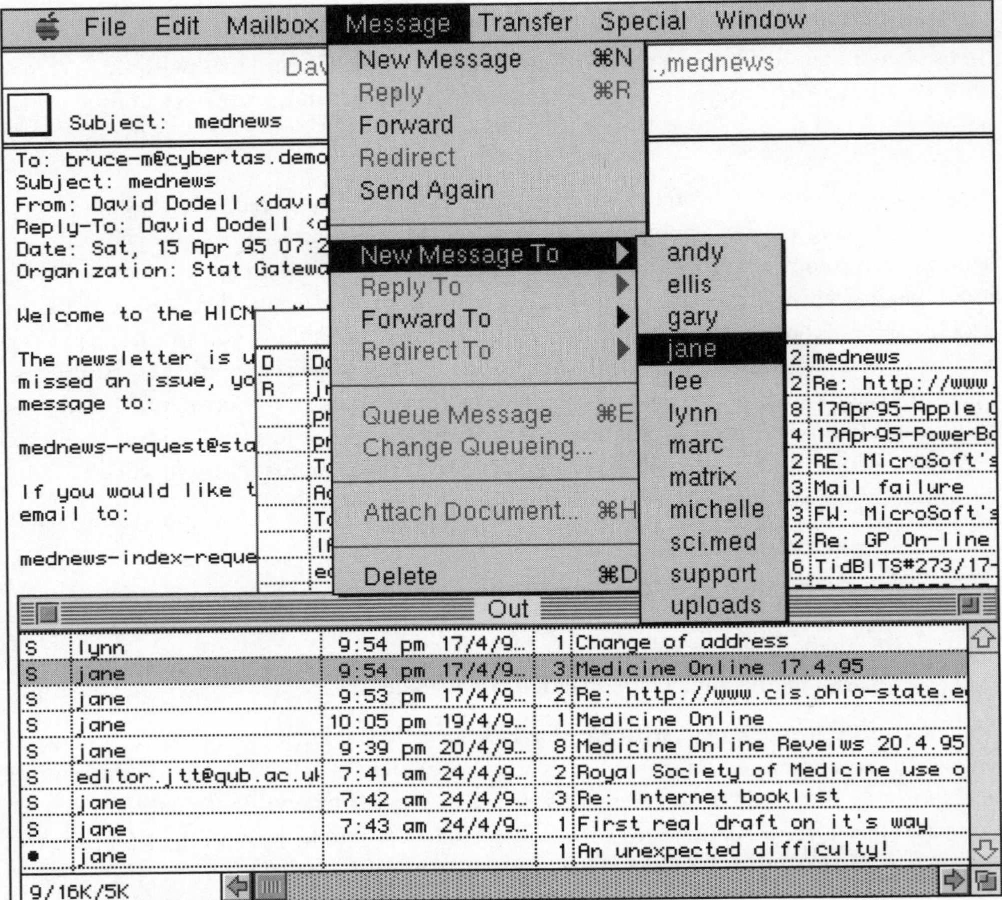

Fig. 17 Using an e-mail client. Popular programs such as Eudora (shown here) feature nicknames or aliases that simplify the process of addressing a message.

JANET

Users on the Joint Academic Network are reached just like anyone at any other Internet site, using the **username@domain.name** address format. Similarly, JANET users can e-mail anyone on the wider Internet using the same standard format. If you have difficulties reaching someone at a JANET site, addressing a message to the **postmaster** may help resolve them. You can obtain the domain name for connected institutions by looking at the list at:

<URL:http://www.ja.net/janet-sites/sites.html>

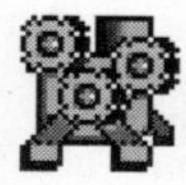

As a historical note, JANET addresses used to be 'back-to-front'. With the advent of SuperJANET and the adoption of TCP/IP standards, JANET sites are now addressed like any other Internet site. Older JANET sites may still use back-to-front addresses which are dealt with by conversion gateways.

CompuServe

To send e-mail to a user with an account on CompuServe the format is **CIS.ID@compuserve.com**. Note that the comma in the CompuServe Member ID number is replaced by a full stop, so **75337,2274** becomes **75337.2274@compuserve.com**. CompuServe users send outgoing mail to the Internet by prefixing it with **INTERNET:** as in:

INTERNET:bruce-m@cybertas.demon.co.uk

FidoNet

FidoNet addresses are complex. As an example, if you wish to send Internet e-mail to someone called Bruce McKenzie on a FidoNet bulletin board denoted by **2:250/232.0**, the format would be **Bruce.McKenzie@p0.f232.n250.z2.fidonet.org**. Here, the **f232** part means *Node 232* (a number in place of **0** would indicate a *Point*); the **n250** means *Network 250*; **z2** means *Zone 2* (Europe), and **fidonet.org** directs the message to a FidoNet gateway. To send mail to the Internet from a FidoNet BBS ask the local SysOp for a 'matrix address', which will route the message to an appropriate gateway.

Finding someone's e-mail address

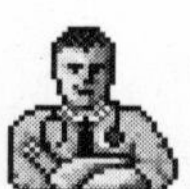

The only reliable way to find out someone's e-mail address is to telephone them and ask for it.

JANET users have access to the X.500 global directory system, and this is a good place to start when looking for a member of the academic staff at a university, for example. Students are not likely to be listed. Some networks, such as CompuServe, have a built-in membership database which can be used to find other people using that service.

There are several projects attempting to build Internet 'white pages' such as WHOIS, the Knowbot Information Service, and the PSInet White Pages. The Knowbot Information Service has the advantage of being able to query several directories from the same interface, including WHOIS and the PSInet White Pages. To query a name type **query (name)** at the following Telnet address:

<URL:telnet://info.cnri.reston.va.us:185>

Perhaps you have read a message in one of the Usenet newsgroups and wish to contact the author but have not retained the message? If the newsgroup is carried by the Massachusetts Institute of Technology you could send a message as follows:

<URL:mailto:mail-server@rtfm.mit.edu> Send: send usenet-addresses/(First name) (Last name)

'Four11' is an e-mail address search-engine on the World-Wide Web at:

<URL:http://www.four11.com/>

For further information about these and other options, refer to Lamb's *FAQ: How to find people's e-mail addresses* at:

<URL:ftp://rtfm.mit.edu/pub/usenet/news.answers/finding-addresses>

Binary files by e-mail

E-mail can be used to send binary files to other users, to reassemble binary files posted to newsgroups, and to retrieve a file from an FTP archive. In Chapter Four we introduced the difference between ASCII (text) files and binary (program) files. Binary files contain 8-bit characters; text files contain only 7-bit ASCII data. The take-home message was that sending binary files as 7-bit characters rendered them unusable.

However, binary files can be converted into ASCII text by a process known as '**ASCII encoding**'. Encoded files can be transferred via e-mail from one computer to another where they can be decoded back into usable program files. As some people are restricted to Internet access by e-mail only, encoding provides them with a way to transfer binary files. There are three common standards for encoding binary files into e-mail (see Table 12).

The uuencode standard

The most frequently encountered standard for ASCII encoding is the UNIX program **uuencode**. Programs that will uuencode (and uudecode) are available for the PC and Mac. These files are said to be 'uuencoded', and can be identified by the suffix **.uu**.

Most e-mail clients will let you attach a uuencoded file to an e-mail message. It is also possible to copy the contents of a uuencoded file using a text editor or word processor, and paste this directly into the body of the message. A common context in which to encounter encoding is when using an 'FTP mail server' to receive binary files when you do not have access to an FTP client (see below).

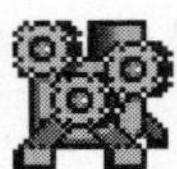

Mac users note: Most uuencode programs will only encode the data fork of a Mac file, missing out vital information in the resource fork (leaving a smaller, useless file). However, files which have no resource fork can be

TABLE 12 Standards for encoding binary files into text for e-mail transmission

Standard	Suffix	Notes
BinHex	.hqx	Macintosh BinHex format for encoding binary files into ASCII. Decoded by Stuffit Expander. Commonly used to retrieve Mac files by e-mail.
MIME	.mime	Multipurpose Internet Mail Extensions (MIME) standard for encoding binary files into ASCII. Encoding/decoding handled automatically by some e-mail clients, or programs such as 'munpack'. Becoming the dominant standard.
uuencode	.uue	Older uuencode standard for encoding binary files into ASCII. Encoding/decoding handled automatically by some e-mail clients, or programs such as Stuffit Expander (Mac) or Wincode (PC). Widely used on Usenet.

uuencoded without losing vital information, such as GIF graphics and compressed archives. This is why you can still use an FTP mail server to receive Mac files as uuencoded archives.

On the other hand, Mac applications make heavy use of the resource fork and cannot be encoded using the standard uuencode (unless they have been made into a compressed archive first, containing only a data fork). Programs like UUTool are aware of the Mac's unique file structure and can perform a 'modified' uuencode operation on Mac application files. Useless to a non-Mac user, the person receiving the file will need UUTool to decode it again. An alternative is to use MIME or BinHex (discussed below).

To uuencode/uudecode on a Windows PC, try Wincode:

<URL:ftp://ftp.demon.co.uk/pub/ibmpc/dos/apps/uucode/wincode.zip>

To uuencode/uudecode on the Mac, try UUTool:

<URL:ftp://sunsite.doc.ic.ac.uk/public/computing/systems/mac/Collections/umich/util/compression/uutool2.4.sit.hqx>

The MIME standard

MIME, an acronym for Multipurpose Internet Mail Extensions, is an alternative and more recent standard for sending binary files by e-mail. MIME can also be used to send US-ASCII files that you do not wish to be altered during the course of the transfer, or files using European character sets for instance. To use MIME your e-mail client has to support the standard, or you can use a special translation program such as 'munpack' (PC and Mac versions):

<URL:ftp://ftp.andrew.cmu.edu/pub/mpack/>

As with uuencoding, MIME works by encoding files within the message body which must be decoded on receipt. Although this is done manually with a program like munpack, it is performed automatically by MIME-compliant mail readers (and other applications that use MIME). MIME allows more than one type of file to be included in the same message. Each part of a MIME message (e.g. graphic, audio clip) is denoted by its 'MIME content type' which is given in a line added to the message header:

MIME-Version: 1.0
Content-Type: text/plain; charset=US-ASCII

The **MIME-Version: 1.0** line indicates a MIME-compliant e-mail client; the above example shows the MIME content type for a plain text file. There are different levels of MIME encoding. If you receive an e-mail message with a MIME content-type line but it contains a number of unreadable characters, it has been partially MIME-encoded. Fully MIME-encoded messages make no sense at all until they are decoded.

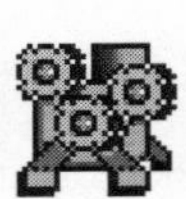

Eight-bit (binary) files can actually be attached to MIME messages without being encoded at all, but only if each system through which the message will pass understands 8-bit data. This is by no means certain on the Internet.

Other content types and further detailed information about MIME is available in *RFC 1521*:

<URL:ftp://src.doc.ic.ac.uk/rfc/rfc1521.txt>

See also Sweet's *comp.mail.mime FAQ* at:

<URL:ftp://rtfm.mit.edu/pub/usenet/news.answers/mail/mime-faq/>

The BinHex standard

BinHex is the Macintosh equivalent of uuencode. Both programs encode binary files into ASCII, but BinHex knows about the Mac's unique file structure (p.31) whereas uuencode does not. Consequently most Mac files on FTP sites are encoded with BinHex (ending with the suffix **.hqx**), although it is possible to uuencode them (see above). Aladdin Systems' shareware Stuffit Expander and DropStuff with Expander Enhancer will create and decode BinHexed files (as well as decode uuencoded files):

<URL:ftp://ftp.aladdinsys.com/pub/>

Encoding/decoding files manually

Fortunately, many recent e-mail clients make encoding and decoding virtually transparent to the user. However, if you do not have a client that will automatically handle this process, it is still possible to do everything manually. The steps involved in transferring binary files by e-mail manually can involve *encoding*, *splicing*, *decoding*, and *decompression*. If you are retrieving a file from an FTP archive, you must also know about FTP mail servers (discussed below).

Encoding

If you wish to receive a file by e-mail from an FTP site, you need to know about uuencoding, whether you use a PC or a Mac. Examples of programs that will uuencode binary files were given above.

If you were to open a uuencoded file in your word processor, you would see a nonsense arrangement of characters that you should recognize from the computer's keyboard. The following (truncated) example shows a file called **MEDBOOKS.ZIP** that has been uuencoded:

```
BEGIN-------cut here-------CUT HERE-------PART 01
begin 644 MEDBOOKS.ZIP
M4$L#!!0````(`#-@CQX0U#/=0J4``/G6`0`,````54Y1D9)0TDN5%A4U?WK
MM8DC6*/@'>`:VNDY:J28IW4:X:_>EJ6YF2K!+E=%7_Z0V2((44";`!4#)S
MC[W?^+S#B1FQKB`IRU7Y?6.<&MUI6R*!=8D5*RXS9ISFX\?D.:ZGT2
M?E2(`0#/%!K^0)DJQA%M_+/K;Y[@[L!?DQE]*9[\9Q#\^[__.[:#>=)D>
`

end
END-------cut here-------CUT HERE-------PART 01
```

If you see lots of very strange-looking non-ASCII characters and symbols mixed in (such as ∫z√îìΠ 5¢´Õ! ¥), you are not looking at an encoded file but have managed to look inside a binary file instead.

Splicing

Many e-mail gateways (and FTP mail servers) break up long encoded files into segments which are received as a series of messages. Some clever e-mail and news-reader programs can automatically splice these parts back together again, but the chances are that you will have to do it manually at some point. Luckily, this isn't hard. Begin by saving each message as a separate text file. Using a word processor, cut the message header from each file. Also remove the **cut here** marks if these are present (as in the above example). The first line in the first message should read **begin 644** (or similar), and the last line in the last message should read **end** when you have finished editing. Next, create a new file in your word processor and paste each message into it in the correct order (i.e. **PART 01** before **PART 02**, etc.) to make one solid block of characters. Finally, save this file as a text file ready for decoding.

Decoding

Once you have reassembled the file you need a program that will decode this ASCII information back into a binary file. Try one of the programs named on p.159. Some e-mail clients and news readers can be configured to decode ASCII encoded messages 'on-the-fly' without further intervention on your part (perhaps using a 'helper' application).

Decompression

Having successfully decoded a file, you should be left with a familiar file format—perhaps a Stuffit or PKZIP archive. If the file needs to be expanded, running one of the programs listed in Table 6 (p.46) should provide you with a file or program which you can use.

FTP mail servers

An FTP mail server is a mail server program that specializes in sending out files in response to the user's requests (as opposed to managing a mailing list, for example), such as 'ftpmail'.

You can ask the ftpmail server to convert binary files into ASCII before sending them. The default encoding is uuencode, but you could use MIME encoding if you prefer. Encoding typically makes the file about 20 per cent larger than its original size.

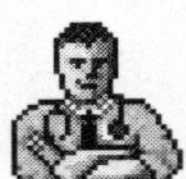

When using FTP by e-mail, make sure you have instructed the FTP mail server to encode the file if it is anything other than plain text. If you don't, you won't be able to use the file.

You can use **ftpmail@doc.ic.ac.uk** for FTP by e-mail (or a closer site if you are not a UK reader e.g. **ftpmail@ftp.uni-stuttgart.de**; **ftpmail@ftp.luth.se**; or **ftpmail@ftp.dartmouth.edu**). The best way to learn about ftpmail is to work through an example (see below). You can get a full list of instructions by sending **help** in the subject line of an e-mail message to one of the ftpmail servers above.

Example

The following commands in the body of a message to an ftpmail server instruct the server to log on to the FTP site **orion.oac.uci.edu**, change to the directory **med-ed/mac/basic-science**, and get the file **anatomiser.demo.sea** after uuencoding it:

```
open orion.oac.uci.edu
chdir med-ed/mac/basic-science
uuencode
get anatomiser.demo.sea
quit
```

Other ways to use e-mail

Although e-mail is used primarily to send and receive private messages, it can be utilized for other purposes. To begin with, e-mail doesn't have to be addressed to a *person*; it can also be addressed to a *mail server,* as is the case with some of the URLs above. Whereas people can usually figure out what it is you are asking of them in an e-mail request, mail servers require *exact* instructions. Using these instructions you can perform tasks such as subscribing to a mailing list (Chapter Nineteen), retrieving files from FTP archives (as above), searching Archie databases (Chapter Twenty three), or browsing Gopher menus (Chapter Twenty four) and WWW pages (Chapter Twenty six). This is however much slower than using a dedicated client over a TCP/IP connection.

In all cases, the body of the message (or sometimes the subject line) contains particular commands understood by the relevant mail server. For example, sending **help** in the body of a message to **cancernet@icicb.nci.nih.gov** will return the contents list to you by e-mail; sending **cn-100013** (obtained from the contents list) will return a file about breast cancer.

CHAPTER NINETEEN
Mailing lists

What is a mailing list?

Sometimes it is more convenient to have messages relating to a particular subject delivered to your electronic mailbox, as opposed to looking in on a newsgroup occasionally. **Mailing lists** are set up to do just this, and don't require users to have full Internet access (just an e-mail account). As with magazines, interested people subscribe to a mailing list covering a particular topic, but unlike magazines, articles on most mailing lists are sent out to all subscribers as they are written. Furthermore, all subscribers are encouraged to contribute articles.

However, some mailing lists do produce digests; they batch a number of articles into a single file and mail it to subscribers at a certain interval. Typically these lists are **moderated**; the **list owner** (p.289) will review each message sent to the list and authorize its distribution to all subscribers. This can improve the quality of the mailings for individual subscribers who do not wish to read erroneous messages sent to the list, or those that wander off the topic. Someone in New Zealand, for instance, may not be interested in Dr Jones's recollection of a party at a Yorkshire junior doctor's mess when the mailing list is an academic one discussing advances in palliative care. The screening out of such 'junk mail' does not amount to censorship.

Not all mailing lists are public either. Although most do allow anybody to subscribe via an automated process (see below), others require the prospective subscriber to contact the list owner and request a subscription personally. Rarely this may require proof of professional status, such as a Medical Council registration number.

Subscribing to a mailing list, therefore, essentially means that you have added your name to a list of e-mail addresses which is accessible to a program (or person) operating the list. In many cases mailing lists require little human intervention once they have been established. The programs that manage mailing lists are known collectively as 'mail servers'. Instead of users sending multiple copies of messages to every other subscriber, a single message is sent to a specific computer running a mail server. The mail server either passes the message on to the moderator for approval, or automatically redistributes the message to other subscribers. Some electronic journals use mail servers for their distribution as well, and so can share the same characteristics as ordinary 'discussion-type' mailing lists.

Using mail servers

Subscribing to a mailing list can be tricky. This is because of the different conventions used by the various mail-server programs on the Internet and other networks. In general, however, using a mailing list involves sending e-mail to one of two different addresses.

The first address is used to send commands to the mail server, such as a subscription message or request for a help file. The second address is used to send a message which will be distributed to subscribers of the list (the 'list address', which is unique to each list). Invariably mistakes are made, but sending an incorrect message to the mail server will sometimes result in the return of a file telling you of the idiosyncrasies of that particular system. On the other hand, commands sent to the list such as 'unsubscribe'—which should be sent to the mail server—tend to annoy people. Practical examples illustrating the use of these two addresses are given below.

When you first subscribe to a list, it is common practice for the mail server to send you a synopsis of the commands needed to use the mail server, and an overview of the aims and guidelines pertaining to the particular mailing list.

Some electronic journal-type mailing lists don't involve sending a subscription message to a list server at all. They will place your name on their mailing list after having received your details and payment by traditional post. Examples are *Journal Watch* from the Massachusetts Medical Society at **jwatch@world.std.com**, and *Health on the Internet* from Healthworks at **sales@d-access.demon.co.uk**.

There are several mail server programs available, running on nearly all computer platforms. Many mailing lists are run by a program called LISTSERV, or by UNIX-based mail server programs. In the UK, academic lists often use the Mailbase Service. These options are discussed individually below.

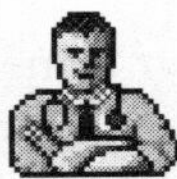

Sending the message **help** to any mail-server address (not to the list itself) is a good place to start in your dealings with mail servers.

BITNET discussion groups and LISTSERV

BITNET is a network that links together many academic sites, primarily in the US. It operates under different protocols to the TCP/IP-based Internet, but gateways between BITNET and the Internet allow the exchange of e-mail. Mailing lists on BITNET are actually called 'discussion groups', but for our purposes 'mailing lists' can be applied to BITNET as well. **LISTSERV** (as in 'list server') is a mail server program that originated on the BITNET network, but has since become more widely distributed.

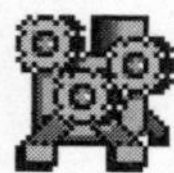

LISTSERV, like many other mail servers, can be used to retrieve mail archives associated with a particular discussion group. Traditionally LISTSERV commands were sent using capital letters since the operating system they were confined to was case-sensitive. In practice this no longer matters.

Many BITNET discussion groups have a two-way gateway to Usenet newsgroups in the **bit.listserv.*** hierarchy. For example, **bit.listserv.mednews** is linked to the BITNET list at **mednews@asuvm.inre.asu.edu**. Sometimes newsgroups outside the **bit.listserv.*** hierarchy are linked to BITNET lists, such as **sci.med.telemedicine** and **hspnet-l%albnydh2@cunyvm.cuny.edu**.

All LISTSERV mailing-list subscription requests are sent to **LISTSERV@domain.name** (substituting the correct domain name). The body of the message to the LISTSERV is usually in the format:

subscribe listname yourname

To send a message to the mailing list subscribers, use the address format:

<URL:mailto:listname@domain.name>

As an example, to subscribe to 'SURGINET', a LISTSERV-based mailing list of interest to general surgeons, I would send the following message:

<URL:mailto:LISTSERV@listserv.utoronto.ca> Send: subscribe SURGINET

To send a message to the list subscribers, I would use the following address:

<URL:mailto:SURGINET@listserv.utoronto.ca>

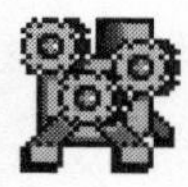

Subscription addresses for LISTSERV lists are sometimes given in BITNET format (e.g. **LISTSERV@ASUACAD**) which is the address that would be used if subscribing from BITNET. Most BITNET machines can be reached from the Internet by adding **.bitnet** to this address, as in **LISTSERV@asuacad.bitnet**. Some of these machines also have a proper Internet address; **LISTSERV@asuvm. inre.asu.edu**, in this case.

Other Internet mail servers

Some UNIX-based mailing lists on the Internet use the following convention for subscription addresses:

<URL:mailto:listname-request@domain.name>

Here, **request** is separated from the name of the list by a hyphen. Sometimes there will be a specific subscription message. Occasionally these lists are managed by people (as opposed to mail servers), in which case a personal message is sent in the body of the message to the list owner. To send a message to the list membership, the following format is used (i.e. the list address):

<URL:mailto:listname@domain.name>

If this doesn't work, or if you happen to know that subscription to a particular list is automated using a mail server program such as Majordomo or ListProcessor, try a LISTSERV-style address:

<URL:mailto:majordomo@domain.name>

<URL:mailto:listproc@domain.name>

To subscribe, use the following in the body of the message as above (substituting **listname** and **yourname** for the name of the list and your name, respectively):

subscribe listname yourname

Mailbase

Mailbase is a UK-based academic mailing list service (see p.288). To join (subscribe to) a list, send a message in the following format:

<URL:mailto:mailbase@mailbase.ac.uk> Send: join listname firstname lastname

To send a message that will be circulated to the list membership, use the format:

<URL:mailto:listname@mailbase.ac.uk>

For example, to join 'GP-UK', a list covering any subject concerning UK General Practice (see Chapter Thirty two) I would send:

<URL:mailto:mailbase@mailbase.ac.uk> Send: join gp-uk Bruce McKenzie

The list address of GP-UK is:

<URL:mailto:gp-uk@mailbase.ac.uk>

Finding medical mailing lists

There are a number of places to look for medical and health-related mailing lists, including frequently asked questions files in Usenet newsgroups, 'lists of lists' on FTP sites, various pointers on WWW pages, and on the mail servers themselves.

To obtain a list of all health and medicine-related mailing lists on BITNET use the following URL (with two lines in the body of the message):

<URL:mailto:LISTSERV@bitnic.cren.net>
Send: list global /medical; list global /health

To retrieve the large multi-part listing of Internet-based mailing lists, use the following URL:

<URL:ftp://rtfm.mit.edu/pub/usenet/news.answers/mail/mailing-lists/>

The subscription procedure for Internet-based lists often varies, so it is best to follow the instructions given in a pointer such as the above document.

'Medical' is one of the special subject groups on Mailbase. To retrieve a list on medical topics available through Mailbase, use this URL:

<URL:mailto:mailbase@mailbase.ac.uk> Send: find lists medical

Alternatively, if you have full Internet access, try the Mailbase WWW server:

<URL:http://www.mailbase.ac.uk/other/medi-class.html>

A quick way to locate medical mailing lists is to try a search on 'health' or 'medicine' (for example) at Scott Southwick's Liszt:

<URL:http://www.liszt.com/>

As mentioned in Chapter Seventeen, the American Medical Informatics Association Internet Working Group supports a list called 'MMatrix-L'. An established list, MMatrix-L discusses the wider issues in medical use of the Internet, in addition to keeping subscribers informed about new medical resources. To subscribe, use this URL:

<URL:mailto:listserv@maelstrom.stjohns.edu> Send: subscribe mmatrix-l Firstname Lastname

The list owners (i.e. people, as opposed to an automated mail server) can be contacted by addressing a message to:

<URL:mailto:mmatrix-l-request@maelstrom.stjohns.edu>

A daily message digest is also available (send **set mmatrix-l digest** to the above address). To send a message to the list subscribers, use:

<URL:mailto:mmatrix-l@maelstrom.stjohns.edu>

CHAPTER TWENTY
Newsgroups

Several large computer networks exchange public electronic messages on a regular basis. These messages are grouped into particular topics, with each grouping known as a newsgroup. In many respects newsgroups are like discussion areas on a bulletin board, although there are hundreds more topics to choose from. People ask questions, others reply. Some newsgroups encourage serious comment, others do not. Some contain files, others do not. Some are 'free-for-all', while discussion on others is guided by a newsgroup moderator. Generally, the term *news*group is something of a misnomer; most groups do not bear 'news' in the usual sense of the word.

Although Usenet newsgroups are the most widely available (see below), other networks operate Internet newsgroups that are entirely separate from Usenet (such as Bionet). As they all use the same protocol (**Network News Transport Protocol**, or **NNTP**) these newsgroups are collectively known as network news.

As new messages (sometimes called articles) are created at one news site, they are passed on to other news sites (if these sites choose to carry that particular newsgroup). In this way, posting a message in England to an international newsgroup like **sci.med** (see below) will see it propagated all around the world by a chain of Usenet sites, each of which in turn provides a 'news feed' to others (such as dial-up users).

What is Usenet?

Usenet, the User's Network, originated as a network of UNIX computers exchanging messages using the UNIX-to-UNIX CoPy (UUCP) program. A number of systems continue to use UUCP to exchange Usenet news, although another protocol (NNTP) is used by machines on the Internet to exchange news over TCP/IP links. Usenet is therefore not strictly an Internet service, but rather a service operating over many types of networks—the TCP/IP-based Internet being one of these. Most JANET sites have access to Usenet news.

A lot has been written about the nature of Usenet and its culture. Starting points for further information include:

What is Usenet? at:

<URL:ftp://rtfm.mit.edu/pub/usenet/news.answers/usenet/what-is/part1>

What is Usenet? A second opinion at:

<URL:ftp://rtfm.mit.edu/pub/usenet/news.answers/usenet/what-is/part2>

Frequently asked questions about Usenet at:

<URL:ftp://rtfm.mit.edu/pub/usenet/news.answers/usenet/faq/part1>

Welcome to news.newusers.questions! at:

<URL:ftp://rtfm.mit.edu/pub/usenet/news.answers/news-newusers-intro>

How to find the right place to post (FAQ) at:

<URL:ftp://rtfm.mit.edu/pub/usenet/news.answers/finding-groups/general>

There are several newsgroups of particular interest to new users, such as **news.announce.newusers** (general new-user information), **news.answers** (FAQs; see below), and **news.newusers.questions** (for new-user questions).

How is Usenet organized?

Usenet newsgroups are organized in a hierarchical fashion, with the name of each group constructed in a way that reveals this hierarchy. The eight broad categories of Usenet newsgroups follow ('*' is a wild card indicating various subgroups):

alt.*	'Alternative', including support newsgroups
comp.*	Computer-related discussions
misc.*	Miscellaneous topics
news.*	Usenet and newsgroup administration
rec.*	Recreation
sci.*	Sciences (including the medical sciences)
soc.*	Issues of social and cultural concern and interest
talk.*	Controversy and debate

Each 'top-level' heading has a number of subtopics. For example, under **sci** comes **sci.med**, and under that several more specific topics such as **sci.med.aids** or **sci.med.radiology.**

The 'alternative' hierarchies tend to be less widely distributed than the remaining 'core' groups. You can obtain a listing of active newsgroups in the core hierarchy, and those in the alternative hierarchy, by FTP using the following URLs:

<URL:ftp://rtfm.mit.edu/pub/usenet/news.answers/active-newsgroups/>

<URL:ftp://rtfm.mit.edu/pub/usenet/news.answers/alt-hierarchies/>

Alternatively, you can use the MIT mail server:

<URL:mailto:mail-server@rtfm.mit.edu> Send: help

Using a news reader

To read the news you require a news feed (i.e. a source of newsgroup articles). This could be a UUCP feed, particularly if you are calling a small bulletin board, although dial-up users typically need to know the domain name of their service provider's NNTP news server.

This information allows NNTP **news readers** on your machine to connect to the news server and download a list of current articles in the newsgroups to which you have 'subscribed'. Rather than download all the articles, the user only needs to click on the subject line of the particular articles that look interesting (Fig. 18). For the most part, news readers behave like e-mail clients, allowing you to create new messages, post replies, save articles to disk, etc. Good news readers will make it easy to follow **threads** (i.e. read the next or previous message relating to a particular topic, rather than follow a chronological sequence of unrelated postings).

Sophisticated news readers simplify the process of downloading (and uploading) binary files in certain Usenet newsgroups. These files, like e-mail messages, must be specially encoded in order to pass through the Internet as an electronic message (see Chapter Eighteen). Offline news readers are also available that retrieve all the articles in a pre-specified newsgroup for reading offline, with the intention of reducing your telephone bill. The main disadvantage of these programs is that you cannot be selective about which articles to retrieve. Popular news readers include:

Free Agent (for the PC):

<URL:ftp://ftp.forteinc.com/pub/forte/free_agent/>

Newswatcher (for the Mac):

<URL:ftp://ftp.acns.nwu.edu/pub/newswatcher/>

Medical Usenet news

There is a wide variety of health-related and medical newsgroups. For a complete listing, extract relevant groups from the full lists using the URLs above.

The sci.med.* hierarchy is the most relevant to the readership of this book. The newsgroup sci.med is a very busy group dealing with general medical topics, with questions and answers about the quality of doctors, new therapies, requests for information and diagnoses, etc. These conferences are open to the public, but health professional contributions are

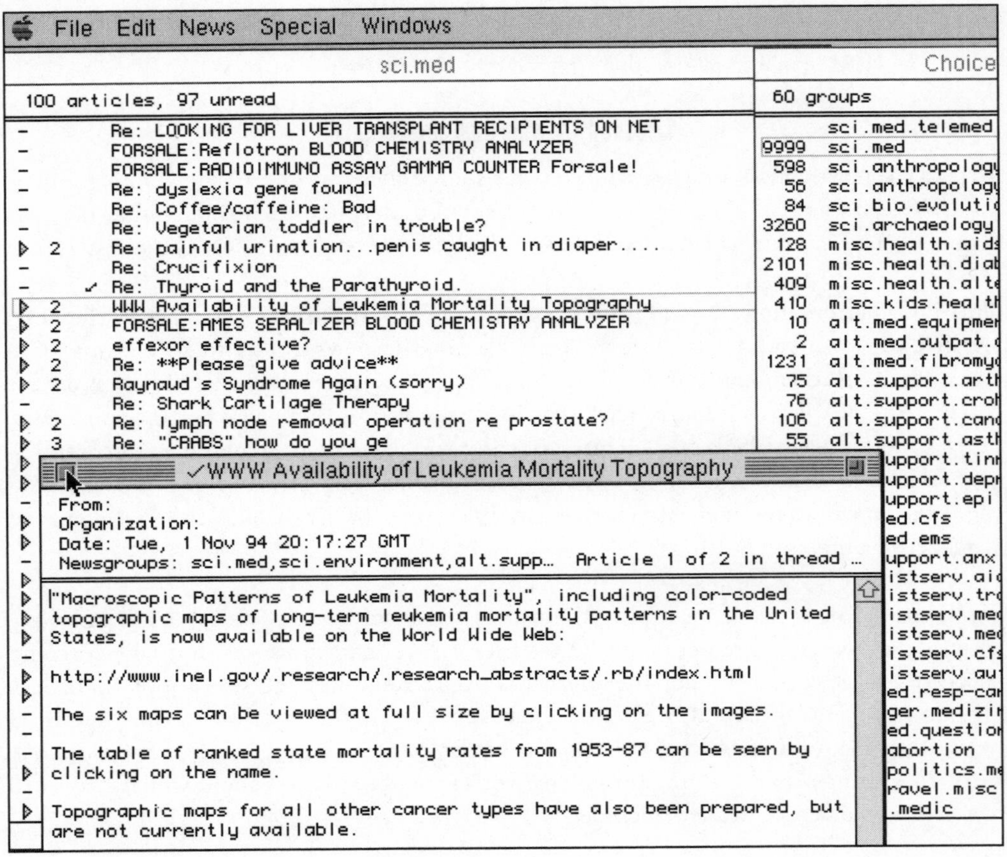

Fig. 18 Using a news reader. Rather than download all the articles in a given newsgroup, some news readers initially retrieve a list of current articles. Clicking on an interesting article in the list causes that article to be retrieved from the news server.

strongly encouraged. Several periodic postings to the **sci.med.*** hierarchy worthy of note include the *Journal Watch* sampler from the Massachusetts Medical Society (picking out the key articles from a range of journals, summarizing them, and pointing out their deficiencies), Dodell's *Health Info-Com Network Medical News Digest*, and the *AIDS Daily Summary* and *Morbidity and Mortality Weekly Report* from the Center for Disease Control. There are also a number of useful FAQs (see below).

The sub-topics available within **sci.med.*** include **sci.med.aids** (HIV and AIDS), **sci.med.diseases.*** (with several lower-level topics such as cancer), and a number of others with self-explanatory names: **sci.med.immunology**, **sci.med.nursing**, **sci.med.informatics**, **sci.med.orthopedics**, **sci.med.pathology**, **sci.med.pharmacy**, **sci.med.radiology**,

sci.med.telemedicine, and **sci.med.vision**, etc.

Aside from **misc.education.medical**, there are several **misc.health.*** newsgroups covering topics such as AIDS, alternative therapies, and diabetes in the **misc.*** hierarchy.

In the **talk.*** hierarchy, **talk.politics.medicine** provides a forum to air views on American medical politics.

The **alt.*** hierarchy includes **alt.image.medical** (medical image formats), **alt.med.*** (e.g. allergy, emergency medical services, fibromyalgia), **alt.health.*** (e.g. haemochromatosis, oxygen therapy), and several **alt.support.*** groups (e.g. support for those people experiencing abortion, anxiety, asthma, cancer, depression, etc.).

Other medical newsgroups

A number of hierarchies that are not part of Usenet also contain newsgroups with a medical or biomedical focus.

The **bit.listserv.*** hierarchy contains several gatewayed BITNET discussion groups (p.166) such as **MEDNEWS**, while the **bionet.*** hierarchy contains **bionet.biology.cardiovascular**, **bionet.diagnostics.prenatal**, **bionet.microbiology**, **bionet.neuroscience**, and many others.

ClariNews is an electronic newspaper implemented in network news format (the **clari.*** groups), with stories written by a paid reporter. Consequently there is a charge to receive the service, including the health newsgroups. If your Internet service provider subscribes to ClariNews, you will have free access. For further information, send e-mail to **info@clarinet.com**.

There are also more localized groups such as **can.med.misc** (Canadian medical discussion), **de.sci.medizin** (German medical discussion), **fj.sci.medical** (Japanese medical discussion), **francom.medical** (French medical discussion), and **no.medisin** (Norwegian medical discussion).

Health-related FAQs and periodicals

Frequently asked questions files (FAQs) were originally lists of commonly asked questions appearing in various newsgroups, together with their answers. Of late almost any periodically posted informational file is dubbed an FAQ, whether it was written as a response to real questions or not. Indeed, many of the FAQs found in the support newsgroups in particular represent an accumulation of a given person's (or newsgroup readership's) knowledge of a particular subject.

FAQs serve several purposes. New users are encouraged to read a newsgroup's FAQ(s) before posting a question. In this way others do not have to read and reply to the same questions, but the discussion in the group can move on to cover new ground. Further, they often contain pointers to other documents available on the Internet, and so help new users find their way about.

There is a growing collection of FAQs on medical subjects. The majority of these are written with an intended audience of health-care consumers rather than health-care providers. While all FAQs can be found by reading Usenet newsgroups on the off chance that an update has been posted, this is not always a convenient tactic. A special newsgroup called **news.answers** serves to collect many of the FAQs into one place. Because this newsgroup is moderated, submission of an FAQ to it requires approval by the *.answers moderation team (see p.253). One benefit of the approval process is that the approved FAQs are then made available on an FTP site (**rtfm.mit.edu**, and various other 'mirrors') from where they can be retrieved at any time. FAQs that have not been approved are sometimes stored by the author on alternative FTP sites (or, increasingly, on WWW sites). A list of approved periodic postings on Usenet is archived at:

<URL:ftp://rtfm.mit.edu/pub/usenet/news.answers/periodic-postings/>

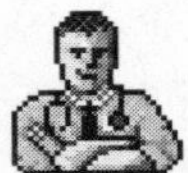

Whenever you see 'Archive-name' in a periodic posting, you will be able to locate an archived copy by using the URL:

<URL:ftp://rtfm.mit.edu/pub/usenet/news.answers/archive-name>

where **archive-name** is the name of the archived document.

For more general information about FAQs, see *FAQs about FAQs* by Hersch at:

<URL:ftp://rtfm.mit.edu/pub/usenet/news.answers/faqs/about-faqs>

Other ways to read the news

By e-mail

There are several ways to read Usenet articles by e-mail, but it is debatable whether they are worth the effort. These are mentioned in Rankin's *Accessing the Internet by e-mail FAQ* (p.149). It is a lot easier to create a new Usenet message by e-mail. To do this from your e-mail client, compose a message as usual and address it to **newsgroup@news.server**, where **newsgroup** is the name of the Usenet group and **news.server** is the domain name of your service provider's news server.

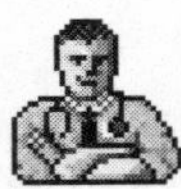

If you ask for a copy of any replies to be sent to your e-mail address, you can post a question to the appropriate audience even if you choose not to (or cannot) read that particular newsgroup.

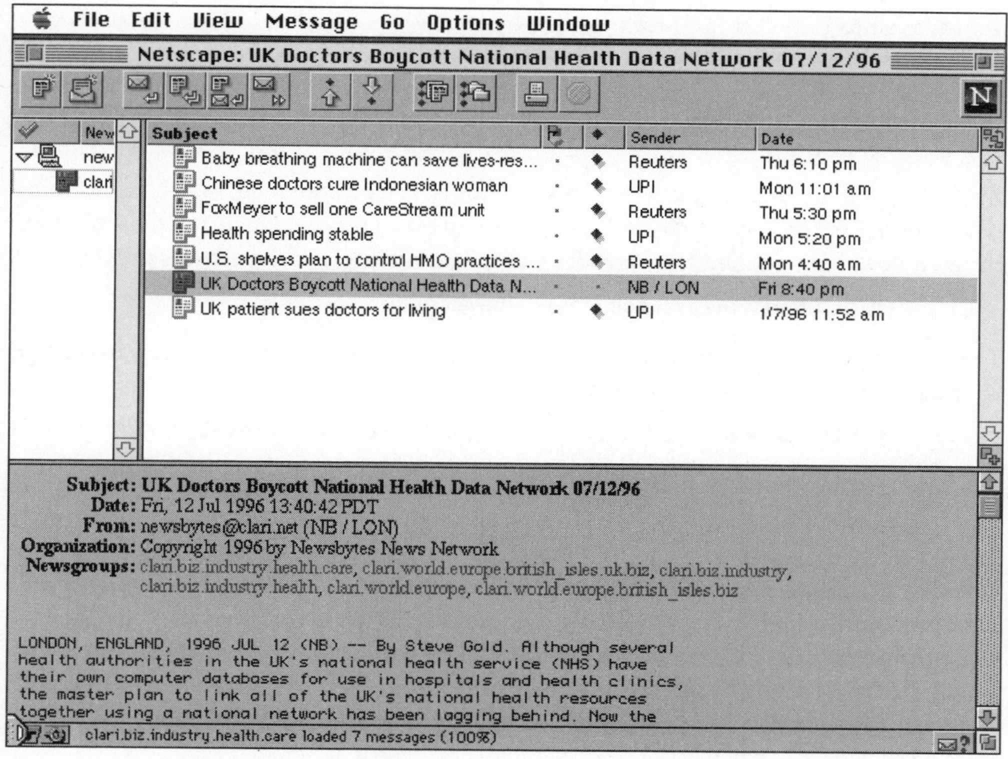

Fig. 19 Using a WWW browser to read the news. Clicking on a newsgroup URL in Navigator will open a connection to your news server and display a list of messages in that group.

By Gopher

The University of Birmingham in the UK operates a Gopher–Usenet interface using Gopher menus to categorize newsgroups and collate threaded articles. The service is read-only, so users cannot post replies or create new articles.

<URL:gopher://news.bham.ac.uk:70/11/Usenet>

Via the WWW

Atkinson's Usenet Info Centre allows you to search for a particular newsgroup from a WWW page. For example, searching for **sci.med.*** returns a listing of the **sci.med.*** hierarchy of newsgroups. Clicking on one of these headings will return a brief description of what the newsgroup is about, whether it is moderated or not, what FAQs and mailing lists are associated with it, and readership statistics. Clicking on the newsgroup name will let you read the current news articles. You access the Usenet Info Centre search page at:

<URL:http://sunsite.unc.edu/usenet-i/search.html>

To read/post to Usenet from these pages, or by typing in a newsgroup URL manually (e.g. **news:sci.med.telemedicine**), your WWW browser must be appropriately configured. Be sure to specify the name of your mail server and news server in the Options/Preferences panel (as supplied by your service provider).

Another quick way to locate relevant newsgroups is to try a search on 'health or medicine' (for example) at Scott Southwick's 'Liszt'. Clicking on a group in Navigator (if configured correctly) will open a connection to your news server and display a list of messages (Fig. 19):

<URL:http://www.liszt.com/cgi-bin/news.cgi>

The University of Ohio and the Libraries Automation Service WWW Server (Oxford University) both maintain a searchable hypertext index to FAQs:

<URL:http://www.cis.ohio-state.edu/hypertext/faq/usenet/FAQ-List.html>

<URL:http://www.lib.ox.ac.uk/internet/news/faq/by_category.index.html>

Via a filtering service

Unless your clinical practice is extremely dull, it is perhaps unlikely that you will be able to peruse newsgroups leisurely looking for infrequent articles of interest. The European Bioinformatics Institute runs a Netnews Filtering Service. A computer will peruse on your behalf, finding articles of interest from biomedical newsgroups, including the **sci.med.*** hierarchy. Users instruct the computer as to which words it should look out for and are notified periodically when articles containing these words are found.

<URL:mailto:netnews@ebi.ac.uk> Send: help

<URL:http://www.ebi.ac.uk:80/sift/>

CHAPTER TWENTY ONE

File Transfer Protocol

Anonymous FTP

File Transfer Protocol (FTP) is the tool for transferring files between computers on the Internet. It doesn't matter what types of computer are involved in handling the file, as long as they all understand TCP/IP protocols. You can use FTP to download files from a remote computer directly to your own machine (if you have a TCP/IP Internet connection). There is an enormous amount of informational files, graphics, and software available that can be obtained in this way.

Anonymous users—anyone without special privileges—can access files on many FTP sites by using 'anonymous' as a user name and their e-mail address as the password. This is called '**anonymous FTP**'. To make things easier for anonymous users, most sites have a top-level directory called **pub** or **public**, containing that site's public or non-confidential files. Anonymous FTP typically gives access to the files in this directory only, and you will be denied permission to open any other directories that you might see. Some FTP sites, however, contain various directories that are all 'public', even if not so named.

For more information about FTP, see Rovers' *Anonymous FTP FAQ list* at:

<URL:ftp://rtfm.mit.edu/pub/usenet/news.answers/ftp-list/faq>

Using an FTP client

Follow the setup instructions that come with your client software, making sure to have specified your e-mail address in the Preferences menu (failing to do so can cause problems retrieving files). A connection to an FTP site can be established by typing in the domain name of the site, or (in some clients) selecting a site from a pre-configured menu.

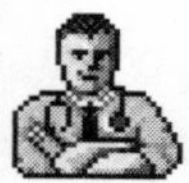

Often a **README** file will be in a prominent location once you have connected; you are supposed to read this if you have not used the site before.

An FTP client lets you browse the various public file directories at an FTP site, and download interesting files by clicking on them or marking them in some way (in a graphical client interface). Some clients display both a local and a remote file directory, with the option of copying a file from one to the other. Thus, using an FTP server is just like reading a floppy disk or another hard drive under Windows.

As on bulletin boards and online services, virtually all files on FTP sites are compressed to save space, which renders them unusable until they have been decompressed. You can use the same programs that you would use on a bulletin board to decompress or expand files downloaded from the Internet. Refer back to Table 6 (p.46) to match the file suffix to the expander program you need. Not listed in Table 6 is the suffix **.hqx**. This indicates a BinHexed file—not a compression format, but rather a form of 'ASCII encoding' commonly applied to Macintosh files stored on the Internet (see p.160).

A few sites allow you to upload your own files to an **incoming** directory where, after approval, they can be made public. The speed at which you can upload and download files depends on several factors, such as the speed of your modem and how many other people have logged on to the same site. If a site is too busy to accept another user the client will let you know.

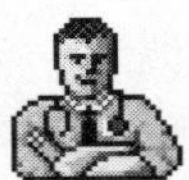

Try and work out when an FTP site is least busy, since your sessions will be a lot faster (and your chances of connecting to the server increase in the first place).

FTP clients work in one of two '**modes**' when downloading or uploading files; ASCII (text) or binary (see Fig. 20). Text files should be transferred in 'ASCII mode', and binary files in 'binary mode'. The important difference between ASCII and binary files was explained on p.30. If you use FTP to retrieve a binary file in ASCII mode it will be unusable. Transferring a text file in binary mode is not so fatal, although the file may contain some odd-looking symbols since differences in the way various operating systems handle text won't be corrected for. If you are uncertain as to the type of file, choose to download it in binary mode, although good clients can automatically determine the appropriate mode.

One of the disadvantages of FTP (compared to Zmodem, for instance—p.31) is that if there is a problem halfway through a file transfer (e.g. due to a dropped connection or software error), you will have to begin the transfer again. FTP does not allow you to resume a partially completed file transfer.

Examples of FTP clients are:

WS-FTP (for the PC):

<URL:ftp://ftp.csra.net/pub/win3/ws_ftp.zip>

Fetch (for the Mac):

<URL:ftp://ftp.dartmouth.edu/pub/mac/>

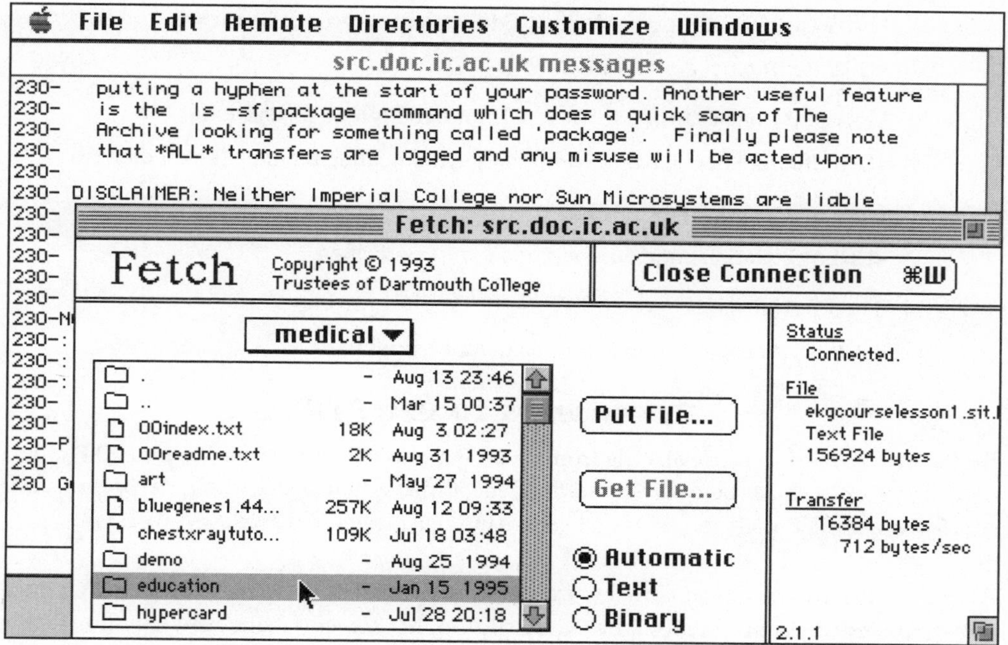

Fig. 20 Using an FTP client. This popular Macintosh client uses pull-down menus and buttons to 'get' files after selecting them with a pointer.

Mirror sites

A **mirror** site is a copy/mirror image of an original site located somewhere else. For example, the **news.answers** FAQ archives are available from several European mirrors of the original American site. Using a local site in preference to a foreign one reduces congestion on transatlantic Internet links. FTP sessions using a local site are nearly always faster than sessions on a distant one.

Medical software archives

There are several repositories for medical programs on the Internet. They include the following:

Gasnet software archive, Yale University:

<URL:ftp://gasnet.med.yale.edu/pub/anes/software/>

University of California Medical Education Software Repository:

<URL:ftp://ftp.uci.edu/med-ed/>

University of Michigan mirror at Imperial College in London:

<URL:ftp://src.doc.ic.ac.uk/computing/systems/mac/umich/misc/medical/>

University of North Carolina:

<URL:ftp://sunsite.unc.edu/pub/academic/medicine>

The Physiological Society FTP repository, Cambridge:

<URL:ftp://physiology.cup.cam.ac.uk/pub/apps/>

Other ways to use FTP

E-mail can be used to retrieve a file from an FTP archive if you do not have an FTP client (or other alternative, as below). The steps of encoding, splicing, decoding, decompression, and the use of FTP mail servers was discussed under *Binary files by e-mail*, p.158.

Archie clients with FTP capabilities are mentioned in Chapter Twenty three. A Gopher only provides access to the files indexed by the Gopher server (Chapter Twenty four). You cannot just launch a Gopher client and hope to connect to any FTP site. Instead, if a Gopher menu happens to lead to a certain file, you will be able to FTP that file using the Gopher client. The same is true of any files that appear in the result window of a search undertaken with a WAIS client (Chapter Twenty five).

WWW browsers, on the other hand, incorporate much more of the functionality of a dedicated FTP client (Chapter Twenty six). You can connect to any anonymous FTP site simply by typing the URL of that site into your browser. 'FTP Search' is a utility with a WWW interface for finding files on FTP sites. It offers a variety of sophisticated search options:

<URL:http://ftpsearch.unit.no/ftpsearch>

CHAPTER TWENTY TWO
Telnet

What is Telnet?

Telnet is a TCP/IP communications protocol that permits interactive access to and control of remote computers on the Internet from your own computer. You can make use of Telnet either by running a Telnet client on your own computer (if you have a TCP/IP link to the Internet), or by using an ordinary terminal emulator to access a Telnet client on someone else's computer. This makes the public resources on the remote machine accessible to you as though your own computer were directly connected to it from a nearby location.

Telnet commonly provides access to library catalogues, university information systems, and other menu-based resources. It also provides access to other programs and Internet services that might not be available on your own computer. For instance, you can use a Telnet interface to navigate Gopher menus and browse WWW pages.

Computers on the Internet that allow users access via Telnet may require you to know a login (log-on) name and password. Sometimes just a login name is necessary, and on other occasions neither are required. You will recall from Chapter Twelve that this information precedes the domain name in Telnet URLs (p.103).

Using a Telnet client

A Telnet client provides a terminal interface to the remote machine (usually emulating a VT100 terminal type—Table 4, p.28). Entering the appropriate URL into the client will open a connection to the remote host and present the user with the login prompt (if there is one). Often it is a good idea to create a capture log at this point (a text file that stores everything you see appearing in the terminal window). This log can then be opened in a word processor when you have closed the connection.

Navigation between different screens of information is normally fairly intuitive, using a minimum of keys (such as the arrow keys to scroll up or down, '**q**' to quit, '**n**' for next page, '**?**' for help, etc.). Systems may vary slightly depending on the program that you are interacting with. Some clients have the ability to retrieve files by FTP. Popular clients are:

CommNet for Windows PCs:
<URL:ftp://ftp.radient.com/>

NCSA Telnet for the Mac:
<URL:ftp://ftp.ncsa.uiuc.edu/Mac/Telnet/>

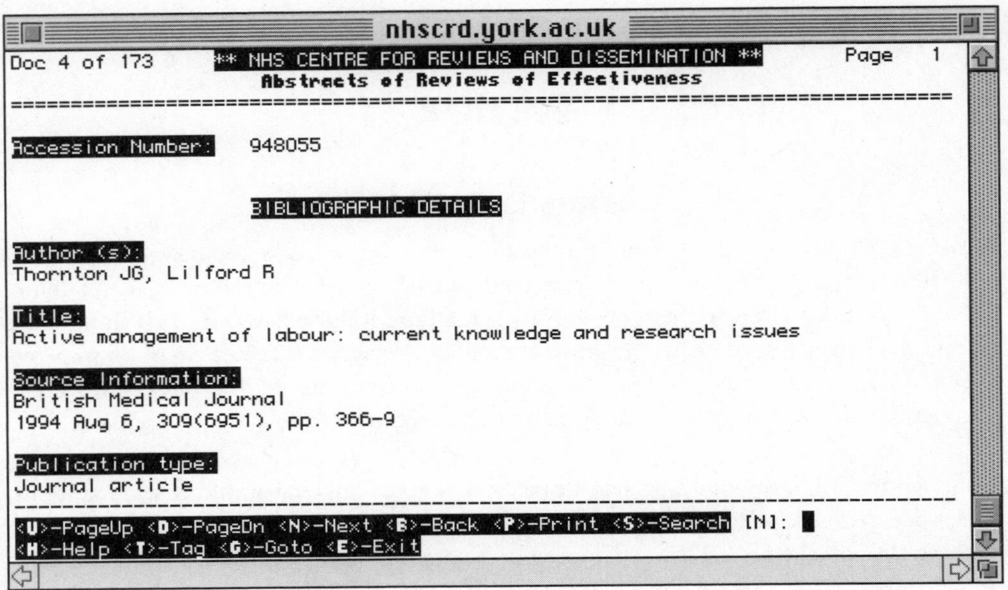

Fig. 21 Using a Telnet client. Telnet provides a simple terminal interface to programs running on other computers. Telnet can provide interactive access to other Internet services without the need for dedicated clients on your own machine. [Reproduced with permission.]

Medical Telnet sites

The following examples allow you to try out the Telnet interface. Perhaps the most common application of Telnet is access to library catalogues. The Library Catalogue Server of St. Bartholomew's and the Royal London School of Medicine and Dentistry additionally allows users to browse undergraduate reading lists:

<URL:telnet://library@lib.barts.qmw.ac.uk>

The NHS Centre for Reviews and Dissemination at the University of York permits the searching of a Database of Abstracts of Reviews of Effectiveness and the NHS Economic Evaluation Database (see Fig. 21):

<URL:telnet://crduser:crduser@nhscrd.york.ac.uk>

Health Services/Technology Assessment Text (HSTAT) from the US National Library of Medicine provides full-text access to AHCPR (Agency for Health Care Policy and Research) clinical-practice guidelines and other information:

<URL:telnet://hstat@text.nlm.nih.gov>

You can find further Telnet sites by telnetting to a program called 'Hytelnet'. This program organizes Telnet sites using menus and provides the URL, login, password, and a site description—as well as letting you connect directly to a site you have selected. Hytelnet is available from a number of sites, including Oxford University:

<URL:telnet://hytelnet@rsl.ox.ac.uk>

Other ways to use Telnet

Because Telnet is an interactive service you cannot access it by e-mail. As mentioned earlier, a Telnet site may, however, provide interactive access to Gopher menus and a text-only WWW client ('Lynx'). For example, you can login at the Oxford University site above using '**gopher**' or '**lynx**' in place of '**hytelnet**'.

CHAPTER TWENTY THREE

Archie

What is Archie?

Archie is a program used to locate files stored on anonymous FTP sites around the world. Archie servers periodically index the contents of FTP sites (Chapter Twenty one) that they know about, which means that some Archie servers index different sites to others. These file indexes are then available to the Archie server when it receives a search request.

Archie requires you to know the name (or a part of the name) of the file you are looking for, but not where it might be found. Archie can then search its database of FTP site directories to find a match for your query. You can access Archie in several ways.

Using an Archie client

Your Archie client may come with a list of Archie servers. Generally, start by connecting to the one which is closest to you. Example servers include **archie.doc.ic.ac.uk** (UK), **archie.rutgers.edu** (US), and **archie.au** (Australia). If a search of one Archie server doesn't turn up what you are looking for, try another server.

Assuming you are using a client on a Windows PC or the Mac, it will be a simple matter to enter the name of the file you wish to look for in the appropriate dialogue window (see Fig. 22). If you know only part of the name, substitute a wild card character (i.e. '*') for the missing part, and this will find all files matching the part that you do know.

The Archie server will return to you the full name of the file on the FTP site, the name of the site, and the path (directory) pointing to the file. With this information you can then obtain the file by FTP. Alternatively, if you are using a client like Anarchie (a combined Archie and FTP client), you will be able to retrieve the file simply by clicking on it in the search result window.

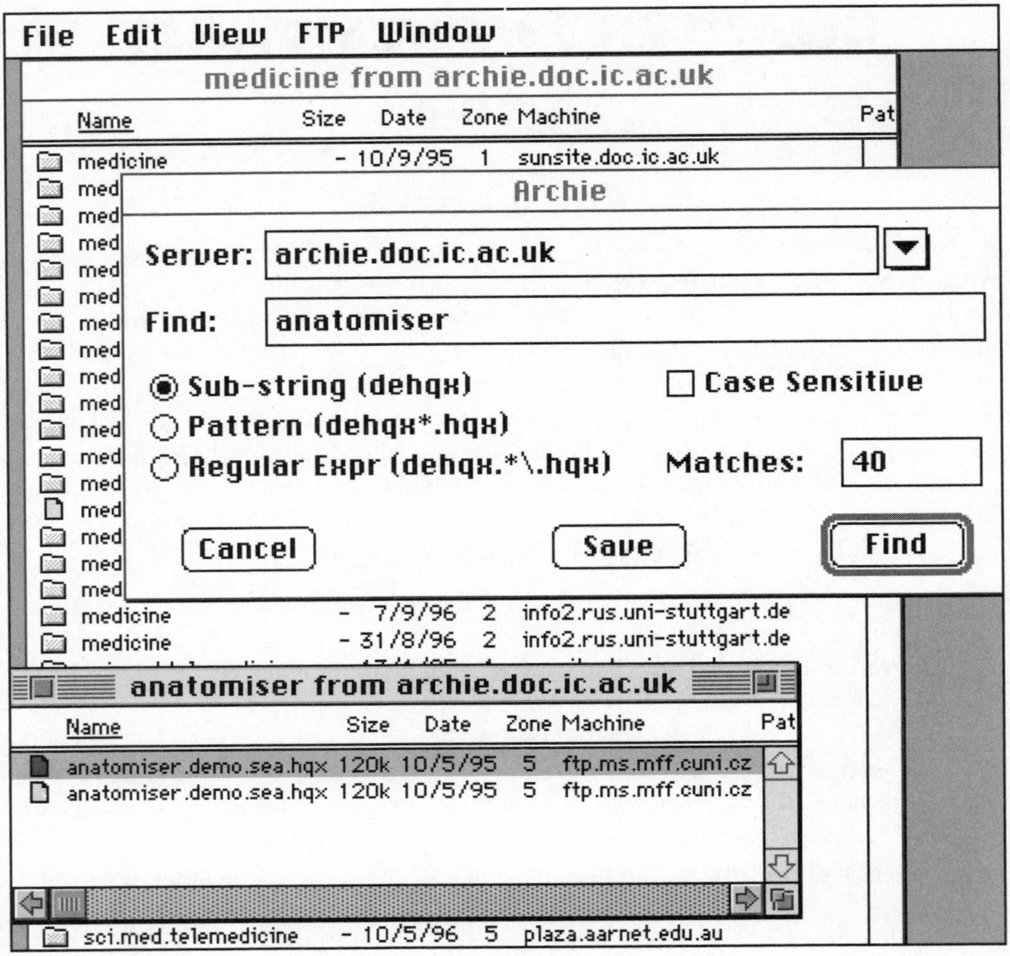

Fig. 22 Using an Archie client. Anarchie for the Macintosh allows the user to search a database of files available from FTP sites. Clicking on a particular file in the result window will retrieve it by FTP.

Archie client software is sometimes available by FTP from sites running Archie servers. The following are examples of popular shareware clients:

WS-Archie (for the PC):

<URL:ftp://ftp.coast.net/SimTel/win3/winsock/>

Anarchie (for the Mac):

<URL:ftp://ftp.share.com/pub/peterlewis/>

Using an Archie mail server

Those who do not have a TCP/IP connection to the Internet, but do have an e-mail account, can still use Archie to find files. A full list of commands that can be included in an e-mail message is available by sending the message **help** to an Archie server. Note that all Archie servers are addressed as 'archie':

<URL:mailto:archie@archie.doc.ic.ac.uk> Send: help

As a simple example, if a student wanted to find a program called 'anatomiser', they could send the following message (remembering to put each command on a separate line in the body of the message):

<URL:mailto:archie@archie.doc.ic.ac.uk> Send: find anatomiser; quit

The '**find**' part asks Archie at Imperial College in London to scan its database for any mention of the string 'anatomiser'. The '**quit**' command tells the server to ignore anything else in the message such as a signature. Archie might return the following (edited) message:

```
>> find anatomiser
# Search type: sub.

Host ftp.ms.mff.cuni.cz    (194.50.16.66)
Last updated 16:11 11 Aug 1996

Location: /OS/Mac/MacSciTech/medicine
FILE    -rw-r--r--  122501 bytes  01:00 10 May 1995  anatomiser.demo.sea.hqx
```

As the student now knows the name of the FTP site (**ftp.ms.mff.cuni.cz**), the directory path (**/OS/Mac/MacSciTech/medicine**), and the name of the file archive (**anatomiser.demo.sea.hqx**), he or she can ask an FTP mail server to fetch the file (p.162). Note that, in this example, the extensions to the file name tell us that this is a demonstration version (**.demo**) in the form of a self-extracting compressed archive (**.sea**) that has been BinHexed (**.hqx**, p.160).

Other ways to use Archie

Aside from using an Archie client or e-mail, you can search Archie via Telnet and the WWW. To try Archie by Telnet (Chapter Twenty two), use the following URL:

<URL:telnet://archie@archie.doc.ic.ac.uk>

Use **archie** as the login name, and the same commands as you would if performing a search by e-mail. A WWW-based Archie interface is described on p.221.

CHAPTER TWENTY FOUR
Gopher

What is Gopher?

The Internet Gopher is a service that lets you 'tunnel' through the Internet to locate information by subject. By presenting various menus and sub-menus to the user, Gopher servers link together related resources, even though these resources may be widely distributed in geographic terms. Having connected to a Gopher server, the user can move from computer to computer, or continent to continent, without having to know any extra commands, domain names, or directory paths.

Opening a Gopher menu may lead to a text or binary file retrievable by FTP, another nested (deeper) menu, a Telnet session (Chapter Twenty two), or a search. Searches from within a Gopher server can include a Veronica search of Gopher menus (see below) and WAIS databases (Chapter Twenty five). Exactly what is available from a given Gopher menu is determined by the interests of the Gopher provider, thus limiting search options to the links they have chosen to offer.

Gopher has been somewhat overshadowed by the WWW, although some information offered through Gopher is not available in hypertext on the Web. Further, Gopher's search capabilities are in competition with sophisticated WWW-based search engines (Chapter Twenty seven). For more information about Gopher, see the (dated) *Gopher FAQ*:

<URL:http://gopher.odu.edu:70/1m/about-odu/gw-faqs/Gopher_FAQ.txt>

Using a Gopher client

Simple text-based clients navigate menus using the arrow keys and the **Enter/Return** key. Under a graphical interface Gopher clients provide point-and-click navigation of menu options. Different icons indicate visually whether an option (known as a 'Gopher object') is a nested menu, file, or search, etc. (see Fig. 23). Double-clicking a file icon will FTP the file to your computer or display it on screen. The icon may even indicate whether it is a text file, graphic, or a binary file for the PC, Mac, or a UNIX machine. If the Gopher object is a search, entering keywords will retrieve a menu of objects containing those words. If the object indicates a Telnet session, double-clicking it will launch a Telnet application, providing access to the services available via Telnet.

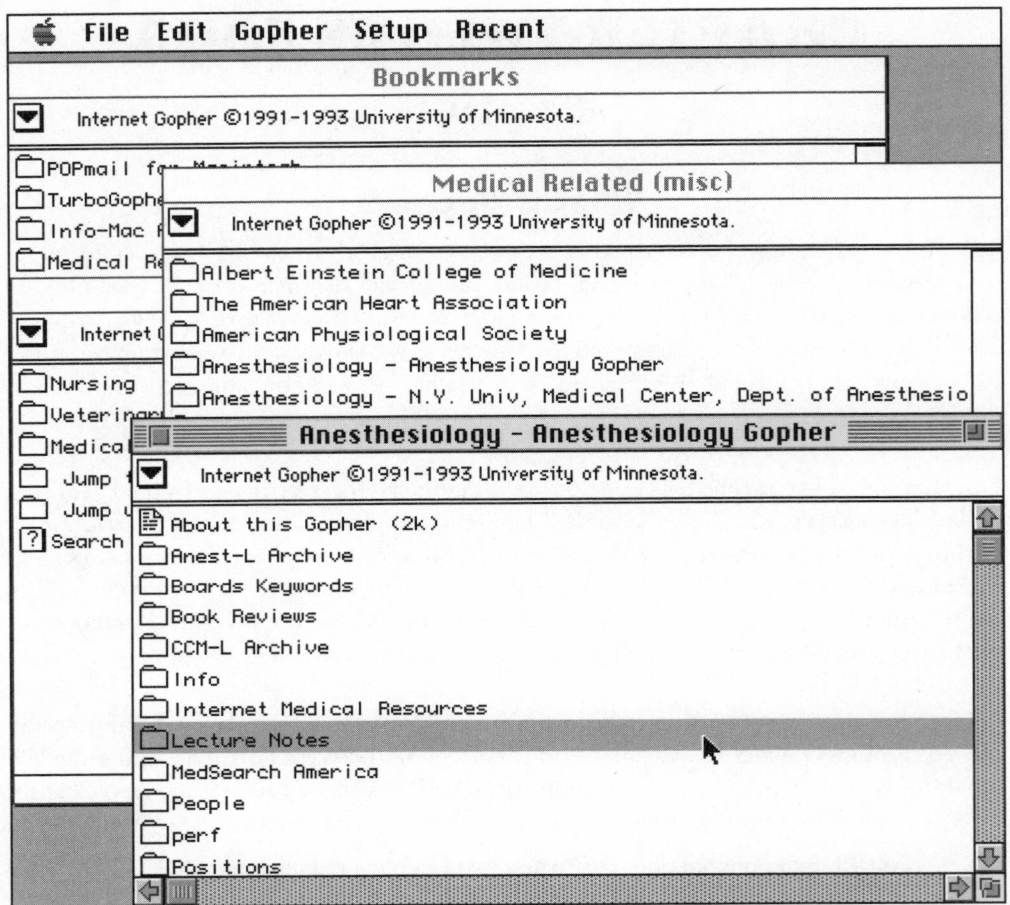

Fig. 23 Using a Gopher client. Point-and-click navigation of nested menus, combined with visual cues as to the nature of objects in each directory and Veronica searches made Gopher an easy-to-use yet powerful tool in locating medical resources. It has been largely superseded by the World-Wide Web.

Your client probably has an option allowing you to find out the domain name of a Gopher object you are interested in. Also, if the server understands the 'Gopher+' protocol you will be able to gather additional information, such as the size of a file you are proposing to download. Good Gopher clients let you create a 'bookmarks' file, providing an easy means to re-access a particular Gopher menu or search result. Example clients are:

WS-Gopher (for the PC):

<URL:ftp://snake.srv.net/pub/windows/archives/wsg-12.exe>

TurboGopher (for the Mac):

<URL:gopher://boombox.micro.umn.edu:70/11/gopher/Macintosh-TurboGopher>

What is Veronica?

Just as Archie locates named files on FTP sites, **Veronica** is a search program that locates Gopher objects on Gopher servers. Veronica is accessed through Gopher, and presents the result of the search as a standard Gopher menu. Clicking on a menu item in the result window likewise opens that object. You can try Veronica at:

<URL:gopher://veronica.scs.unr.edu:70/11/veronica>

A Veronica search uses keywords to find object *titles*; it does not look inside documents. In addition, each kind of Gopher object has a 'type ID', and this can be used by Veronica to narrow down the search. For example, type 1 is a directory, and type 8 is a Telnet session. Boolean operators (i.e. 'and', 'or', 'not') and limited wild cards (i.e. '*') are also permitted. Combining these alternatives can create a search term such as **-t1 pulmonary or lung**, where '**-t**' means Gopher object type and '**1**' indicates that the type is a directory. This search would look for Gopher objects of the directory type containing the words 'pulmonary' or 'lung'. See also:

Veronica FAQ:

<URL:gopher://futique.scs.unr.edu:70/00/veronica/veronica-faq>

How to query Veronica:

<URL:gopher://futique.scs.unr.edu:70/00/veronica/how-to-query-veronica>

Medical Gophers

The following Gopher sites are given below by way of example. For other medicine-related Gophers, try a Veronica search as above.

University of Southampton Biomedical Gopher:

<URL:gopher://medstats.soton.ac.uk:70/>

US National Institutes of Health Gopher:

<URL:gopher://gopher.nih.gov/>

World Health Organization Gopher:

<URL:gopher://gopher.who.ch/>

Other ways to use Gopher

Gophermail provides limited access to Gopher objects by e-mail. For instructions, send the following message:

<URL:mailto:gophermail@eunet.cz> Send: help

Briefly, if you wanted to access the World Health Organization Gopher, you would send '**gopher.who.ch**' in the subject line of an e-mail message to Gophermail. This returns the Gopher menu, and you can make a selection from it by putting an '**x**' next to your choice and mailing the menu back. Keep doing this until you arrive at what you want.

Gophers and Veronica can also be used via Telnet or a WWW client. Many Telnet sites provide Gopher menus which can be selected using the arrow and **Enter/Return** keys. In such an interface, a forward slash (/) next to a menu item indicates that further resources are nested beneath it.

You can type any Gopher URL into a WWW client such as Netscape or Internet Explorer and see its various menus listed, with different Gopher objects indicated by distinct icons in Netscape. For example, searches are marked by a pair of binoculars. See also p.221.

CHAPTER TWENTY FIVE
Wide Area Information Servers

What is WAIS?

A Wide Area Information Server, or WAIS, is a server program used to support information retrieval on the Internet. WAIS servers can index the contents of text files in public file archives, and clients can interrogate the resulting database using keywords. The database might hold every word appearing in a text file, for example. The server returns a list of documents containing the keyword, and the client can ask the server to send a copy of any relevant documents found.

Each database covers a particular topic or topics, although several databases can be searched at once. This means the user can start a search without knowing which specific database might lead to a relevant document.

How does WAIS work?

In using a WAIS client, users first need to nominate a source (or sources). A **source** is a short text file that describes how to access the database (see below). Questions are sent to the WAIS server using a single word (e.g. pain), a question (how do I control pain?), or a phrase (pain control in cancer). You can also use 'and', 'or', 'not' (to exclude something from the search), and 'adj' (to find words adjacent to each other) in the question. Common words (e.g. 'in') and punctuation are ignored.

When a WAIS server receives a question it searches its database for references to documents containing those words, and displays the search result as a list of documents. The documents are listed by the client in order of how relevant the server thinks they are to your request, with a score assigned to each document (with 1000 being the most relevant, and 1 the least). This is called 'relevance feedback', and uses several criteria to compose the score.

If that document or any others are relevant, they can be marked and the search re-run to find more documents that are 'similar' (essentially on the basis of the number of common words). Some will be more similar to the original documents than others, and thus listed higher in the new result window. The user can download any of these documents or view them on screen.

Descriptions of individual databases (i.e. source files) can be found in various locations on the Internet. These source descriptions, usually ending with the suffix **.src**, can be used with a WAIS client to query a particular database. Alternatively, client software allows you to create a new source file. The information needed to do this is in the URL for each WAIS server/database. For example, you might know that the URL for a WAIS search of the CANCERLIT abstracts database is:

<URL:wais://imsdd.meb.uni-bonn.de:210/CancerLit_MedLine>

This information can then be given to the WAIS client, where **CancerLit_MedLine** is the name of the database, **imsdd.meb.uni-bonn.de** is the host (domain) name, and **210** is the port used to address the server.

Medical WAIS databases

There are relatively few medicine-related sources—which may seem a little surprising, given the potential of WAIS to index medical research and literature. However, the growth of the World-Wide Web saw a flood of alternative searching and indexing tools, all accessible through simple hypertext links (see Chapter Twenty seven). WAIS has to a large extent been relegated to a back-end role, not especially distinguished among the ranks of other search tools—all of which are virtually invisible to the end-user with a WWW browser.

Other ways to use WAIS

The Gophermail service (p.193) can be used to search WAIS databases by e-mail. However, as mentioned above, the most common way to access a WAIS index today is using a forms-compatible Web browser, which in practice is very similar to using any other WWW search engine. For example, the University of Bonn Medical Center hosts a full-text WAIS index of the US National Cancer Institute's Cancernet database at:

<URL:http://imsdd.meb.uni-bonn.de/cancernet/>

CHAPTER TWENTY SIX

The World-Wide Web

What is the WWW?

The World-Wide Web and the Internet are virtually synonymous for many people. Developed at the CERN Institute for Particle Physics in Geneva, the World-Wide Web ('the Web', or WWW) is so popular because it is so easy to use. It also manages to provide the functionality of many other Internet services in one simple 'point-and-click' interface.

The nature of hypertext

This interface uses the metaphor of a page to present information. Within a page there may be text and pictures just like in a book, although Web pages can also contain sounds, animations, video, or even small interactive programs. Whereas pages in a book are fixed together by a spine, Web pages are connected to each other by something called '**hypertext**'. In a book, the spine dictates that one page must follow the next in a certain sequence. Hypertext changes all that.

Hypertext simply implies that clicking on a highlighted word with your mouse causes you to 'jump' to related information on another page (or elsewhere on the same page). The word (or words) that you click on are known as 'hypertext links'. Thus, hypertext breaks away from the 'linear' approach to information retrieval where you might read something from beginning to end. You can instead 'jump sideways' to associated information as and when you choose, and return to the point where you jumped from. Hypertext will already be familiar to readers who have used the online Help feature of Microsoft Windows or an Apple Macintosh (it is used in HyperCard and the Apple Guide).

In a Web page hypertext links are usually identified by text that is a different colour and/or underlined. However, it isn't just text that can link to information elsewhere. Other page elements, especially pictures, can also be links. For this reason 'hypermedia' is sometimes used to describe all kinds of links within and between Web pages.

How are these links made?

Hypertext links are actually described by URLs (p.102), although the user need not be aware of them. A WWW client can therefore connect to or display any Internet resource that can be described by a URL (although sometimes it needs plug-ins or helper applications—see below).

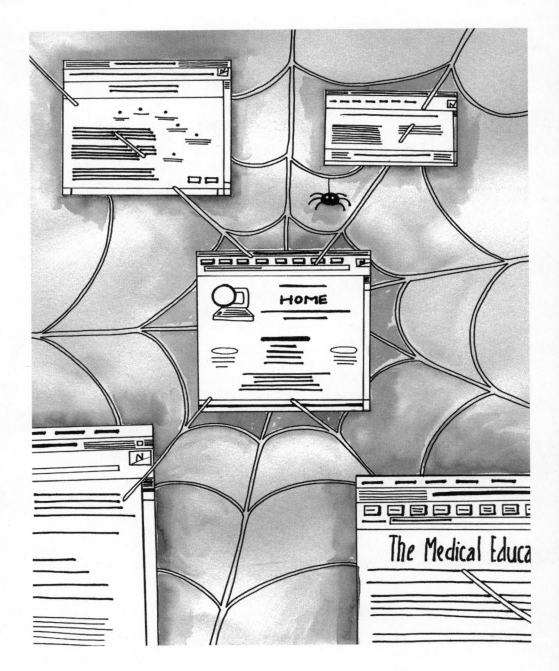

Fig. 24 Hypertext links weave the World-Wide Web. To move from page to page, users need only point-and-click with a mouse. Each page may contain text, pictures, sounds, animations, or interactive mini-programs.

It isn't difficult to imagine an intricate web of links between a huge number of resources at various Internet addresses (i.e. URLs). In fact it is possible to traverse the globe without knowing which computer, country, or continent is providing a particular page of information—hence, the *world-wide* WEB (Fig. 24).

A URL is connected to a hypertext link by means of a code called **Hypertext Markup Language** (HTML). HTML also determines what a WWW page looks like.

What is HTML?

HTML is a 'markup language' used to create hypertext pages that can be used on different types of computer. A markup language is a standard set of rules for bringing structure and meaning to parts of a document. HTML documents are indicated by an **.html** extension to the file name (or **.htm** on PCs).

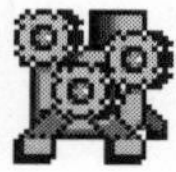

HTML uses '**tags**' to assign meaning to particular segments of text. These tags are analogous to the annotations a copy editor makes to instruct a typesetter how a page is to be laid out, and what fonts and styles should be used. Thus, there are tags to indicate relative heading sizes, new paragraphs, italics, underlines, quotes, and lists for example. Other tags indicate the position of images within the page and where hypertext links are, etc.

Note that **Hypertext Transport Protocol** (HTTP) is used by Web servers to send pages to Web clients. This is why WWW universal resource locators begin with '**http://**'. To learn more about HTML, see *Creating a Web page* (Chapter Thirty one). For more general information about the WWW, the following online resources may be useful:

Boutell's *WWW FAQ*:

<URL:http://info.ox.ac.uk/help/wwwfaq/index.html>

Hughes' *Entering the World-Wide Web: A guide to cyberspace*:

<URL:http://www.eit.com/web/www.guide>

Choosing a WWW browser

A WWW client (or browser, as it is commonly known) establishes a connection to the server described by the URL associated with a particular hypertext link. HTML documents are retrieved and the embedded tags are interpreted. Graphics and other page elements, perhaps from another host, are likewise retrieved and loaded by the browser to create a complete WWW page.

The Mosaic client from the National Center for Supercomputer Applications (NCSA) takes the credit for popularizing the WWW. Mosaic was further developed by Netscape Communications Corporation into Netscape Navigator, and by Microsoft into Internet Explorer. All of these browsers require a TCP/IP Internet connection, although other text-only browsers can be used via ordinary terminal emulation (p.27) or Telnet. By deviating from ratified standards Navigator's release caused some disquiet, although it went on to take the WWW by storm.

The drive for innovation soon deteriorated into an all-out 'features war' between Netscape and Microsoft. Web page authors face the dilemma of choosing between ratified HTML, or proprietary HTML and other technologies from both Netscape and Microsoft to create their pages—undermining the philosophy of a 'universal experience' on the WWW. While this may bring cutting-edge technology into the hands of Web users, it does mean a given version of any client is effectively obsolete within months. For this reason, I will discuss browser features in general terms only.

Some browsers are free to all or just to non-profit users. Others are shareware or sold commercially. Some Internet service providers offer Navigator and others Internet Explorer as their preferred browser. Those accessing the Web through a LAN or WAN (p.93) may have no choice but to use whatever is provided. Because many Web sites are designed or 'optimized' with a particular browser in mind, some home users choose to have a copy of both Navigator and Internet Explorer available. Both are available for Windows PCs and the Mac. Information about hardware requirements and downloading the software is available at:

> Netscape Navigator:
>
> **<URL:http://home.netscape.com/>**
>
> Microsoft Internet Explorer:
>
> **<URL:http://www.microsoft.com/ie/>**

Browser features

Which ever browser you are using, it is likely to support a core set of features, established as part of a shared heritage. Many of these features are illustrated in Fig. 25.

Menu options

The menu bar is the strip across the top of a program window that contains various pull-down menus. The menu bar of a WWW client is not too different from that of a word processor or any other program. The **File** menu contains options to open and save files. Browsers give users the choice of opening a local file (a file on the computers hard disk) or

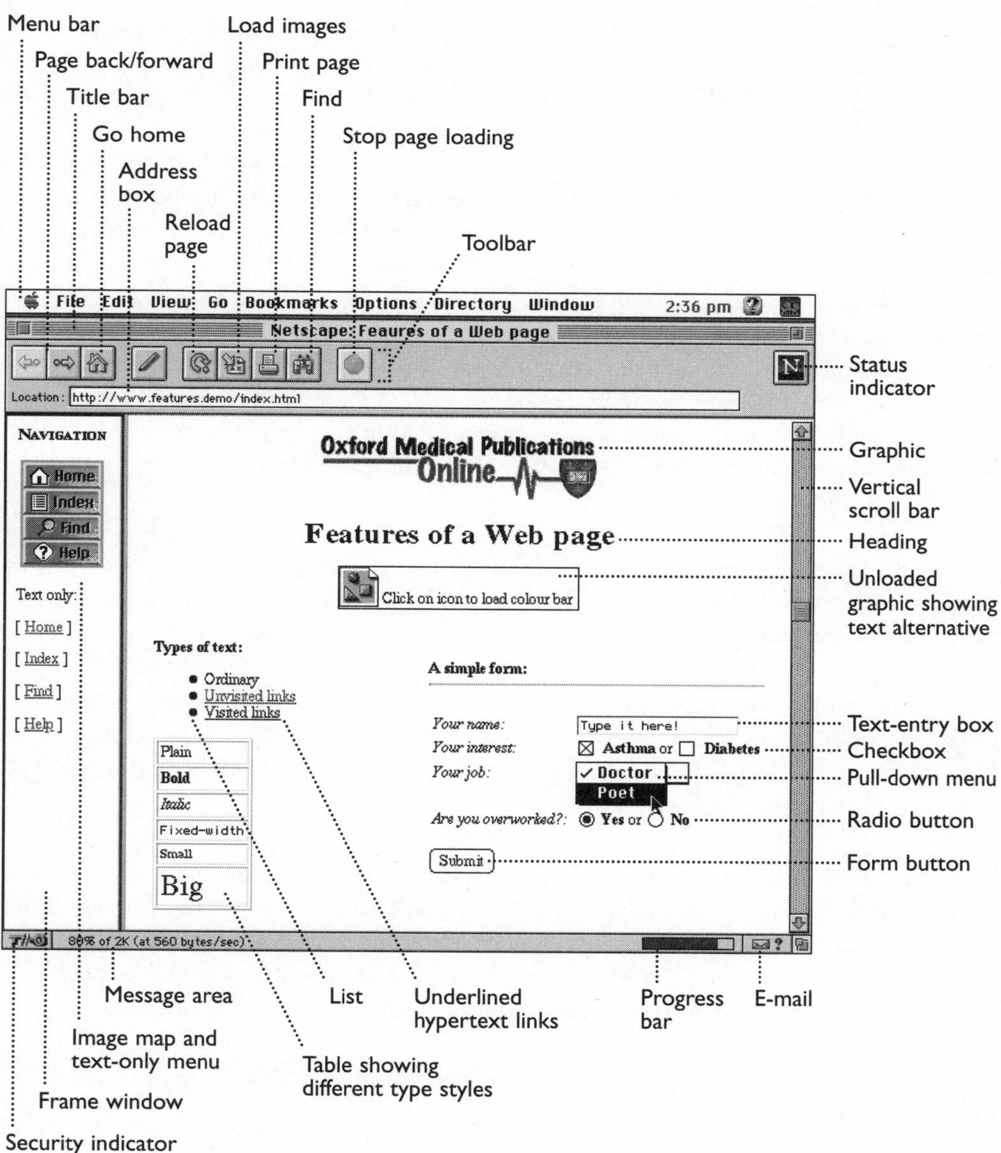

Fig. 25 Common features of a WWW browser and page. Because today's browsers share a common heritage, the user interface is essentially the same across all platforms and individual clients. Likewise, despite increasing use of proprietary technologies, a given Web page looks similar irrespective of the program or computer type being used to access it.

opening a file located on another computer (described by its URL). Web pages can be saved as text files or as source (HTML) files. Saving a Web page as a text file takes out the hypertext links and produces a file in which all the text is the same style and the same size—only basic formatting is retained. Saving a page as a source file, however, renders an exact copy of the page you are viewing minus any images.

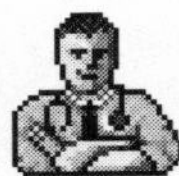

To save time online and cut the cost of telephone calls, users can read WWW pages offline. In this way it is very easy to keep personal copies of any medical information you come across on the Web. Save the WWW page you wish to copy to disk as a source file (i.e. in HTML format), and open it at your leisure with your browser as a local file. If you wish to save any images, holding the mouse button down over an image will display a pop-up menu with an option allowing you to do this. An alternative is to print the page while still online with the images displayed in their proper place. Bear in mind that although it may be free, electronic information is still protected by copyright.

By default, your browser will automatically display (load) any images embedded within a Web page. Pages with lots of images consume available bandwidth and image-intensive pages take longer to load.

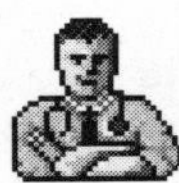

Disabling the automatic loading of images is a useful trick to improve the time it takes to download a Web page. The menu bar provides a means to load the images on individual pages if they are an essential part of a particular page (under the **View** menu).

The **Bookmarks** menu (or **Favourites** in Internet Explorer) provides a means of storing the URLs of WWW pages which you might like to visit again. When a page is saved as a **Bookmark**, it is added to a hierarchical menu from where it can be selected the next time you wish to visit that site. Browsers typically allow you to save your Bookmarks to a separate file so you can swap your list of favourite medical sites with a colleague.

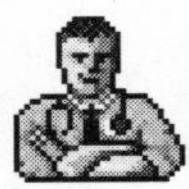

It is not too difficult to create your own customized WWW page to store favourite URLs. See Chapter Thirty one.

Both Navigator and Internet Explorer have a **Go** menu, which is used to navigate back and forth between recently visited Web pages and a '**home page**'. Unless otherwise configured, clients attempt to connect to a default Web page when launched. This so-called home page can be changed to any page at the user's discretion, even to a personalized one on their own machine (set using the **Options** menu).

The **Options** menu serves to set many other preferences. These include page appearance (colours, whether hypertext links should be underlined, etc.); which fonts should be used; which helper applications and plug-ins should be called upon; cache size; proxy servers, and options for managing news, mail, and security (see below).

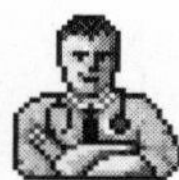

A local **disk cache** on your hard disk can be used for storing Web pages on your own computer, rather than fetching them via the modem when you return to a given WWW page. If your computer has the disk space and you often revisit pages, a cache of several megabytes can significantly speed up your sessions on the WWW. Similarly, using a local **proxy server**—a large cache on the Internet for frequently accessed pages—ensures that pages are loaded from a more local source where possible.

Browser buttons (the toolbar)

Often commonly used functions available through the menu bar will be duplicated in the toolbar for easy access. A **toolbar** is a row of distinctive buttons across the top of the browser window. Pictures on the buttons depict their function. See Fig. 26.

Address box

The address box (see Fig. 25) displays the URL of the page that is currently being displayed. Deleting this address and manually typing in a new URL (then pressing **Return/Enter**) will connect to the new site. Alternatively, choose a site from a pull-down menu (**Bookmarks**, **Favourites**, or recently visited sites).

Indicators

When the pointer hovers over a hypertext link, the associated URL is displayed in a small message area at the bottom of the browser window. This area is also used to display status messages during the retrieval of a page, such as 'Contacting host...'. Next to the message area, a progress bar indicates graphically what percentage of a page or file has been retrieved. An animated logo in the top right-hand corner of the browser window provides a more general indication that the client is actively communicating with a server (Web clients don't remain connected to the server in between requests from the client). Lastly, Navigator users will have noticed a broken key in the bottom left corner of the browser window. This indicates an insecure connection between the client and Web server. When depicted as an intact key, this indicates that information (such as credit card details) you submit to the server via a form is securely encrypted. Internet Explorer uses a lock icon instead.

Handling different file formats

Browsers differ in their capabilities for handling different file formats (Table 7, p.45), although all can of course interpret HTML. Other files can be handled by your browser in one of three ways:

Internally:

Browsers such as Navigator and Internet Explorer have the built-in ability to display/play back a variety of image, audio, and other file formats. Formats handled by some Web browsers internally include GIF, JPEG, Java, and Wave files.

Helper applications:

If the file you are loading is not one that your browser can handle internally, nor one that can be handled by a plug-in (see below), it will need help to view/play the file. You can specify such '**helper applications**' to be launched alongside your browser when these types of file are encountered. Programs to handle compressed file archives, such as WinZip or Stuffit Expander, are typical examples of helper applications. Freeware and shareware helpers are available from numerous FTP sites. Netscape maintain a list of recommendations for each computer type at:

<URL:http://home.netscape.com/assist/helper_apps/index.html>

Plug-ins:

Plug-ins turn your Web browser into a 'bells and whistles' multimedia player. Devised by Netscape, plug-ins are supported by both Navigator and Internet Explorer. Plug-ins for our purposes are similar to helper applications—they enable us to handle certain file types—but they do this seamlessly from within the Web browser itself. Plug-ins exist for a wide variety of applications, including 3-D (see below) and animations (such as the Shockwave for Director plug-in, from Macromedia); portable document formats (such as Acrobat Reader from Adobe); a Word Viewer (from Inso Corporation); a PowerPoint Animation Player (from Microsoft); and audio and video players (such as RealAudio from Progressive Networks, and QuickTime from Apple).

Be aware that the added memory requirements of some of these plug-ins can be very taxing on your machine. You can locate plug-ins directly using a search engine (Chapter Twenty seven), although Netscape maintain a list of plug-ins at their Web site:

<URL:http://home.netscape.com/comprod/products/navigator/version_2.0/plugins/index.html>

Mail and news

Navigator is a fully integrated e-mail client and news reader. Internet Explorer 3.0 introduced an Internet Mail and News add-on which, like Navigator, formats e-mail messages and news articles in HTML so they contain active hypertext links. Dedicated clients may provide a better interface and more specialized features, but a fully integrated system does mean users have to learn the quirks of only one program. Using a Web client for e-mail and accessing newsgroups is discussed further toward the end of this chapter.

Other features

At the very top of the browser window a title bar contains the name of the document currently being displayed. Vertical and horizontal scroll bars are used to view areas of a Web page that don't fit into the browser window on a small computer screen. The re-size box is used to make the browser window fit the dimensions of a page automatically. Most other features are particular to a given client. You are advised to familiarize yourself with the documentation accompanying your client in order to get the most out of the software.

The browser will let you know if it has problems connecting to a Web site or retrieving a particular page. Some troubleshooting advice is given in Table 13 (below).

TABLE 13 Having problems?

Problem	Solution
The server cannot be found.	Have you spelt the URL wrong? Check that every letter, slash, special symbol, and full stop is in the right place.
The server doesn't respond.	Are you using the right URL prefix? Files on FTP sites begin with ftp://; those on Web sites begin http://.
	Has your modem lost the connection, or is the computer you are calling offline? Try connecting to another site, or try again later.
You get a message saying 'Connection refused by host'.	Too many people may be accessing that site. Try again later.
You get a message saying that a file can't be found.	It may no longer exist, or could have been moved. Try the URL without the filename or sub-directory, or use a search facility (if there is one).
A Web page seems to stop loading half-way through.	Use the browser's 'Reload' button to re-connect to the server. Connections sometimes 'hang'.
You cannot playback/view certain files (e.g. video or sound).	Ensure that your browser Preferences are configured to launch an appropriate helper application, or that any necessary plug-ins are installed. There may be insufficient memory available to launch a player/viewer.

Web page content

The content on Web pages is more important than the browser you use to access it. Web pages may feature text; images and other media; tables; forms; and frames. These features are also shown in Fig. 25.

Text

There are three types of text in a WWW page, usually indicated in different colours. The majority of Web pages are composed largely of ordinary text. Parts of this text will be hypertext links to information elsewhere. Linked text is by default underlined, and *unvisited* links (i.e. links that haven't been clicked on) typically change colour when they have been explored (i.e. they become *visited* links).

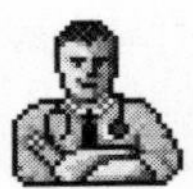

How do you know when text on a page has been updated? Many pages indicate a revision date in the footer of the page. An easier solution is to use 'URL-minder' from NetMind. This service lets you register your e-mail address to receive e-mail when the content of a page at a certain URL changes.

<URL:http://www.netmind.com/URL-minder/URL-minder.html>

Images and other media

Some images are purely decorative. Links to other resources can also be indicated by coloured boxes around images, or by graphics that look like buttons, for example. A single click with your mouse on any such object will activate the link, and call up the next WWW page (or download a file). The same is true of image maps (p.273).

As mentioned previously, you can stop the automatic loading of images—but what if the graphics themselves are links to other resources? Most sites provide a text alternative describing the image next to a small image icon. Clicking on the image icon will load that image only (although the text alternative may be a hypertext link itself).

Some browsers can display 'interlaced' images which means they are initially a blurred outline, but clarity improves as the rest of the image loads. This enables you to carry on reading the page while this happens, or alternatively if the page doesn't look interesting there is no need to wait for the images to become fully resolved—you can still click on a blurred outline image to activate a hypertext link.

As you now know, Web pages can contain much more than text and images. Browsers like Navigator and Internet Explorer use MIME content types (p.160) and/or the file suffix (p.44) to determine whether a file can be displayed by the browser itself or handled in another way (see *Handling different file formats*, above).

Tables

Information can be tabulated using certain HTML tags that describe rows and columns (p.274). More often, however, these tags are used by Web page designers to create more interesting page layouts. In the later case, the data cells making up the table are often invisible.

Forms

Pages can feature fill-out forms containing elements that allow the user to send data such as a password or search term to the host computer. Filling out a form may involve entering text, checking boxes, or using pull-down menus and buttons. Browsers that support this facility are said to be 'forms compatible'.

Frames

A 'frame' is a feature that divides the browser window into separate areas, each displaying a different HTML file. Frames can cause confusion and many sites avoid using them for this reason.

Java, NCs, and friends

Java is a cross-platform programming language (a complex character-based code for writing programs) from Sun Microsystems. Small applications (known as **applets**) written in Java code can be linked into an HTML page so they are downloaded and run when that page is displayed by a Java-aware browser (see Fig. 26, p.209). This happens irrespective of what operating system your computer is running. The 'Java Virtual Machine' (p.16) built into Web browsers (or operating systems) will ensure that the same applet will run regardless.

Rather than store Java applets on your local hard disk like conventional applications, the latest versions could be downloaded as required from the Internet and run without using much RAM (p.8). It is possible to run applets using a computer without a hard disk and fitted with minimal RAM, a simple operating system, a built-in Web browser, and an inexpensive CPU. In fact this is Oracle's concept of the **network computer** (NC)—a 'cut-down' PC, in effect. In another departure from the conventional way of working, ongoing projects could be stored on the network rather than on a local disk; completed ones could be sent directly to a printer. NCs may find a niche on intranets (p.113) and in the home entertainment market, but are unlikely to replace the multi-functional PC.

Despite the hype, truly useful applets have been slow to materialize. Initial experiments with brief animations and sound have been joined more recently by applets aimed at health-care professionals. Part of the reason for the slow takeoff in medical applications is the level of expertise required to create Java applets. Medical utilization and acceptance of Java as a useful tool is in any case likely to lag behind general acceptance (as it has with the WWW itself). Furthermore, in practice applets can prove painfully slow over dial-up Internet connections by comparison with applications stored on hard disk. Early examples of medical Java applets (dominated by radiology) are:

Pregnancy Calculator (R. Giffen):

<URL:http://fox.nstn.ca/~rgiffen/PregnancyCalculator.html>

Volume Slicer Applet Demos (A. Barclay):

<URL:http://www.cc.emory.edu/CRL/java/slicer/>

The Whole Brain Atlas Navigator (K. Johnson and J.A. Becker):

<URL:http://www.med.harvard.edu/AANLIB/cases/java/case.html>

The NPAC Visible Human Viewer (Northeast Parallel Architectures Center, Syracuse University):

<URL:http://www.npac.syr.edu/projects/vishuman/VisibleHuman.html>

Radiologic Anatomy Quiz (Gold Standard Multimedia, Inc.):

<URL:http://www.gsm.com/resources/raquiz/>

Although the most prominent, Java is not the only 'Internet programming language' seeking to make Web pages more interactive. Others include **ActiveX**, **JavaScript**, and **VBScript**. Your Web browser itself must understand each language before it can handle content written in these languages.

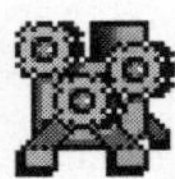

Netscape's JavaScript is a scripting language (a kind of mini-programming language using English-like statements instead of incomprehensible codes). Based on Java, these scripts can be written directly into an HTML page (in contrast to external applets), and provide for less ambitious interaction and enhancements than Java itself. VBScript (a subset of the Visual Basic programming language) is Microsoft's answer to JavaScript.

Microsoft's ActiveX technology can be used to create small applications (called ActiveX controls) that can be downloaded over the Internet when the Web page they are linked to is displayed by an ActiveX-aware browser. ActiveX controls can be considered equivalent to Java applets.

For more information about Java (including an FAQ), see the Java home page at:

<URL:http://java.sun.com/>

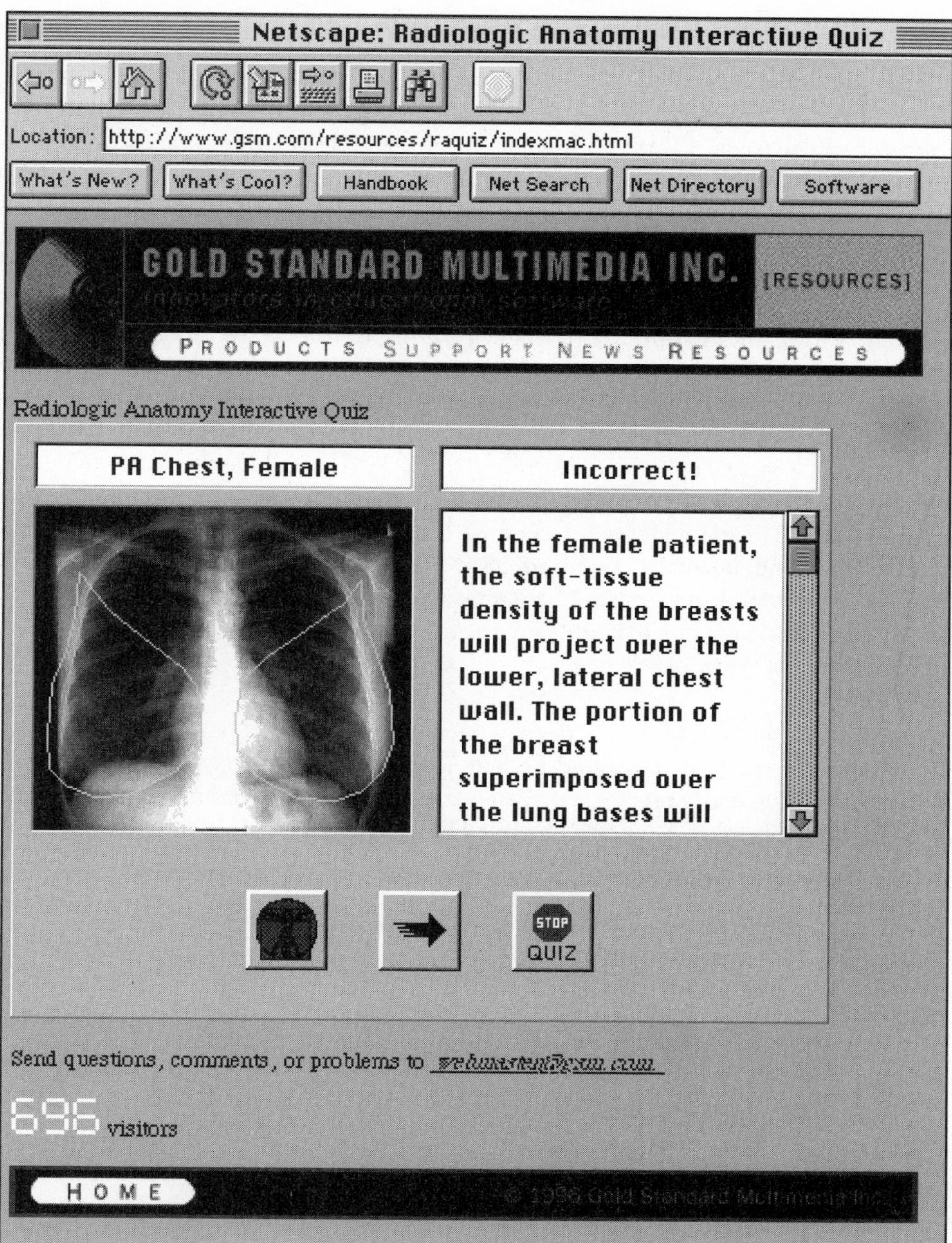

Fig. 26 How Java works. Small programs (applets) are embedded into an HTML page for display by Java-aware browsers. Java promises to make the Web much more interactive. [Screen capture: Prof. R.L. Brown. Reproduced with permission.]

Virtual reality and VRML

Despite the similar acronym, **Virtual Reality Modelling Language** (VRML) is quite different from HTML. Whereas HTML is interpreted by a Web browser to describe two-dimensional Web pages, VRML is a graphics file format that describes a three-dimensional scene—or at least the *illusion* thereof. Although there are several competing VRML standards, 'Moving Worlds' from Silicon Graphics and collaborators has been adopted as the official VRML 2.0 standard:

<URL:http://vrml.sgi.com/>

Although VRML files (identified by the **.wrl** suffix) can be viewed by an independent VRML player, they can also be embedded into WWW pages in a similar way to Java applets/ActiveX controls. The 'Cosmo Player' from Silicon Graphics and 'Live3D' from Netscape are example plug-ins (see above) that enable the embedding of VRML files into a Web page. The virtual environments created by VRML can include the ability to interact with 'virtual objects', and may feature integrated sounds, animations, Java applets, and hypertext links. This technology is too new to describe any serious medical applications at the time of writing, but its potential can be glimpsed from the entertainment-orientated VRML worlds that already exist. With almost unlimited interactivity on the WWW, health-care professionals should be able to partake in remote collaborative projects, teaching, and simulations as never before.

Virtual reality technologies can also offer new perspectives on clinical problems. Considerable interest is being directed into building three-dimensional medical images that can be manipulated and used in diagnostic and therapeutic simulations. An example on the Internet is the National Library of Medicine's Visible Human Project:

<URL:http://www.nlm.nih.gov/research/visible/visible_human.html>

This project is creating three-dimensional representations of the male and female body, using digitized cadaver photographs, magnetic resonance scans, and computer tomography data.

Medical WWW sites

In contrast to the traditional medical publishing industry there are no widely recognized 'authoritative' WWW publishing houses. The range in quality of information is thus greater than that seen between paper-based medical books and journals. For most publishers the WWW remains something of a novelty, although there are now many examples of professional sites which offer a tantalizing view of the future.

As more and more medical content finds its way on to the Web, it has the potential to develop into a 'virtual medical textbook' sharing the best of an institution's knowledge

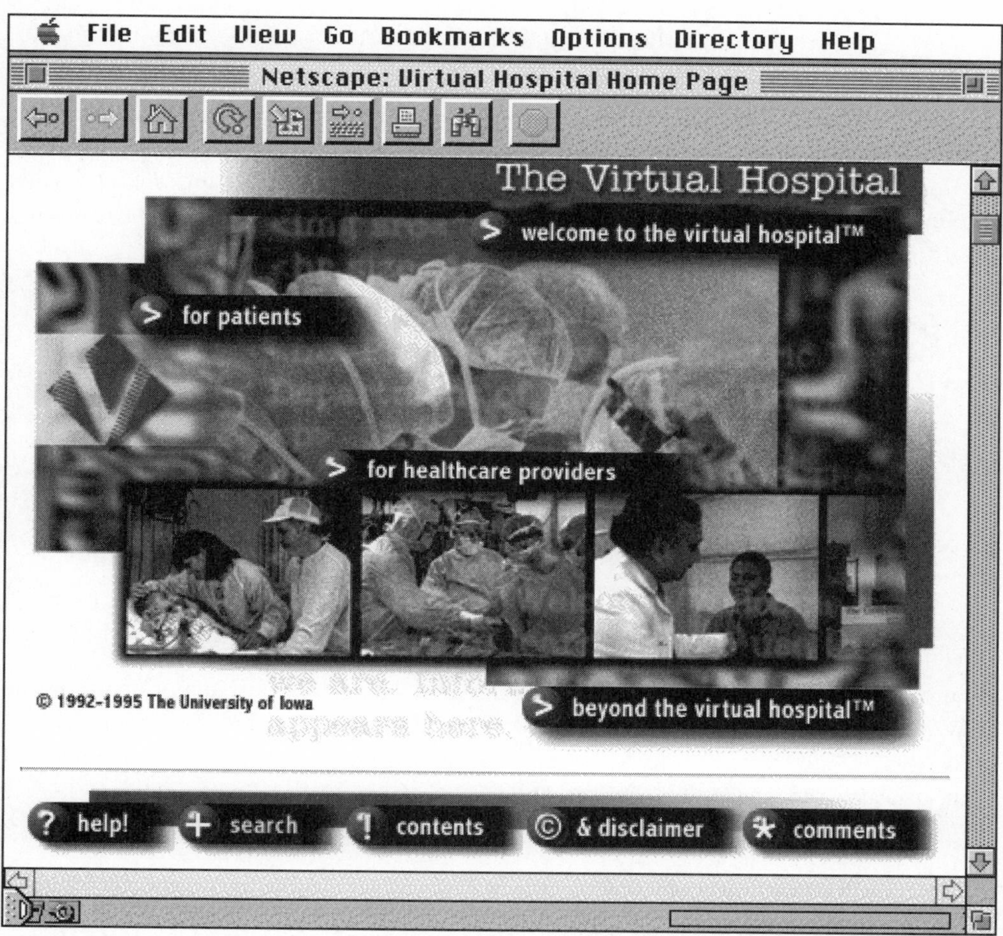

Fig. 27 The Virtual Hospital contains multimedia textbooks and teaching modules, patient simulations, clinical practice guidelines, a formulary and clinical laboratory reference manual, continuing medical education information, and patient handouts and guides.

and teaching skills with the best of others. The Virtual Hospital from the University of Iowa College of Medicine is one of the earliest well-known sites. It features a wide range of services for both physicians and patients (Fig. 27).

Today there are literally pages and pages of medical information available on the WWW. The only practical way to approach this volume of information in a book such as this is to select a few examples of the many types of medical and health-related resources available. Although many resources originate in the US, it is increasingly easy to find those with a more local perspective.

Advertising and recruitment

The commercial possibilities afforded by the Web were quickly realized, and it is not difficult to locate a site wanting to sell you something—including medical vacancies. Several sites, some from the major journals and others from opportunistic new companies, provide job listings by specialty and/or location, notice of practices for sale, and other employment-related information. Examples include:

BMJ Classified:

<URL:http://www.bmj.com/bmj/>

CareerLinks (*New England Journal of Medicine*):

<URL:http://www2.nejm.org/>

Medical Ad-Mart (Russell Johns Associates, Ltd.):

<URL:www.medical-admart.com/>

MedSearch America (MedSearch America, Inc.):

<URL:www.medsearch.com/>

Agencies

A number of governmental and international health agencies maintain a presence on the WWW. These can be a valuable source of authoritative statements on health-care policy, press releases, and statistics, etc. Some information is directed at health professionals, and some at health-care consumers. For example:

World Health Organization:

<URL:http://www.who.ch/>

UK Department of Health:

<URL:http://www.open.gov.uk/doh/dhhome.htm>

US National Library of Medicine:

<URL:http://www.nlm.nih.gov/>

Clinical cases

A number of sites feature clinical cases on a regular basis. The user may be presented with a simple discussion, or alternatively must work progressively through the clinical history, examination findings, and investigation results before coming to a diagnosis. Issues raised by the case are then discussed:

Case of the Month (Medical Network, Inc.):

<URL:http://www.medconnect.com/home-cas.htm>

MedRounds (University of Colorado):

<URL:http://www.uchsc.edu/sm/pmb/medrounds/index.html>

Reuters Clinical Challenge (Reuters Health Information Services):

<URL:http://www.reutershealth.com/clinchal/>

Clinical pharmacology

Although sourced from the American pharmaceutical industry, prescribing information is available on the Internet in an accessible and (sometimes) authoritative form:

Clinical Pharmacology (Gold Standard Multimedia, Inc.):

<URL:http://www.gsm.com/resources/cponline/>

PharmInfoNet (VirSci Corp.):

<URL:http://pharminfo.com>

Physicians GenRx (Mosby-Year Book, Inc.):

<URL:http://www.mosby.com/>

Clinical specialties

WWW pages now exist for virtually every clinical specialty and sub-specialty. A selection of specialty index sites is presented in the *Appendix*, p.303. WWW-based directories and search engines are also useful in locating specialty sites (see Chapter Twenty seven, *Searching the medical Web*).

Commercial sites for health-care consumers

As Chapter Thirteen revealed, the Internet (and the WWW in particular) soon became home to a significant amount of self-help and support information. Voluntary efforts have been joined more recently by commercial interest in filling the information void. Some sites offer information about risk factors, explanations of investigations and treatments, glossaries of medical jargon, and 'ask the expert' facilities, etc. Examples are:

HealthGate (HealthGate Data Corp.):

<URL:http://www.healthgate.com/>

MedicineNet (Information Network, Inc.):

<URL:http://www.medicinenet.com/>

WellnessWeb (WellnessWeb):

<URL:http://www.wellweb.com/>

Commercial sites for health professionals

Commercial sites for health professionals also exist, aiming to become a 'one-stop shop' for peer-reviewed medical information. This may be achieved by way of advertising revenue or subscription which in turn permits high-quality databases and other services to be offered:

Healthworks Online (Healthworks Ltd.):

<URL:http://www.healthworks.co.uk/>

Health Online Service (Burda Medien GmbH):

<URL:http://www.hos.de/>

Medscape (Medscape, Inc.):

<URL:http://www.medscape.com/>

The Physicians' Home Page (p.249) and BioMedNet (Chapter Thirty three) are further examples. The Health Online Service is illustrated in Fig. 28.

Comparative image databases

A meeting of doctors can result in an exchange of slides—in effect sharing clinical encounters. And sometimes pictures are more valuable than a description when preparing lecture material or educating oneself. The Internet can offer libraries of images that can be compared with each other, or with a particular case you may have in mind. Such a facility is especially suited to specialties like dermatology, pathology, and radiology where visualization is important. Examples include:

Atlas of Hematology (T. Ichihashi):

<URL:http://www.med.nagoya-u.ac.jp/pathy/Pictures/atlas.html>

Dermatology Online Atlas (A. Bittorf):

<URL:http://www.rrze.uni-erlangen.de/docs/FAU/fakultaet/med/kli/derma/bilddb/db.htm>

The Whole Brain Atlas (K.A. Johnson and J.A. Becker):

<URL:http://count51.med.harvard.edu/AANLIB/home.html>

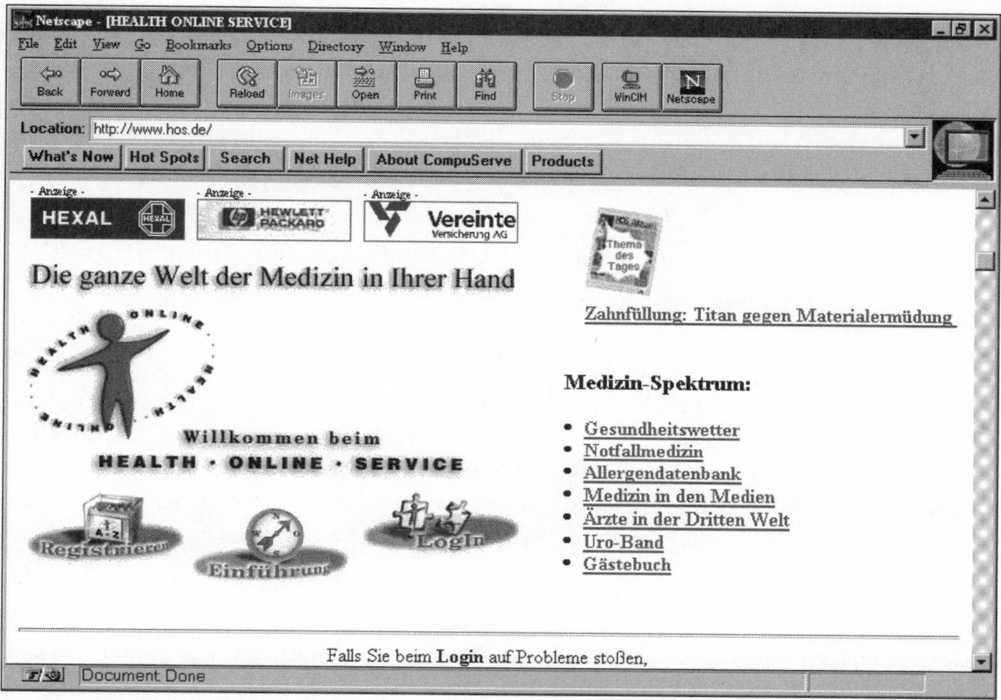

Fig. 28 Germany's Health Online Service. Commercial interests are improving the quality of medical information available to health-care professionals and consumers. Successful Web sites must also provide users with the incentive to return. [Reproduced with permission.]

Continuing medical education

Many sites listed under other categories could be said to offer a form of continuing medical education (CME). Some American sites, however, actually offer CME credit towards the Physicians' Recognition Award of the American Medical Association (for a fee). These include:

Medconnect (Medical Network, Inc.):

<URL:http://www.medconnect.com/>

Pathology Cases for Diagnosis (Uniformed Services University of the Health Sciences):

<URL:http://wwwpath.usuf2.usuhs.mil/surg_path/surg_path.html>

Radiology teaching files (University of Washington):

<URL:http://www.rad.washington.edu/>

Databases

One of the foremost freely available and authoritative databases on the Internet as of writing is Cancernet from the US National Cancer Institute. Significant databases are not yet widely deployed on the Web, due partly to fear of lost revenue and technical difficulties in converting them into hypertext. Other notable exceptions are Physicians GenRx (see above) and MEDLINE (see Chapter Twenty nine).

Cancernet (US National Cancer Institute and University of Bonn):

<URL:http://www.meb.uni-bonn.de/cancernet/>

Directories of medical sites

Many medical pages point to other sites, as is the nature of hypertext. Some pages take this to the extreme, focusing on the organization of links to other resources rather than providing clinical information themselves. These 'entry points' to medicine on the Internet play a valuable role in indexing the growing collection of resources. Directories of medical specialty and disease-categorized resources are discussed in Chapter Twenty seven.

Journals

Chapter Thirteen introduced the concept of Web-based medical journals. Some of these sites are maintained by long-established journal publishers; others have been conceived in recent times on the WWW. No doubt some of these journals are dabbling in what they see as a potential source of revenue, and what is currently 'free' may be a prelude to a subscription-based service. Examples include:

British Medical Journal (British Medical Association):

<URL:http://www.bmj.com/bmj/>

General Practice On-Line (Priory Lodge Education Ltd.):

<URL:http://www.priory.co.uk/journals/gp.htm>

Journal of the American Medical Association (American Medical Association):

<URL:http://www.ama-assn.org/journals/standing/jama/jamahome.htm>

New England Journal of Medicine (Massachusetts Medical Society):

<URL:http://www.nejm.org/JHome.htm>

The Annals of Internal Medicine (American College of Physicians):

<URL:http://www.acponline.org/journals/annals/annaltoc.htm>

The Lancet (Elsevier Science Ltd.):

<URL:http://www.thelancet.com>

For a more complete listing of medical journals on the Web, see 'Electronic Newsletters and Journals' at MedWeb:

<URL:http://www.cc.emory.edu/WHSCL/medweb.ejs.html>

Medical news

Although some online medical journals contain a news section, health-care industry news is also available from respected news agencies:

CNN-Health (Cable Network News, Inc.):

<URL:http://www.cnn.com/HEALTH/index.html>

Reuters Health Information Services (Reuters Ltd.):

<URL:http://www.reutershealth.com/news/>

Medical schools

Refer back to Chapter Thirteen for URLs pointing to worldwide medical schools and pages of particular interest to medical students (p.121). Many medical school pages offer local curricula, student information, and teaching files of their own. UK examples include:

MedWeb (University of Birmingham):

<URL:http://medweb.bham.ac.uk/>

United Medical and Dental Schools of Guy's and St. Thomas's Hospitals:

<URL:http://www.umds.ac.uk/>

University of Cambridge Clinical School Home Page:

<URL:http://fester.his.path.cam.ac.uk/cshp.html>

Patient education

The plethora of self-help information disseminated over the Internet in the form of Usenet news and mailing lists has been alluded to previously. The WWW is also an attractive medium for providing preventive health advice, support, and general information. Examples are:

Internet Based Patient Education Program (Group Health Cooperative):

<URL:http://weber.u.washington.edu/~ghcfpr/netpep/>

Healthtouch (Medical Strategies, Inc.):

<URL:http://www.healthtouch.com/>

Patient Education Materials (American Academy of Family Physicians):

<URL:http://www.housecall.com/sponsors/aafp/aafp.front.html>

Practice guidelines

Practice guidelines have grown out of need to improve quality of care, to satisfy others and ourselves that we are practising evidence-based medicine (p.241), and to reduce the risk of malpractice. Practice guidelines on the Internet include:

Clinical Practice Guidelines (Agency for Health Policy and Research):

<URL:http://text.nlm.nih.gov/ahcpr/guidesc.html>

CPG Infobase (Canadian Medical Association):

<URL:http://www.cma.ca/cpgs/>

Practice Guidelines (American College of Cardiology):

<URL:http://www.acc.org/publications/index.html>

Pre-clinical sciences

Several universities have placed multimedia learning modules on the WWW. This enables the sharing of course material in subjects such as anatomy, biochemistry, and physiology:

Computer Enhanced Learning Linkage (University of Arizona):

<URL:http://www.physiol.arizona.edu/CELL/CELLHomePage.html>

NetBiochem (University of Utah):

<URL:http://www-medlib.med.utah.edu/NetBiochem/NetWelco.htm>

Medical Education (Loyola University):

<URL:http://bsd.meddean.luc.edu:80/lumen/MedEd/Medpage.html>

Professional and academic organizations

Many of the world's major professional and academic medical organizations now promote their activities, publications, and/or examinations on the WWW. These include:

American College of Physicians:

<URL:http://www.acponline.org/>

American Medical Association:

<URL:http://www.ama-assn.org/>

The Royal College of General Practitioners:

<URL:http://www.rcgp.org.uk/>

The Royal College of Surgeons of England:

<URL:http://www.rcseng.ac.uk/>

Research

Other sites focus on research and the dissemination of evidence-based health care information. Examples include:

Centre for Evidence-Based Medicine:

<URL:http://cebm.jr2.ox.ac.uk/>

Cochrane Collaboration (Cochrane Collaboration Informatics Methods Group and McMaster University):

<URL:http://hiru.mcmaster.ca/cochrane/default.htm>

Medical Research Council:

<URL:http://www.nimr.mrc.ac.uk/MRC/>

Special-interest sites

Doctors with interests in the application of new technologies, non-clinical sciences, and other aspects of medicine can explore these interests online:

Primary Health Care Specialist Group (British Computer Society):

<URL:http://www.ncl.ac.uk/~nphcare/PHCSG/phcsg1.htm>

OnLine Images from the History of Medicine (US National Library of Medicine):

<URL:http://wwwoli.nlm.nih.gov/databases/olihmd/olihmd.html>

Textbooks and handbooks online

The advantages of providing medical content on the Web are discussed in Chapter Thirty, *Becoming an information provider*. Many of these advantages, such as full-text searching and hypertext cross-referencing, can be realized through the implementation of online 'books'. The conversion of traditional reference manuals and texts into electronic form, together with the provision of Web-based updates to printed works, is likely to accelerate as doctors latch on to the Internet in greater numbers. Examples are:

Neurosurgery Resident's Online Handbook (University of North Carolina):

<URL:http://sunsite.unc.edu/Neuro/handbook/handbook.html>

The Family Practice Handbook (Mosby-Year Book, Inc. and University of Iowa College of Medicine):

<URL:http://vh.radiology.uiowa.edu/Providers/ClinRef/FPHandbook/FPHomepage.html>

The Merck Manual (Merck & Co., Inc.):

<URL:http://www.merck.com/>

Undergraduate clinical education

Just as educational modules are available for pre-clinical sciences, the clinical sciences are also served. The WWW should not become a substitute for, but rather a supplement to, existing teaching methods:

Primary Care Teaching Modules (Stanford University and University of California at San Francisco):

<URL:http://www.med.stanford.edu/school/DGIM/Teaching/Modules-index.html>

The Online Course in Medical Bacteriology (M. Pallen):

<URL:http://www.qmw.ac.uk/~rhbm001/intro.html>

What is Orthopaedics? (Queen's University, Belfast):

<URL:http://brigit.os.qub.ac.uk/whatis/>

Other ways to use the WWW

To make full use of your browser's features you must specify the name of your mail server and news server in the **Options** panel. You can then send (and perhaps receive) e-mail, subscribe to mailing lists, retrieve files by FTP, read newsgroups, navigate Gopher menus, and search WAIS databases—all from within the comfort of your browser. For all but heavy users of a particular Internet service, Navigator and Internet Explorer are competent enough to negate the need for several dedicated clients if you want to stick to one program.

E-mail and newsgroups

The WWW by e-mail is possible but not recommended if you have access to an interactive alternative such as a WWW client or Telnet. If you are limited to receiving WWW pages by e-mail, try the Webmail service ('**url**' is replaced by the URL of the page you wish to retrieve):

<URL:mailto:webmail@curia.ucc.ie> Send: go url

For information about using WWW search engines such as Lycos and WebCrawler by electronic mail, see Rankin's *Accessing the Internet by e-mail* at:

<URL:mailto:mailbase@mailbase.ac.uk> Send: send lis-iis e-access-inet.txt

As mentioned earlier (p.205), the leading browsers offer e-mail and news-reading facilities. This means you can send messages to anybody whether you are connected to their Web page or not. E-mail was discussed in Chapter Eighteen.

The newsgroup interface provided by current versions of Navigator and Internet Explorer also supports message threading, quotation of articles, and allows you to attach a document to any message you send. Newsgroups were discussed in Chapter Twenty. Fig. 19 shows a news article being read via a Web browser (p.177).

FTP

When you use a Web browser to connect to an FTP site, it presents the file directory as a list of hypertext links. If the link is a file, clicking on it will display or download it. If it is a menu, clicking on the link will change the current directory. Sometimes files are accompanied by an indication of their size, or a brief description. See also Chapter Twenty one.

Telnet

Current WWW browsers do not operate as Telnet clients. To use Telnet (Chapter Twenty two) via your browser, you need to assign a Telnet helper application (p.204). If you have Telnet but not a WWW client, you can Telnet to a text-based WWW client at:

<URL:telnet://lynx@sun1.bham.ac.uk>

Archie

ArchiePlex from NEXOR is an Archie–WWW gateway that finds files on FTP sites:

<URL:http://pubweb.nexor.co.uk/public/archie/servers.html>

Gopher

Like directories on FTP sites, Gopher menus are displayed by WWW browsers as a list of hypertext links and are navigated in the same way. To access a Gopher's search capabilities, forms-compatible WWW browsers display a field into which a search term can be entered. The result of a search is returned as another list of hypertext links. See also Chapter Twenty four.

WAIS

You can search WAIS databases from the WWW using a WAIS–WWW gateway (p.196). You cannot type the URL for a WAIS database directly into the address box using PC or Mac Web clients (this is possible on UNIX systems).

Web-based conferencing

The use of the WWW to support conferencing is discussed in Chapter Twenty eight, p.236.

CHAPTER TWENTY SEVEN

Searching the medical Web

For most people, 'Internet' and 'World-Wide Web' are synonymous. Indeed, it would not be untrue to say that if you cannot find something through the WWW, then that something is not on the Internet. The WWW provides an interface to various forms of medical information on the Internet in many ingenious ways. Broadly speaking, it does this through different kinds of catalogues or directories, and search engines.

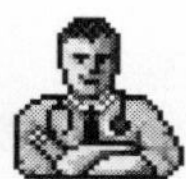

If you are looking for nonspecific resources or general information, a directory is a good place to start. For a more focused search, start with a search engine.

WWW-based directories

There are several large multi-subject catalogues of Internet resources that cover medical topics, often dividing resources by clinical specialty or general health and medical subject headings. Most are also linked to powerful search engines (programs that look for information in response to a query). Search engines are covered under the next subheading; directories characteristically lend themselves to 'casual browsing'. The biggest advantage of manually created directories is the ability to include an annotation describing the resource—although not all directories choose to do this. When present, such annotations constitute a rudimentary form of peer review (see also *Standards and peer review*, p.116).

Other directories focus specifically on medicine and health care, again, usually indexing resources by medical specialty or broad subject. In general, these catalogues are more discriminating about which sites they index. Some medical catalogues aim to provide features such as annotations, fast search engines, more effective subject organization, or even training and documentation.

The most developed specialist index in the UK is OMNI (Organizing Medical Networked Information), funded by the Joint Information Systems Committee (JISC) and operated by a consortium including the British Medical Association Library, Medical Research Council, Wellcome Centre for Medical Science, and others. It is a searchable subject-based catalogue of UK and global medical education and research resources, providing a brief description of each resource:

<URL:http://omni.ac.uk/>

The NHSweb Directory is being developed for NHSnet (p.137) users, indexing resources on NHSweb (the NHS intranet, p.113) and the Internet.

Medical Matrix from Healthtel Corporation, with the support of the Internet Working Group of the American Medical Informatics Association, categorizes clinical Internet resources into specialties, journals, education resources, etc., that can be used free at the point of care. It can be browsed or searched at:

<URL:http://www.slackinc.com/matrix>

Another popular and well-supported North American resource is MedWeb from the Emory University Health Sciences Center Library:

<URL:http://www.emory.edu/WHSCL/medweb.html>

CIC HealthWeb (Committee for Institutional Cooperation) is a cooperative project by the 'Big Ten' US university health-science libraries cataloguing medical specialty resources, and those in health and basic sciences:

<URL:http://www.ghsl.nwu.edu/healthweb/>

Alternatives to annotation

Another approach has been to attempt to map individual Web pages to the MeSH terms (p.241) used to index articles in MEDLINE. Although MeSH indexing can be done manually, Fowler *et al.* (1995) have described their experiments using a 'Web-MeSH Medibot', an automated tool for assigning MeSH terms to WWW pages. Although further development is needed, such a Medibot could be used to create a static index for organizing information, or as a search engine operated via a WWW browser. The Internet could eventually become a 'second MEDLINE' in its own right, complete with familiar options to refine and combine searches, etc.

CliniWeb, from the Oregon Health Sciences University, is a browsable index of clinically relevant information at the level of individual WWW pages, using the MeSH disease tree. Searches are mapped to the closest available MeSH term:

<URL:http://www.ohsu.edu/cliniweb/>

In Europe a similar service is provided by the Library and Medical Information Center at the Karolinska Institute in Stockholm:

<URL:http://www.mic.ki.se/Diseases/index.html>

Meta-directories

There are now so many catalogues that, in true Internet fashion, catalogues of catalogues have become necessary (known as meta-directories). An example is the Hardin Meta-Directory from the Hardin Library for the Health Sciences, University of Iowa:

<URL:http://www.arcade.uiowa.edu/hardin-www/md.html>

WWW-based search engines

Search engines accessed via a Web page use fill-out forms (p.207) to enter the search terms and criteria. Typically terms are entered into a text box, with modifications to search parameters made via pull-down menus, check boxes, etc. Clicking on the 'Search' button (or equivalent) will return a hypertext page of links to files meeting your search criteria (known as 'hits'). Rather than a simple list of file names or URLs, many search engines provide a small extract or other information about the file. Hits can be ranked in order of relevancy, calculated by the frequency with which the terms appear in a document, their proximity to one another, or their relative position in a Web page (e.g. in a header).

There are numerous individual search engines available. Each search engine operates differently and consequently has different strengths and weaknesses depending on what you are looking for. These tools may index WWW page titles, URLs, existing indexes, and often the actual content of documents (see Fig. 29). Some include newsgroup postings, files in FTP archives, and Gopher menu items—perhaps even by way of a multilingual search form. Some search for individual keywords, others for phrases or the co-occurrence of terms. Some allow searches with wild cards or Boolean operators. Some engines allow limited searches for free, with further functionality available upon subscription. Example search engines follow; all of these tools will tell you about themselves, so these details have been omitted here:

AltaVista (Digital Equipment Corporation):

<URL:http://altavista.digital.com/>

Excite (Excite, Inc.):

<URL:http://www.excite.com/>

Infoseek (InfoSeek Corporation):

<URL:http://www.infoseek.com/>

Lycos (Carnegie Mellon University):

<URL:http://www.lycos.com/>

Open Text (Open Text Corporation):

<URL:http://www.opentext.com>

WebCrawler (America Online, Inc.):

<URL:http://webcrawler.com/>

Yahoo! (Yahoo!):

<URL:http://www.yahoo.com/>

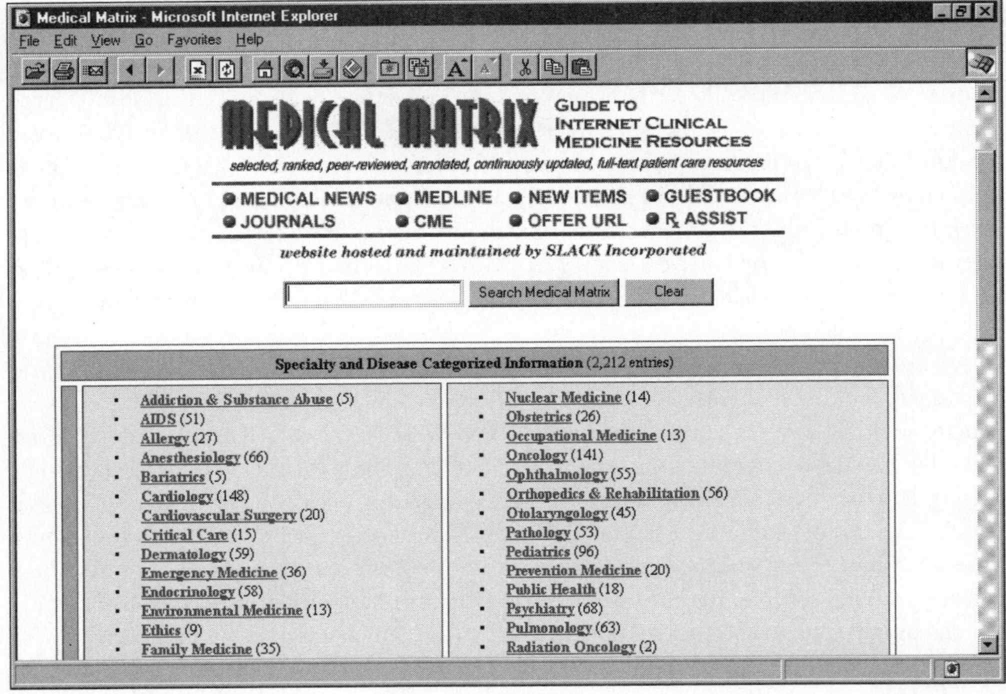

Fig. 29 Searching the medical Web. Some search engines such as Medical Matrix (shown) are integrated with a browsable directory. [Reproduced with permission.]

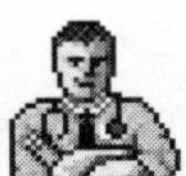

Familiarize yourself with the capabilities of the index you choose; all have help pages explaining the various search options. This author has found AltaVista and Open Text to be particularly useful tools.

There are also search engines that confine themselves to medical information. Many of the specialist medical directories mentioned above are also searchable. WWW-based MEDLINE searches are considered in Chapter Twenty nine. Another example is MediS from Docnet, a search facility for manually indexed abstracts and articles from major medical journals such as the *BMJ*, *Journal of the American Medical Association*, and the *New England Journal of Medicine*:

<URL:http://www.docnet.org.uk/medis/search.html>

In yet another approach, Health On the Net Foundation's Marvin search engine employs a 12 000 word medical dictionary to search out documents containing medical terms, using word weighting and word counts to determine relevance. Users search the resultant smaller (yet hopefully more specific) database, rather than the Internet at large. A database of reviewed sites is also available:

MedHunt (Health On the Net Foundation):

<URL:http://www.hon.ch/cgi-bin/find>

Meta-search engines

An easy way to access multiple search engines is to use a 'meta-search engine', or a page that allows you to search several individual engines simultaneously. Although convenient, such searches don't offer the flexibility to alter search criteria as would an individual engine. Example meta-search engines are:

All-in-one Search Page (William Cross):

<URL:http://www.albany.net/allinone/>

CUSI (NEXOR):

<URL:http://pubweb.nexor.co.uk/public/cusi/cusi.html>

SavvySearch (Daniel Drelinger):

<URL:http://guaraldi.cs.colostate.edu:2000/>

Other ways to locate information

Remember that not all information on the Internet is located on the WWW. However, the WWW can provide a familiar interface to help you find relevant newsgroup postings (p.177), Gopher items (p.194), frequently asked questions files (p.178), people (p.158), files in FTP archives (p.182), and information indexed by WAIS (p.196).

Intelligent agents

In the near future so-called 'intelligent agents' (information-seeking programs) could be directed to roam the Internet scanning for items of interest on the user's behalf. Their 'artificial intelligence' lies in the ability to adapt subsequent search patterns based on the results of earlier searches. With such an agent looking for items matching the users individual information requirements with a high degree of specificity, the clinician need concentrate only on absorbing information—not finding it.

Reference

Fowler, J., Kouramajian, V., Maram, S., and Devadhar, V. (1995). Automated MeSH indexing of the World Wide Web. In *Proceedings of the Nineteenth Annual Symposium on Computer Applications in Medical Care*, pp.893–7. American Medical Informatics Association, Bethesda.

CHAPTER TWENTY EIGHT

Other ways to communicate

Internet Relay Chat

Internet Relay Chat, or IRC, is a means of communicating with other people over the Internet using messages typed on your keyboard. Unlike e-mail, this communication takes place in real time (i.e. it is 'live'). Both parties require a Telnet facility or an IRC client and must be connected to an IRC server (such as **irc.demon.co.uk**).

Early IRC clients used simple text-only windows and users were required to learn a number of IRC commands. Newer clients use a more graphically orientated interface featuring pull-down menus and buttons, and come in many varieties.

Some clients (such as WorldsAway) allow participants in a conversation to interact in the form of an animated online persona known as an **avatar**, enabling facial expressions and gestures, as they roam around a virtual environment.

Other clients work as helper applications (p.204) in conjunction with your Web browser so that hypertext links within a Web page will launch the IRC client and connect to the appropriate chat server and channel (see below). Global Chat from Quarterdeck Corporation is an example of such an IRC helper application. PC and Mac versions can be downloaded from:

<URL:http://www.qdeck.com/chat/>

The Netscape plug-in (p.204) ichat, from ichat Inc., integrates IRC directly into a frame (p.207) within the WWW page itself. PC and Mac versions can be downloaded from:

<URL:http://www.ichat.com/>

The WebDoctor Chat Room from Gretmar Communications provides a chat window in the form of a Java applet (p.207):

<URL:http://www.gretmar.com/webdoctor/chat.html>

Configuring a conventional IRC client typically requires you to specify your real name, a nickname, the domain name of the server, and its port number (usually **6667**). IRC servers carry many global **channels** with names prefixed by **#**, one of which you must join before you can participate in or initiate a conversation. Public channels, open to anyone, are joined using the **/join** command (for example, **/join #irchelp**—the help channel). You can see what channels are available by typing **/list**. Once you have joined a channel just type a message and hit the **Enter/Return** key: your message will appear in the channel window (see Fig. 30). Popular channels can be extremely confusing, with lines of text from many simultaneous conversations intermingled.

Luckily anyone can set up a new channel in order to hold a more focused discussion. This is done simply by typing **/join #channelname**, where **channelname** is any unique name you choose. The dialogue can be recorded and saved on to disk as a text file. Note that you can send a private message (visible only to the recipient) on any channel by typing **/msg nickname**, substituting the nickname of the person to whom you wish to chat. Clients that support DCC (Direct Client-to-Client) can be used to exchange files or private messages by establishing a direct link between two IRC clients. For instructions, type **/help dcc**.

IRC potentially provides a very inexpensive means for geographically isolated or distant health professionals to talk in real time. This is especially true in relation to doctors from the underdeveloped world who could converse with distant colleagues in real time without prohibitive communications costs. While most channels host impromptu conversations, others occur at prearranged times. Informal chat is available on Undernet (one of the IRC networks) most of the time for people with chronic fatigue syndrome/myalgic encephalomyelitis, although there are also scheduled 'meetings' (**eu.undernet.org**, port **6667**, channel **#CFS**).

> *FAQ: CFS IRC Internet Relay Chat*:
> **<URL:ftp://rtfm.mit.edu/pub/usenet/news.answers/medicine/chronic-fatigue-syndrome/cfs-irc>**

Undernet also plays host to an international paediatric chat session. The 'International pediatric chat home instruction page' is at:

> **<URL:http://www.peds.umn.edu/deptinfo/irc.html>**

For more general information about IRC, see *IRC Frequently Asked Questions*:

> **<URL:http://www.kei.com/irc.html>**

MOOs

Multi-User Dungeons (MUDs, sometimes called Multi-User Dimensions) originated as a text-based role-playing game in which any number of users could register a 'character' and interact with each other in a virtual environment. **MOOs** (MUD, Object-Oriented) evolved from MUDs and, as the name suggests, treat everything (including characters) as a virtual object that can be examined or manipulated within a virtual room. La Porte *et al*. (1995) envisage a MOO where health researchers can browse articles in a public health room, strike up conversations, and take classes in which they interact and exchange research communications with others.

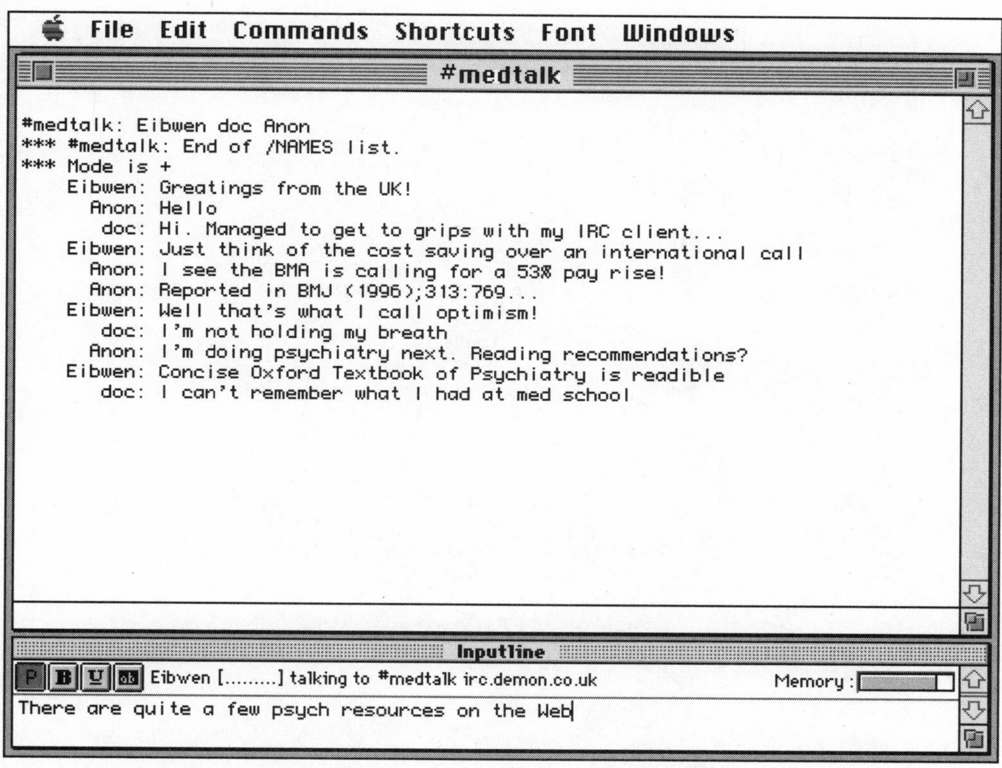

Fig. 30 Internet Relay Chat (IRC) permits distant users to communicate in real-time typing for the cost of a local telephone call.

MOOs already exist to support real-time electronic conferencing and virtual classrooms on the Internet, and users can record all conversations which they have participated in. MOOs can be accessed by Telnet (p.183) or with a dedicated MUD client. A well-known example is BioMOO from the Bioinformatics Unit at the Weizmann Institute of Science in Israel. BioMOO also has a gateway for concomitant Web access, allowing multimedia attachments to MOO objects such as graphics or sound clips. This provides for point-and-click exploration of the virtual BioCenter building (see Fig. 31), although Telnet is still required for real-time interaction between characters (users).

BioMOO:

<URL:telnet://bioinfo.weizmann.ac.il 8888>

<URL:http://bioinformatics.weizmann.ac.il/BioMOO>

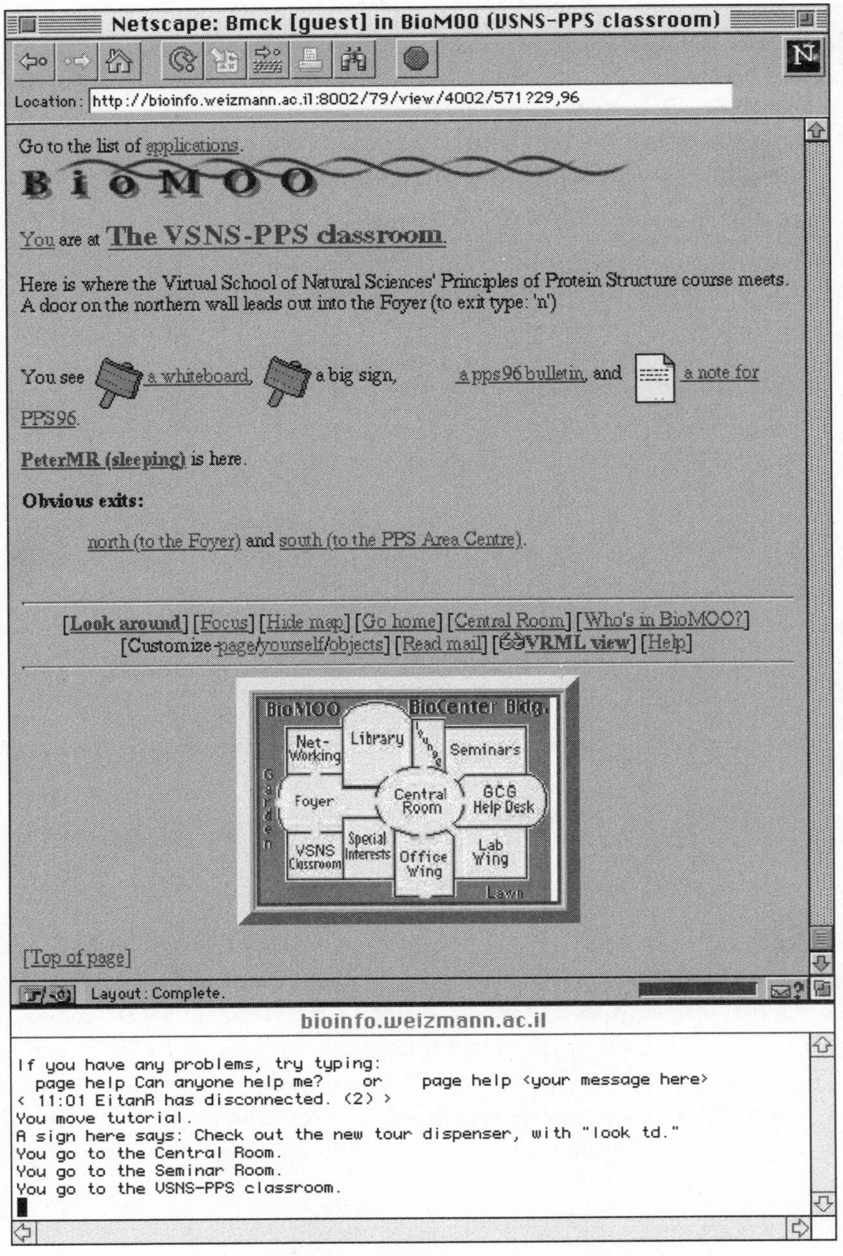

Fig. 31 Exploring BioMOO. After initiating a text-only Telnet connection to BioMOO, users can opt to open a multimedia Web window. Telnet is used for real-time conversations, while the 'virtual environment' can easily be manipulated using point-and-click (e.g. click on the map to 'teleport' to a different room). [Reproduced with permission.]

Streaming audio

Several technologies now exist that change the way we can use sound on the Internet. RealAudio from Progressive Networks is a well-known example that provides on-demand **streaming audio**. Sound is heard throughout transmission (downloading) as a continuously processed stream of data, much like sound transmitted by a radio station (it is not necessary to wait until the entire clip has been transmitted before it can be played). It is 'on-demand' because unlike a radio station, audio clips can be played in any order at any time as determined by listener selection. The RealAudio Player includes a plug-in to enable the reception of streaming audio while you simultaneously browse the WWW:

<URL:http://www.realaudio.com>

Streaming audio over the Internet has many potential applications in medicine. It has been used to narrate an online slide presentation about radiotherapy in paediatric brain tumours (see Fig. 32), to deliver commentary on reproductive health issues, and may permit distance learning through 'on-demand' broadcasting of tutorials, etc:

Radiation Therapy for Pediatric Brain Tumors (J.W. Goldwein, University of Pennsylvania Cancer Center):

<URL:http://goldwein1.xrt.upenn.edu/ASTRO95/framed.htm>

Atlanta Reproductive Health Centre WWW home page (M. Perloe):

<URL:http://www.ivf.com/>

Even over relatively slow Internet connections this technology can provide sound quality comparable to AM radio; this may degrade over transatlantic links but is often still at least as good as short wave radio. Perhaps the biggest advantage is that it avoids the need to download large files.

Internet telephony and videoconferencing

Internet users with a multimedia computer (i.e. sound card, speakers, and a microphone) can use it like a telephone—but without international call charges. Somewhat more complicated than using a real telephone, **Internet telephony** works by digitizing and compressing speech for transmission to users with similar software that will decompress and play it back in real time. There are also online equivalents of telephone address books. The receiver must, however, be online at the same time as the sender to take the call, unless he or she has a product offering a 'virtual answerphone'.

Software for Internet telephony is available in free and commercial forms for all platforms. Note that a full-duplex sound card is required for simultaneous two-way conversation. A half-duplex sound card (more common) will permit one person to speak at a time. The use

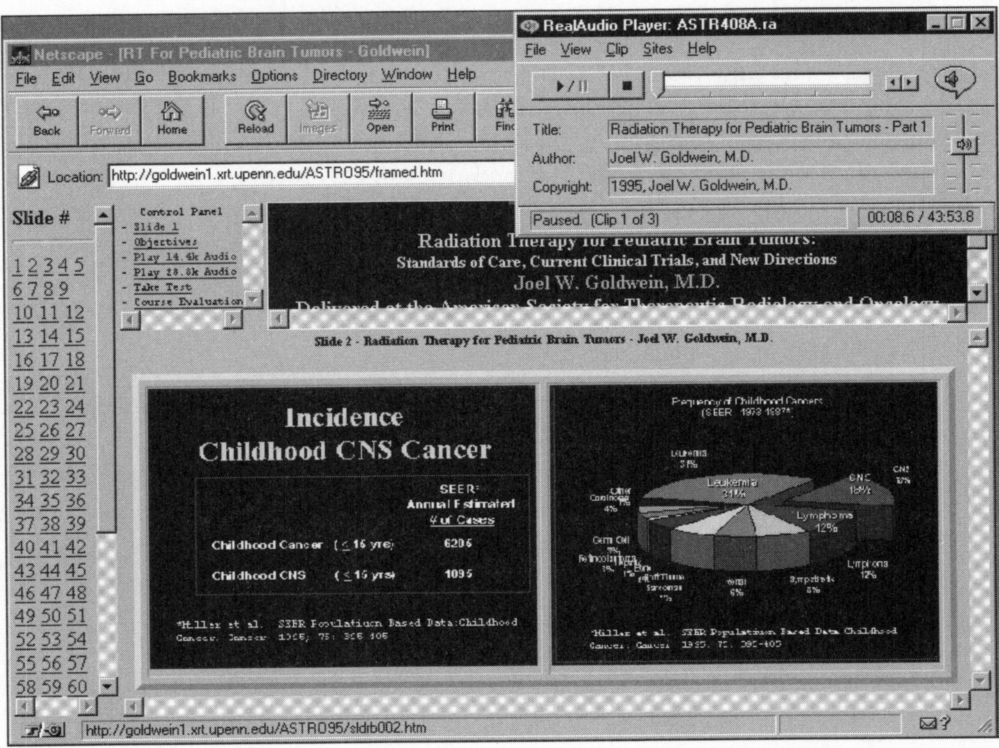

Fig. 32 Using streaming audio to narrate an online slide presentation about radiotherapy in paediatric brain tumours. The 'slides' are changed automatically to keep pace with the narration. [Screen capture: Assoc. Prof. Joel W. Goldwein.]

of a product with a 'whiteboarding' feature (a window that two or more users can draw in) enables users to illustrate points more clearly. VocalTec's Internet Phone software is shown in Fig. 33.

<URL:http://www.vocaltec.com/>

Some Internet telephony products allow one user to speak to several others simultaneously for conferencing. With the added ability to handle video, a small inexpensive video camera, and a high-bandwidth Internet connection (i.e. ISDN or better), videoconferencing is possible. An example videoconferencing program is Cu-SeeMe from White Pine Software:

<URL:http://www.cu-seeme.com/>

Because some of these products use different standards to digitize and compress voice and video, conversations between users of different products may not be possible. Sound and video quality is highly variable, but such products provide remote collaboration at a fraction of the cost of direct ISDN links or satellite link ups. For more information, see *FAQ: How do I use the Internet as a telephone?* (K. Savetz):

<URL:http://www.northcoast.com/savetz/voice-faq.html>

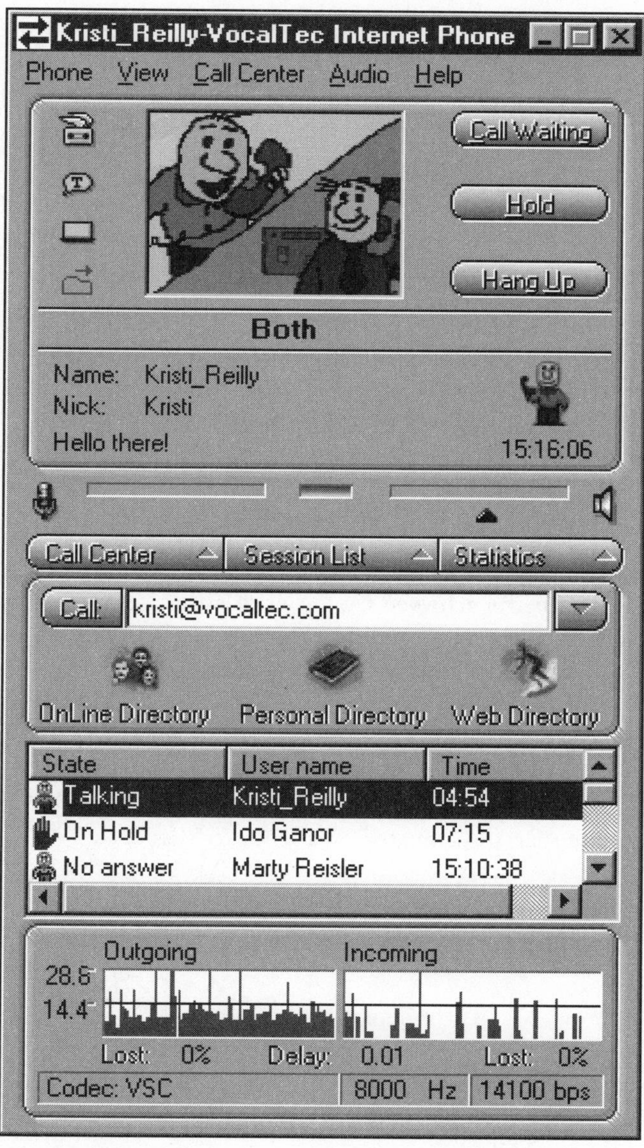

Fig. 33 Internet telephony using VocalTec's Internet Phone software. [Screen capture: VocalTec.]

In addition to the Internet Protocol (IP) service, the JANET infrastructure (p.136) supports ATM and Mbone, both of which can be used for videoconferencing. Asynchronous Transfer Mode (**ATM**) networks are used by the Interactive Teaching Project in Surgery to allow students to watch operations and interact with their teachers in real time from remote locations:

<URL:http://av.avc.ucl.ac.uk/tltp/insurrect.html>

The Multicast Backbone of the Internet (**Mbone**) was used by the Multimedia Integrated Conferencing for Europe (MICE) project in 1994 to demonstrate live video of minimally-invasive surgery over the Internet (Bennett 1996). Although the variable bandwidth typical of Internet connections does not provide the guaranteed bandwidth of a direct connection, the results were encouraging enough to secure ongoing development:

<URL:http://www-mice.cs.ucl.ac.uk/merci/>

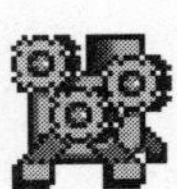

ATM networks use 'virtual channels' within a shared physical link to distribute data to several sites simultaneously (a technique called 'multiplexing'). Mbone is a 'virtual network' running over the Internet using its own **routers** to 'tunnel' data from one network to many simultaneously (a technique known as '**multicasting**').

Web-based conferencing

Conferencing need not rely on telephony or audiovisual communication; in many cases effective collaberation is better achieved via the written word. Some systems based on real-time typing (such as IRC plug-ins, or Telnet applets) are so closely integrated with the WWW that it is tempting to include them under the heading of Web-based conferencing. However, Web-based conferencing is generally taken to involve **asynchronous** messaging (along the lines of bulletin-board forums or newsgroups, for example). This is important to doctors who can then participate in ongoing discussions without the necessity to be online at a particular time (or to meet travel costs). It also means that exchanges are, in general, less impulsive than those made in real-time discussion.

A number of Web-based conferencing systems have recently become available. These systems address some of the shortcomings in communicating by mailing lists or newsgroups. It is very difficult to follow dialogue on a range of topics posted to a single list, and the propagation of multiple copies of newsgroup postings around the world wastes Internet bandwidth and hard disk space. In contrast, multi-topic conferences can be hosted on a single Web server.

A basic tenet of any conferencing system is the ability to organize messages into topics with threaded replies (see p.173). Using forms (p.207) to generate and manage messages, Web-based conferencing presents a familiar cross-platform interface and provides for several enhancements via hypertext. For example, LARG*net uses the Caucus package (from Screen Porch) to host a nuclear medicine discussion (among others). Users can dress-up a message with HTML (p.199) and thereby incoporate images, tables, and links to files for downloading or to other Web sites, etc. The system tracks which messages have been read by a given user through the use of a log-in password. The E.D.iscuss conferencing system based at Massachusetts General Hospital (using WebBoard from O'Reilly & Associations, Inc.) is another example:

LARG*net conferencing system (University of Western Ontario):

<URL:http://johns.largnet.uwo.ca/~caucus/LARGNET/>

E.D.iscuss (MGH Department of Emergency Medicine):

<URL:http://emergency.mgh.harvard.edu/ediscuss.html>

Conferencing on the Web is arguably present in more limited forms such as Hypermail, which converts mailing list articles into hypertext Web pages, and the Navigator browser, which does the same for newsgroup postings (see Fig.19, p.177).

Internet fax

Several services, both free and commercial, offer a facility to convert e-mail into fax format. In this way faxes can be sent without international call rates to those who have a fax machine but not a connection to the Internet. For more information, see *FAQ: How can I send a fax from the Internet?* (K. Savetz):

<URL:http://www.northcoast.com/savetz/fax-faq.html>

References

Bennett, R. (1996). In *Demonstrating minimal invasive therapy over the Internet*, European Congress of the Internet in Medicine Programme and Abstracts, (ed. Arvanitis, T.N., Baldock, C., Lutkin, J., Vincent, R. and Watson, D.), pp. 40–1. University of Sussex, Brighton.

La Porte, R.E., Marler, E., Akazawa, S., Sauer, F., Gamboa, C., Shenton, C., *et al.* (1995). The death of biomedical journals. *BMJ*, **310**, 1387–90.

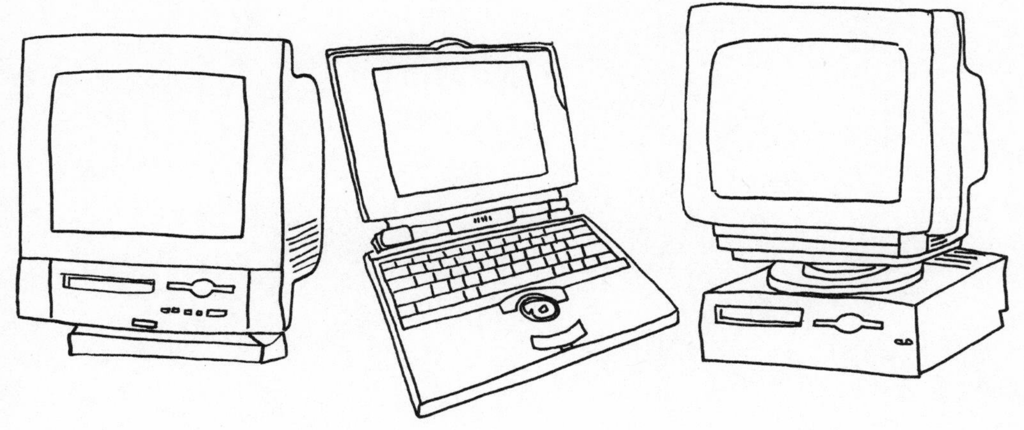

PART 5

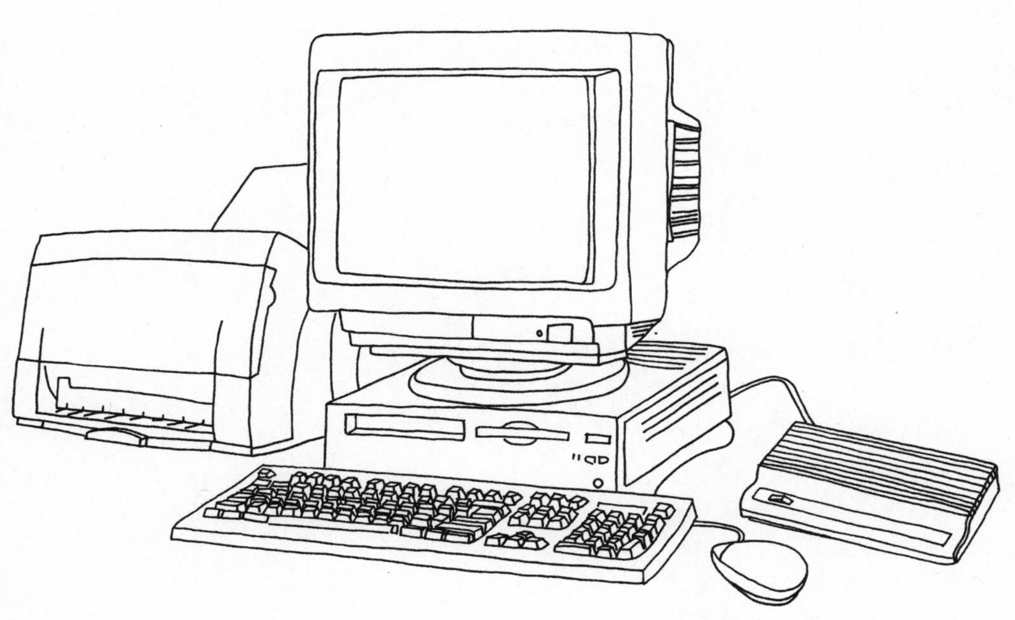

CHAPTER TWENTY NINE
MEDLINE by modem

Many readers will have thumbed through the heavy tomes of *Index Medicus*, the printed biomedical bibliography from the National Library of Medicine (NLM) in the United States. Others will have used MEDLINE on CD-ROM. Students and clinicians alike are increasingly required to back their decisions with reference to peer-reviewed literature, particularly since the advent of evidence-based medicine—'the process of systematically finding, appraising, and using contemporaneous research findings as the basis for clinical decisions' (Rosenberg and Donald 1995). Indeed, it has been said that 'rapid and effective access to the biomedical literature via MEDLINE is at times critical to sound patient care and favorably influences patient outcomes' (Lindberg *et al.* 1993). Rather than visit your local university campus or hospital to conduct such a search, it is possible to achieve the same result from your home or surgery PC.

MEDLARS

The MEDical Literature Analysis and Retrieval System (MEDLARS) is a collection of over forty databases from the National Library of Medicine (NLM). MEDLARS itself is divided into two subsystems, called ELHILL (which includes MEDLINE) and TOXNET.

MEDLINE

MEDLINE (MEDlars onLINE) is the largest biomedical bibliographic database, incorporating the printed Index Medicus, Index to Dental Literature, and the International Nursing Index. It covers almost 4000 international journals from 1966 to date. These journals cover all medical and surgical specialities and preclinical sciences, in addition to dentistry, nursing, pharmacology, nutrition, and health-service administration. About seventy per cent of the records include abstracts. MEDLINE searches can be printed, stored on disk, or imported into a bibliographic management program such as EndNote or Pro-Cite.

Searches automatically make use of the **MeSH** (Medical Subject Headings) thesaurus, a 'keyword' system which maps the users own words to terms in the MeSH index for searching. The MeSH thesaurus can also be used manually by the operator to narrow or widen the search on the basis of very specific criteria. For example, 'shock' could be further qualified with 'cardiogenic'.

A more recent development is the Unified Medical Language System (UMLS) Metathesaurus:

<URL:http://www.nlm.nih.gov/publications/factsheets/umls_metathesaurus.html>

The NLM's Metathesaurus contains information about terms and their co-occurrence in numerous classification systems or 'controlled vocabularies' (such as the *Diagnostic and Statistical Manual of Mental Disorders*, *International Classification of Diseases*, etc.)—in addition to those in the familiar MeSH hierarchy. A user's search term can thus be mapped to the equivalent term(s) in any of the indexed vocabularies, providing even greater control over search parameters. For example, a psychiatrist might enter familiar terms from the DSM vocabulary which could be mapped to MeSH equivalents.

Why MEDLINE by modem?

Searching MEDLINE over telecommunications links has a number of distinct advantages. Compared to a locally available system based on CD-ROM, MEDLINE by modem requires less investment in hardware (since all that is required is a fairly basic PC and modem) and consequently, perhaps, in technical support. A remotely updated database does away with reliance on a regular supply of updates on CD-ROM. Because it can be accessed from a variety of locations (work, home, library, etc.) it is available to a wider audience. As a twenty-four hour service, it can be utilized when most convenient. Furthermore, search results can be saved directly on to the user's own computer.

British Medical Association MEDLINE service

Aside from the cost of British Medical Association membership and usual telephone charges, this MEDLINE service is otherwise free.

The service is based on the Ovid MEDLINE interface. Basic navigation (if using terminal emulation to access the service) requires the use of arrow keys to move up and down a list of choices, a single key to select and deselect items, and several two-key combination commands. Search results may be downloaded to disk. A detailed Ovid user guide is supplied as part of a start-up Information Pack. Photocopies can be requested by e-mail, fax, or phone.

Almost any terminal emulation package can be used to access the service (Fig. 34). The BMA Library has produced a detailed guide to configuring several popular PC and Mac terminal communications packages for use with the service. The following settings should work with any package: Speed to 28 800 bps, 8 data bits, no parity, 1 stop bit, hardware handshake, full duplex, VT100 terminal type, and local echo off. ASCII, Kermit, Xmodem, Ymodem, and Zmodem are all supported for downloading search results. Unfortunately some VT100 emulators are not 100 per cent compatible with the system.

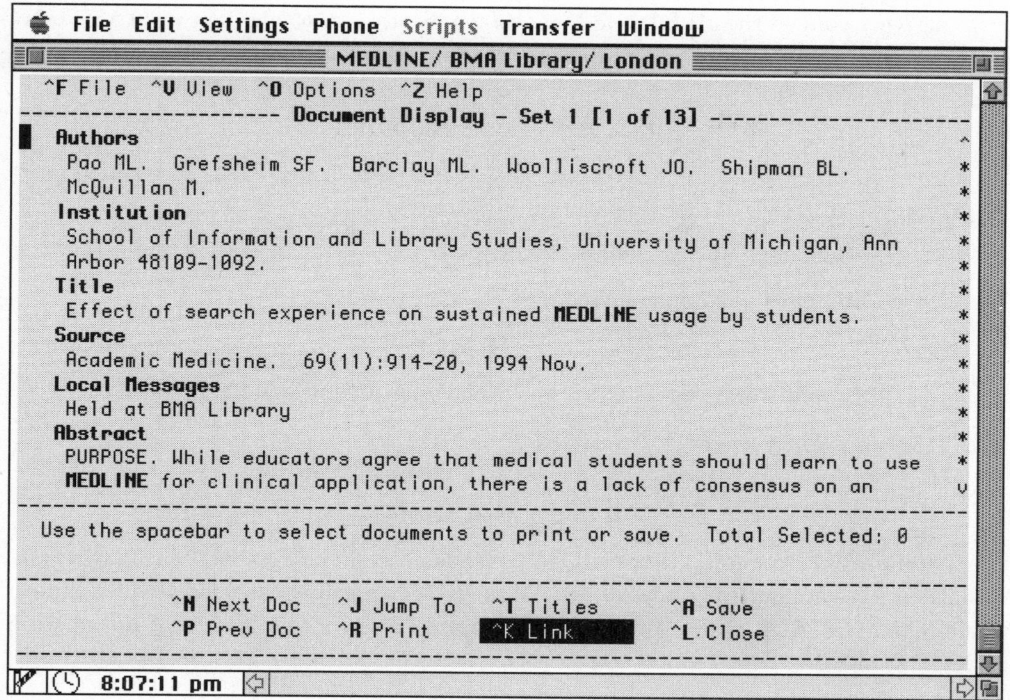

Fig. 34 Using VT100 terminal emulation to access the BMA's OVID 3.0 DOS MEDLINE service. Citations can be saved to your local disk or printed. [Reproduced with permission.]

Access via the Internet using Ovid client software for Windows is currently available. Access using your preferred WWW browser, and online ordering of photocopy requests, is also planned.

For further information, contact the BMA Library, BMA House, Tavistock Square, London WC1H 9JP (tel. 0171 383 6224 or fax 0171 388 2544), or send e-mail to **bma-library@bma.org.uk**.

National Library of Medicine services

The NLM offers three types of account to US customers, each requiring an access code. They are the MEDLARS, AIDS, and Student (half-price access to MEDLARS) codes. The application forms for all three accounts (and Grateful Med software—see below) can be retrieved from:

<URL:http://www.nlm.nih.gov/top_level.dir/accounts.html>

Alternatively, contact the MEDLARS Management Section, National Library of Medicine, Bethesda, MD 20894, USA (where completed applications should be sent).

MEDLARS code accounts

This gives access to all of the ELHILL databases, TOXNET, and PDQ. Registered users can access the NLM via Telnet. You can do this directly:

<URL:telnet://login@medlars.nlm.nih.gov>

<URL:telnet://toxnet.nlm.nih.gov>

Alternatively, establish a connection via the NLM's WWW pages (called HyperDOC) at:

<URL:http://www.nlm.nih.gov/top_level.dir/nlm_online_info.html>

This URL also works for the AIDS databases.

AIDS code accounts

The NLM provides free access to the AIDS-related databases. These are AIDSLINE (research, clinical aspects and health policy issues), AIDSDRUGS (agents being evaluated in clinical trials), AIDSTRIALS (clinical trials), and an online directory of sources of information called DIRLINE.

<URL:telnet://login@medlars.nlm.nih.gov>

Grateful Med

The NLM's Grateful Med software can be used over the Internet (or a direct connection) to improve on the basic Telnet interface to a MEDLARS/TOXNET/PDQ account. Search terms for MEDLINE (and most other databases) can be pre-selected before opening a connection to the NLM. The search result is downloaded to your computer for offline viewing within the program, which allows the marking of relevant articles and will suggest MeSH terms to employ in a subsequent search. A 'Loansome Doc' facility allows US users to request copies of relevant papers from participating libraries. Clients are available for the PC and Mac at $US29.95, and searches are charged at a rate of approximately $US18 per hour. Help is available by sending e-mail to **gmhelp@gmedserv.nlm.nih.gov**.

Internet Grateful Med

Internet Grateful Med is a gateway to MEDLINE with a WWW interface, requiring a MEDLARS account ID and password (Fig. 35).

<URL:http://igm.nlm.nih.gov/>

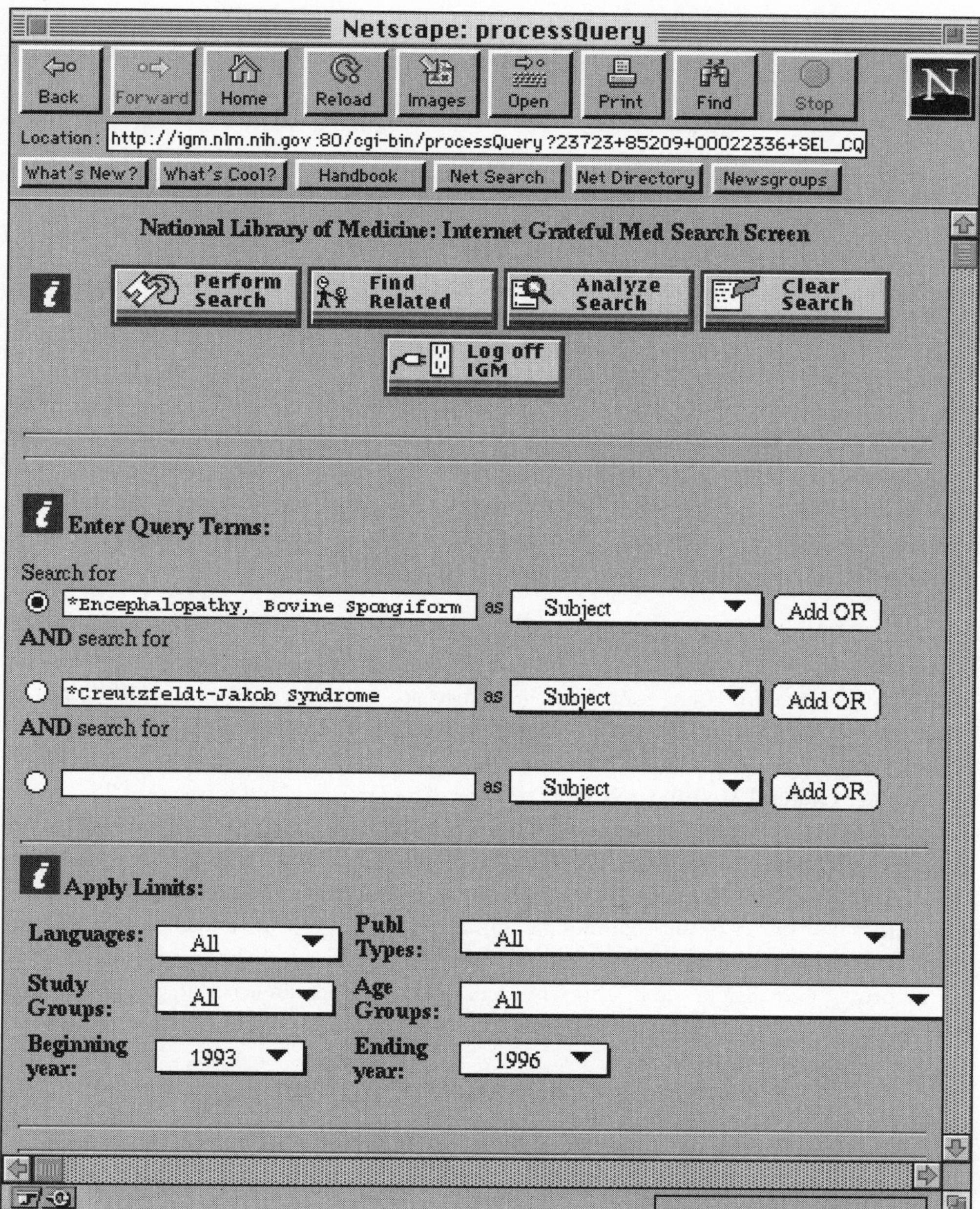

Fig. 35 Internet Grateful Med, a WWW-based interface to MEDLINE. [Screen capture: National library of Medicine.]

As well as the usual MEDLINE search options, the system can map a user's search term (such as mad cow disease) to terms indexed by the UMLS Metathesaurus (in this case—Encephalopathy, Bovine Spongiform).

The Metathesaurus also produces hypertext links to other online databases, including Agency for Health Care Policy and Research *Clinical Practice Guidelines* and online images from the History of Medicine Division at the NLM. Search results can be sent direct to a printer (from the Web browser menu), saved to disk, or sent to an e-mail address. For more information, contact the Internet Grateful Med Development Team at **access@nlm.nih.gov**.

Access to NLM databases for international customers

The National Library of Medicine (NLM) does not presently allow non-US users to open direct accounts, although this is expected to change (requiring a TCP/IP connection and credit card). Details will be available from the MEDLARS Management Section at **mms@nlm.nih.gov**. Currently, indirect access outside of the US is coordinated by International MEDLARS Centers. A list of these centres is available on the HyperDOC Web pages.

The British Library is one of these centres. In the UK the service is called BLAISE-LINK. It involves running a terminal emulator or Grateful Med on your local computer, and establishing a modem connection to an intermediatory network (Mercury 5000 or BT's DIALPLUS). When the link is established, the call is routed to the NLM in the US. Alternatively, if you have TCP/IP Internet access you can Telnet directly to the NLM, or use Internet Grateful Med and a WWW browser. The Grateful Med software (£55 + VAT) and a BLAISE-LINK password can be obtained from The Health Care Information Service, The British Library, Science Reference and Information Service, Boston Spa, Wetherby, West Yorkshire LS23 7BQ, tel. 01937 546 364, e-mail **BLINK-helpdesk@bl.uk**. Pricing structure is complicated, but includes an annual subscription (£61 + VAT), connect-time fee (£20 per hour + VAT for MEDLINE), and other charges based on the number of citations, offline prints, and searches, etc. You would also need to open an account with a network provider.

Ovid Online and Ovid Web Gateway

Ovid Technologies, Inc., offer a number of databases (including MEDLINE) through its Ovid Online service. Customers can choose between fixed-fee or pay-as-you-go access using either VT100 emulation (Table 4, p.28) and a carrier such as SprintNet or MCI (see also the BMA's service, above), or the Internet. The Ovid Web Gateway interface consists of a series of Web pages containing text fields and buttons that are used to send search requests and commands to the Ovid server. Thus, a forms-compatible Web browser (p.207) is necessary to use the service.

<URL:http://www.ovid.com/>

The Web interface (Fig. 36) closely matches the existing Ovid client interface, featuring the ability to search by keyword, author, title, or journal, to combine or limit searches, and online help. As of writing it is not possible to use the MeSH thesaurus although this omission is expected to be addressed in a future version of the Gateway.

Displayed MEDLINE references may link directly to searchable full-text articles with an outline and references in hypertext, complete with linked high-resolution illustrations (where Ovid have permission from the copyright owner). These articles/graphics can then be saved on to your hard disk as normal (p.202). Alternatively, users can click the appropriate button to have the citation and abstracts of articles they have selected sent to them by electronic mail in a choice of format (or simply display them on screen or save them to disk).

For further information, contact Ovid Technologies Ltd., 1 Lamington Street, London W6 0HU, tel. 0181 748 3777, or e-mail **london@ovid.co.uk**.

PaperChase

PaperChase was developed at Boston's Beth Israel Hospital, part of Harvard Medical School. It provides an interface to the MEDLINE, *Health Planning and Administration* (HealthSTAR), and AIDSLINE databases from the NLM, and to the National Cancer Institute's CANCERLIT database, in addition to the *Cumulative Index to Nursing and Allied Health Literature* (CINAHL). Because the interface is menu based, there are few commands to remember. PaperChase offers the most common criterion for narrowing a search simply by typing **LIMIT** at the **LOOK FOR:** prompt. A WWW interface is under development.

All databases (including article abstracts) can be searched simultaneously, past searches are automatically saved, and search terms are mapped to MeSH headings. Search results can be combined, viewed online, printed, or saved to disk. Photocopies or faxed articles can be supplied. Further information is available from PaperChase, 350 Longwood Avenue, Boston, MA 02115, USA, or send e-mail to **info@www.paperchase.com**.

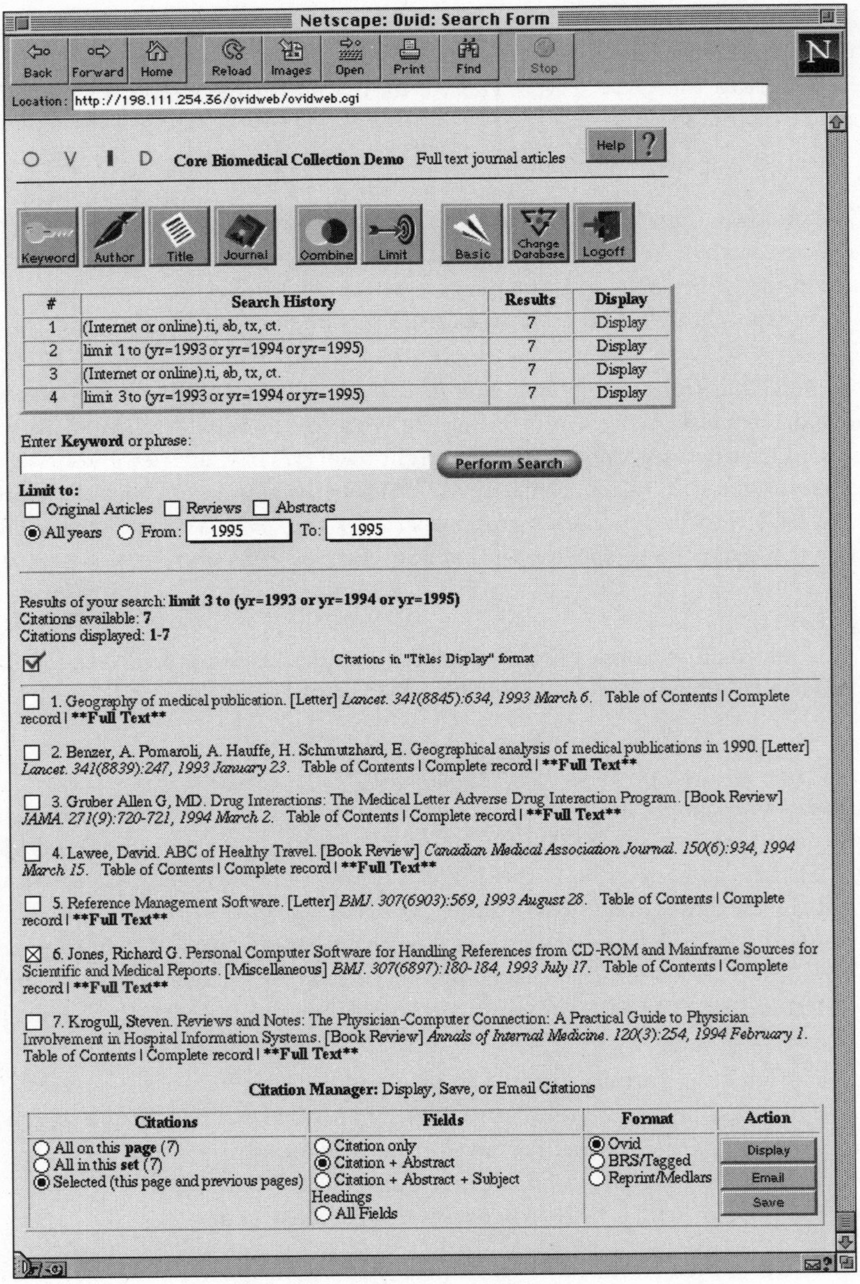

Netscape: Ovid: Search Form

Back | Forward | Home | Reload | Images | Open | Print | Find | Stop

Location: http://198.111.254.36/ovidweb/ovidweb.cgi

O V I D **Core Biomedical Collection Demo** Full text journal articles Help ?

Keyword | Author | Title | Journal | Combine | Limit | Basic | Change Database | Logoff

#	Search History	Results	Display
1	(Internet or online).ti, ab, tx, ct.	7	Display
2	limit 1 to (yr=1993 or yr=1994 or yr=1995)	7	Display
3	(Internet or online).ti, ab, tx, ct.	7	Display
4	limit 3 to (yr=1993 or yr=1994 or yr=1995)	7	Display

Enter **Keyword** or phrase:

Perform Search

Limit to:
☐ Original Articles ☐ Reviews ☐ Abstracts
◉ All years ○ From: 1995 To: 1995

Results of your search: **limit 3 to (yr=1993 or yr=1994 or yr=1995)**
Citations available: **7**
Citations displayed: **1-7**

Citations in "Titles Display" format

☐ 1. Geography of medical publication. [Letter] *Lancet. 341(8845):634, 1993 March 6.* Table of Contents | Complete record | ****Full Text****

☐ 2. Benzer, A. Pomaroli, A. Hauffe, H. Schmutzhard, E. Geographical analysis of medical publications in 1990. [Letter] *Lancet. 341(8839):247, 1993 January 23.* Table of Contents | Complete record | ****Full Text****

☐ 3. Gruber Allen G, MD. Drug Interactions: The Medical Letter Adverse Drug Interaction Program. [Book Review] *JAMA. 271(9):720-721, 1994 March 2.* Table of Contents | Complete record | ****Full Text****

☐ 4. Lawee, David. ABC of Healthy Travel. [Book Review] *Canadian Medical Association Journal. 150(6):934, 1994 March 15.* Table of Contents | Complete record | ****Full Text****

☐ 5. Reference Management Software. [Letter] *BMJ. 307(6903):569, 1993 August 28.* Table of Contents | Complete record | ****Full Text****

☒ 6. Jones, Richard G. Personal Computer Software for Handling References from CD-ROM and Mainframe Sources for Scientific and Medical Reports. [Miscellaneous] *BMJ. 307(6897):180-184, 1993 July 17.* Table of Contents | Complete record | ****Full Text****

☐ 7. Krogull, Steven. Reviews and Notes: The Physician-Computer Connection: A Practical Guide to Physician Involvement in Hospital Information Systems. [Book Review] *Annals of Internal Medicine. 120(3):254, 1994 February 1.* Table of Contents | Complete record | ****Full Text****

Citation Manager: Display, Save, or Email Citations

Citations	Fields	Format	Action
○ All on this **page** (7) ○ All in this **set** (7) ◉ Selected (this page and previous pages)	○ Citation only ◉ Citation + Abstract ○ Citation + Abstract + Subject Headings ○ All Fields	◉ Ovid ○ BRS/Tagged ○ Reprint/Medlars	Display Email Save

Fig. 36 The Ovid Web Gateway, which provides hypertext links to full-text articles from a core journal collection (where available). [Reproduced with permission.]

PaperChase by Telnet

To access PaperChase directly, Telnet to the following URL (using **PCH,SIGNUP** at the password prompt):

<URL:telnet://pch.bih.harvard.edu>

To use the service via the PaperChase World-Wide Web home page, a Telnet helper application must be assigned to your WWW browser. Clicking on the hypertext link in the page below will launch the Telnet client and open a connection to the computers at Boston's Beth Israel Hospital:

<URL:http://www.paperchase.com/>

You will be asked for your name, address, and credit card details and then be assigned a password to begin using the service immediately. Using PaperCase by Telnet incurs a charge of $US16 per hour connect-time, plus 10¢ per reference displayed or printed, 10¢ per abstract displayed or printed, 10¢ per search statement or list created, and 5¢ per abbreviated reference displayed. Alternatively, type **PCH,go150** at the password prompt for a $US150 per year flat-fee account.

PaperChase on CompuServe

To access PaperChase via CompuServe, type **GO PCH** (or **GO PCH100** to bypass introductory and help information). Using PaperChase via CompuServe incurs a flat charge of $US18 per hour (7 pm to 8 am local time weekdays and weekends) or $US24 per hour (8 am to 7 pm local time weekdays), with billing at 1 second intervals. This is in addition to normal CompuServe charges, but there are no extra charges on the basis of number of references, abstracts, or searches obtained.

SilverPlatter Education MEDLINE

SilverPlatter Education offer MEDLINE over the Internet with weekly updates through their World-Wide Web service, Physicians' Home Page. Launched in early 1996, Physicians' Home Page provides unlimited access to MEDLINE and other databases via *MD Answers*. In addition to a monthly subscription, users pay an initial sign-up fee (plus a one-off US National Library of Medicine International Users fee for non-US customers).

The service uses WebSPIRS-PHP, a Web-based interface to MEDLINE and other databases, rather than a proprietary client. A basic search involves selecting a database, entering one or more search terms which can be combined with a separator term, and clicking on the 'Search' button. Wild cards and parentheses can also be used, as in '(bloggs in au) and (an*emia near diagnosis)'. Searches can be refined using the MeSH index. In some instances it is possible to view full-text articles using your browser; when not available a copy can be requested by fax at extra cost.

The Home Page also links to other subscriber-only services, but other services—*MD Opinions* (a moderated question-and-answer forum) and *MD Digests* (article summaries from major medical journals)—can be freely browsed:

<URL:http://www.silverplatter.com/physicians>

For further information, write to SilverPlatter Education, Physicians' Home Page, 246 Walnut Street, Suite 302, Newton, MA 02160, USA, or send e-mail to php@silverplatter.com.

Other MEDLINE services

The number of Web sites offering free, registration-only, and subscription-based MEDLINE searches over the Internet is proliferating (aided by advertising revenue and sponsorship). A list of many of these sites is maintained at:

<URL:http://www.oup.co.uk/scimed/medint/search.html>

Bibliography

Lindberg, D.A.B, Siegel, E.R., Rapp, B.A., Wallingford, K.T., and Wilson, S.R. (1993). Use of MEDLINE by physicians for clinical problem solving. *Journal of the American Medical Association*, 269, 3124–9.

National Library of Medicine. (1996, Feb.) *Unified Medical Language System*, [Online]. <URL:http://www.nlm.nih.gov/publications/factsheets/umls.html>.

Rosenberg, W. and Donald, A. (1995). Evidence based medicine: an approach to clinical problem-solving. *BMJ*, 310, 1122–6.

Rowlands, J., Morrow, T., Lee, N., and Millman, A. (1995). ABC of medical computing: online searching. *BMJ*, 311, 500–4.

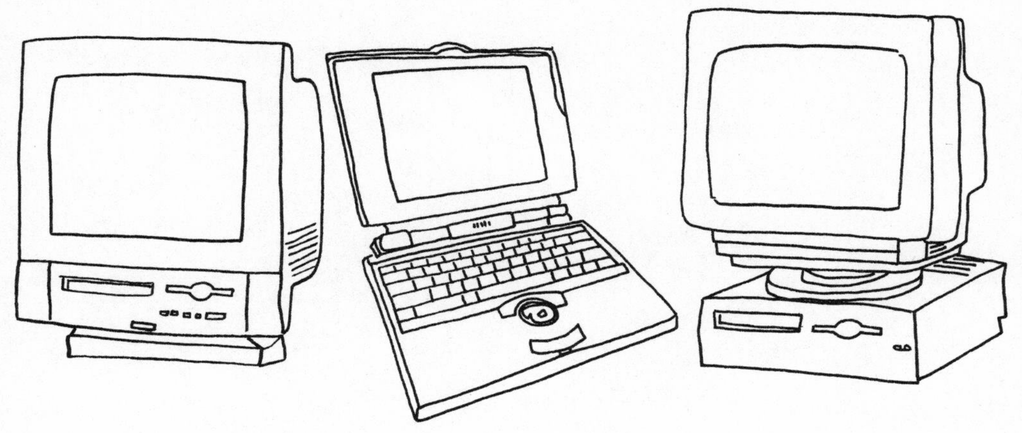

PART 6

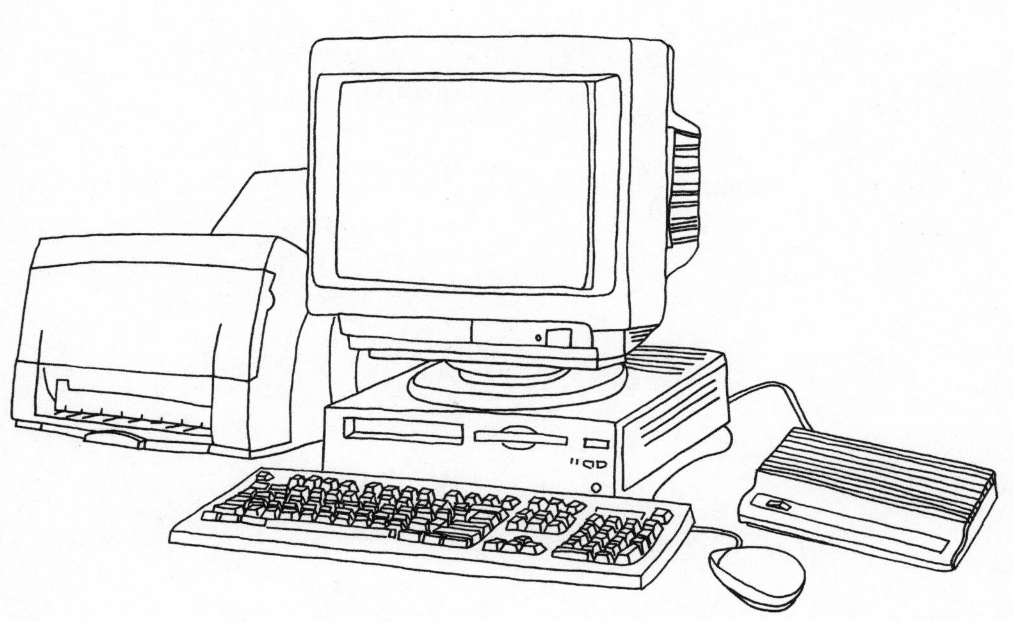

CHAPTER THIRTY
Becoming an information provider

Individuals and institutions of all sizes can easily become information providers on the Internet. Goals may vary from the desire to disseminate research findings, practice guidelines, press releases, clinical newsletters, and other information, or promotion of online education, to the establishment a discussion group.

This chapter provides a brief introduction to writing frequently asked questions (FAQ) files, creating newsgroups, and using or running an Internet server. Using a mailing list is discussed separately in Chapter Thirty two. For most readers, however, the WWW presents the most attractive and readily available option. Consequently, discussion on providing information on the WWW forms the bulk of this chapter. Chapter Thirty one follows with guidance on how to create your own WWW page. The final two chapters in this Part illustrate the practical aspects of information provision through the use of case studies (the GP-UK mailing list, and the BioMedNet Web site).

Using newsgroups

Write an FAQ

Although it is possible for anyone to write and post an FAQ (p.175) to most newsgroups, postings to **news.answers** and other ***.answers** Usenet newsgroups require approval. With this approval, your FAQ can become an 'official' periodic Usenet posting, archived on the *.answers FAQ server. Approval is carried out by the *.answers moderation team based at Massachusetts Institute of Technology. You will need to obtain the *.answers submission guidelines:

By e-mail:

<URL:mailto:mail-server@rtfm.mit.edu> Send: send usenet/news.answers/ news-answers/guidelines

By FTP:

<URL:ftp://rtfm.mit.edu/pub/usenet/news.answers/news-answers/guidelines>

If you do write an FAQ, remember that your e-mail address becomes very public, so be prepared to field questions a little 'off topic', and to receive junk e-mail from advertisers who have culled your address from Usenet.

Create a newsgroup

Taking things one step further, you could create a new newsgroup. If you want to create a new Usenet newsgroup, useful places to start include:

*Guidelines for group creation for *.uk*:

<URL:http://www.usenet.org.uk/guidelines.html>

Usenet newsgroup creation companion:

<URL:ftp://rtfm.mit.edu/pub/usenet/news.answers/usenet/creating-newsgroups/helper>

How to create a new Usenet newsgroup:

<URL:ftp://rtfm.mit.edu/pub/usenet/news.answers/news/creating-newsgroups/part1>

So you want to create an alt newsgroup?:

<URL:ftp://rtfm.mit.edu/pub/usenet/news.answers/alt-creation-guide>

If you want to create a local newsgroup, contact your service provider or local network administrator. You could even set up your own news server to carry relevant newsgroups, including those created by you specifically for your own purposes. Refer to *How to become a Usenet site* at:

<URL:ftp://rtfm.mit.edu/pub/usenet/news.answers/usenet/site-setup>

Use or rent server space

Many public FTP sites have an incoming directory where anyone can upload informational files or software. Contact the uploads administrator, who will probably expect a description of the file you intend to upload and suggestions as to in which directory it should be placed. Some Internet service providers offer individual subscribers free space on their World-Wide Web servers to put up a collection of Web pages (p.146). This is certainly the easiest option for most people. Many providers also rent out space on the server to those who have something more ambitious in mind. Medical students and academics may find it worthwhile taking any proposals to the Computing Service at their university or institution, who may be able to help. Providing information on the WWW is discussed in more detail below.

Run your own Internet server

If you are to go to the expense of installing a leased line to the Internet (p.135), giving you a permanent IP address and a constant connection, your options broaden. However, this is also likely to incur significant cost in terms of hardware, administration, and technical support time. Server software for mail, FTP, Gopher, WAIS, and the WWW is available for most computer platforms. The following examples point to sources of further information about server software:

Mail archive server software list:

<URL:ftp://rtfm.mit.edu/pub/usenet/news.answers/mail/archive-servers/faq>

Anonymous FTP: frequently asked questions list:

<URL:ftp://rtfm.mit.edu/pub/usenet/news.answers/ftp-list/faq>

Gopher FAQ:

<URL:gopher://mudhoney.micro.umn.edu:70/00/Gopher.FAQ>

freeWAIS-sf frequently asked questions:

<URL:ftp://rtfm.mit.edu/pub/usenet/news.answers/wais-faq/freeWAIS-sf>

Setting up your own Internet server requires you to register a domain name (p.100). Many companies can do this for you; have a look at the *Domain name registration FAQ*:

<URL:http://rs.internic.net/domain-info/registration-FAQ.html>

Providing information on the WWW

The need for local information providers

The rapid growth of the Internet has seen the appearance of numerous medical resources. Most of these are based on the World-Wide Web (WWW), an Internet service noted for its unparalleled ease of use. However, because of the low cost of access to the network and the ease with which individuals or groups can self-publish on the WWW, there is great variation in the quality of these resources. The lack of adequate copy-editing, peer review, and publishing experience means that little can presently be regarded as 'authoritative' information. The medical profession can help address this imbalance.

Furthermore, much of the material that is available is US-sourced. Not only is the style of medicine practised across the Atlantic different in many respects to European medicine, but the retrieval of US material is hampered by slow intercontinental communications links. Even among US-sourced material there is a relative deficiency in resources that can be utilized in a clinical setting, although clinically orientated material has begun to appear (see Chapter Twenty six).

The need for locally sourced content on the Internet will grow as hospitals and general practices join the recently implemented NHSnet (p.137). This network will enable all connected NHS institutions to 'dial out' and access global WWW-based information. The uptake of Internet access by the local population (which again includes health professionals) is also steadily increasing.

Indeed, the need for local content to reflect this has been widely recognized. For example, the OMNI project (Organizing Networked Medical Information, p.223) is seeking to develop a relationship with information providers in the UK. OMNI is also committed to the provision of documentation and training in accessing these resources.

In this environment medical publishers, academic departments, research organizations, pharmaceutical companies, and others are in a good position to employ the WWW as a means of improving the delivery of information to the point of care over the next few years; the growing interest in and ease of WWW publishing is being matched by improved access to WWW-based resources for health professionals.

What type of information can be provided?

The most obvious applications of the WWW to clinical medicine include the provision of current information and/or supplemental multimedia.

Current information:

One of the hurdles for both practising doctors and medical students is finding up-to-date information. Traditional paper-based publications lag significantly behind emerging clinical trends and new developments. We are now entering a climate where information technology is expected to deliver current information to clinicians. The WWW presents an effective solution as a means of disseminating online updates to printed works, in addition to current information in new electronic formats.

Supplemental multimedia:

Traditional medical books and papers contain only text and still images. The WWW enables this to be supplemented with animations, movie clips, and audio. These multimedia elements enable an author to convey much more useful and realistic descriptions of a clinical presentation or practical procedure. With the advent of Netscape's plug-in technology, ActiveX, and Java in particular, the WWW promises an integrated multimedia environment utilizing a variety of file formats—all glued together by HTML (p.199) Examples of medical multimedia can be found at the Multimedia Medical Reference Library:

<URL:http://www.tiac.net/users/jtward/>

Hybrid CD-ROM/WWW publishing:

The majority of medical knowledge is relatively static; it would be false to suggest that we need to download essentially unchanged information afresh each time we need to investigate a clinical problem. In addition, the Internet's limited bandwidth (p.99) makes the retrieval of large video clips of ultrasound scans (for

> example) decidedly unappealing. One solution is to create a hybrid CD-ROM/WWW product, as pioneered by Microsoft (Pitchford 1995). A CD-ROM might contain relatively static information in the form of text, high-resolution images, and video, while hypertext links from this material take users to a source of updates on the WWW, which can be downloaded and stored on a local disk. In addition to current information, such a solution would provide cross-platform compatibility (i.e. no need to develop separate PC/Mac versions). It would be possible to enable such a hybrid product to update itself automatically by periodically initiating a connection to the Internet.

As a flick through Chapter Twenty six will demonstrate, there are numerous other niches for medical information providers on the WWW.

Advantages of the WWW medium

The WWW may offer information providers the following advantages:

Currency

WWW-based material can be made available within hours of copy-editing being completed. The current peer review system employed by journals can incur a 12–16 month gap between submission and publication (La Porte *et al.* 1995). There is then a further delay in incorporating this information in medical textbooks. Electronic publication could partially overcome this delay, and does not need to have an adverse effect on the process of peer review (p.116).

International availability

A WWW-based resource could become available simultaneously in many countries including those, for example, who do not have such ready access to printed material. A wider prospective audience brings with it a more international flavour and appeal, particularly where readers are offered the choice of accessing information in their local language or in association with additional material emphasizing local relevance.

Reader-directed learning

Hypertext linking between information increases the ease and speed with which the reader can locate relevant material. Inserting links to additional information or providing built-in cross-references does not disrupt the flow of the information being presented, but offers the choice of gaining deeper knowledge of a particular subject or sticking with an overview. No printed material can offer such freedom.

Ease of use

To use WWW-based information, the reader need only be aware how to point-and-click with a mouse. All WWW pages have the same basic structure, and all browser software the same basic features (p.200). This enables access to many diverse information resources via one familiar user interface.

Monitoring

WWW server software can gather statistics about who is using the service, when, and what content is accessed most often (especially if registration is required—see below).

User feedback

The use of an online feedback page and a page for comments should encourage constructive feedback that will help guide subsequent versions of the pages to the requirements of the audience. A comments page also provides for the publication of additional material and/or debate on certain topics that for reasons of economy were excluded from a printed work, and offers readers a unique two-way interaction with the authors. This author has found, incidentally, that a simple linked e-mail address attracts significantly more comment than a fill-in form for feedback (and requires less technical knowledge to create).

Protection of investment

Online updates can protect the buyer's investment in a printed book (or CD-ROM). These updates can be saved to disk and printed for the user to add to his or her copy. The reader does not have to type in the updates manually, nor decipher their own handwriting.

Ease of revision

Major errors (or developments) in printed material sometimes have to wait for a subsequent print run, or be followed by errata which may not reach many readers. WWW-based information can be revised within minutes in the knowledge that all who subsequently view the page will be viewing the correct version; flawed copies are less likely to remain in circulation. Furthermore, if online updates are provided for a printed work, the process of revision of that work is much simpler (since most of the digesting/reviewing/writing has been spread across the online updates).

Multimedia and interactivity

Incorporation of moving images and/or sound enhances an author's ability to convey information (see above). The ability to download Java applets and ActiveX controls (for example) enables all kinds of interactive applications (see p.207).

Searchability

The entire content of a WWW-based publication or Web site can be searched quickly using an extremely simple interface and without any requirement for manual indexing.

Cost-effectiveness

From the end-users point of view, electronic information can be transmitted/distributed and reproduced/duplicated very cheaply. Home computers are costing less and cheap high-speed modems further decrease the cost of digital transmission. Sophisticated client software is widely available for little or no cost to users from third parties (reducing development and support overheads for information providers). Whether WWW publishing is in practice truly cost-effective for medical journal publishers (and others) has yet to be determined.

Platform independence

The same HTML page can be viewed on virtually all types of computer and will have the same basic structure.

Future proofing

HTML describes only the role of each element within a Web page and their inter-relationships, but the actual page layout is determined by the WWW browser. Thus hypertext publications need not be written with a particular reader program in mind (although this needs qualification—see p.200). HTML—by its definition as a structured mark-up language—inherently supports translation into other current and future document formats without loss of information.

Disadvantages of the WWW medium

While providing information on the WWW may boast many attractions, it also incurs some compromise. Web pages typically incorporate fairly low-resolution images and, because HTML is not as flexible as desktop publishing (DTP) software, publishers have poor control over fonts (the typeface) and layout; each Web browser can display the same document differently. The importance of these factors is, however, debatable where content is far more important than preservation of layout, and it may not in fact be desirable for online material to mirror a printed document. However, new technologies such as OpenType from Adobe/Microsoft for embedding font descriptions within HTML pages, and Bitstream's TrueDoc, are addressing this.

It may be more time-consuming to produce paper and WWW versions of the same document. A possible solution is to use the high-powered SGML (Standard Generalized Mark-up Language) which can be interpreted by both HTML and DTP software (Pallen

1995). Alternatively, some products (such as Adobe PageMaker) can export to both HTML and Adobe Acrobat format (see below). While this may save some time, the exported HTML will probably still need further work to overcome the limitations of an 'automatic' translation.

A number of publications are published on the WWW in Acrobat PDF format rather than HTML. Acrobat is the most widely-known portable document format (i.e. a reader program can be used to view the files on different computer types while preserving the appearance of fonts, images, and layout). An example is the *Mortality and Morbidity Weekly Review* from the Center for Disease Control in Atlanta:

<URL:http://www.cdc.gov/epo/mmwr/mmwr.html>

What does WWW publishing require?

Below are a number of considerations that any prospective WWW publishing project will need to make provision for. Internet connectivity is discussed in Chapter Fifteen.

Hardware

WWW publishing requires a computer acting as a WWW server with a permanent IP address and a permanent connection to the Internet. This may be your own machine, or somebody else's.

Most types of computer can be used as a WWW server. Originally all Web sites were run on UNIX computers, but these can prove unfriendly (UNIX isn't known for ease of use) and the machines were (and remain) generally expensive. PC and Mac-based Internet server solutions have since addressed both these faults.

Software

For as little as a $US10 shareware fee, almost any Macintosh can be turned into a fully fledged Web server in a matter of minutes, and a free add-on for Windows NT users (Internet Information Server) is available from Microsoft. There are also a number of competing commercial WWW server products on the market such as WebSTAR from Quarterdeck and Netsite from Netscape. More information about WWW server products can be found in Boutell's *World-Wide Web frequently asked questions*:

<URL:http://info.ox.ac.uk/help/wwwfaq/index.html>

Aside from Web server (and connectivity) software on the developers computer, a small set of readily available tools is needed to manipulate original content into a form suitable for publication on the WWW. These include a text editor, HTML-editing software (see Chapter Thirty one), a Web browser, and graphics programs for manipulating images. An FTP client (p.179) may be required to upload finished pages to a remote computer if the Web server you are using is run on another machine.

Original content

Authors willing to provide content will need to be found. Written material should be copy-edited and subject to the same standards as would be expected of material destined for print publication. Written material could be supplied by the authors electronically in a file format suitable for encoding into HTML. All common image formats can be converted into the GIF standard. Small digital cameras can be used to capture clinical signs, for example. Moving images or animations can be supplied on disk or on a video cassette ready for digitization. Sound samples can easily be recorded and supplied on a pocket memo recorder (readily available to clinical staff). With these simple tools, almost any doctor can provide material for a multimedia Web site.

An HTML encoder

Someone will (obviously) have to know how to write WWW pages. Creating Web pages is discussed in the following chapter. This person may also need to know how to convert existing documents into HTML, as well as be familiar with the file formats of any multimedia elements that will be a part of the site (such as audio and video clips, or animations and Java applets).

A graphic designer

A professional-looking site may need the skills of a graphic designer to produce quality logos and other graphic elements such as navigation buttons, etc.

A programmer

Expertise may be required to write custom CGI scripts (p.279) to work with fill-in forms, etc. This person may in fact be responsible for the entire technical side of running the Web server. In addition to skills in CGI programming (often requiring a knowledge of the Perl language), the programmer may be called upon to build Java applets or ActiveX controls, or write JavaScripts, for example (see p.207).

Editorial input and copy-editing

With respect, programmers are not always good candidates for the task of ensuring that content on a Web site is of a high standard; an editor best fulfils this role. As happens with paper-based publications, ideally a copy-editor should check the content of the Web pages for structure, spelling and grammatical errors, inconsistencies and (where appropriate) general compliance with a prescribed style. Review by medical peers may also be important here (see p.116).

A publication mechanism

A mechanism for handling publication of content generated remotely will need to be considered if you are providing information via someone else's server. Usually this involves using FTP to transfer material to an uploads directory on an FTP server. This can then be made available to the Web server automatically, or it may require manual intervention by someone at the remote site (such as transfer to a different machine, de-archiving, etc.).

Funding

A Web site may offer free unrestricted access, free access for registered users, or subscriber-only access. Registration enables information providers to gather information about users which can be used to review the service (see below). Registration commonly involves the completion of an online fill-out form. Once registered, users access the service via another form or dialogue box requiring a user name and/or password. The experience of large online services like CompuServe has clearly demonstrated that people are willing to pay for quality information with commercial potential. A growing number of services offer the delivery of online journal articles via the Internet on a pay-as-you-go basis, including BioMedNet (see Chapter Thirty two). These services address the hesitancy of medical journal publishers to offer journal services over the Internet for free because of the anticipated loss of revenue this would incur. Ultimately, in order to be self-sustaining, any substantive WWW publishing project would need to be funded by a modest subscription, advertising revenue, or some form of sponsorship.

A strategy and review process

A successful Web site has to be visibly well-tended. A good strategy will demonstrate that this is so by seekxing to:

- ensure a regular supply of new content
- estimate the number of person-hours involved in maintaining the service
- estimate the suitability of current hardware and software to ensure the longer-term viability of the service
- act on user feedback to refine the service
- ensure that the service is stable (e.g. not subject to computer down-time)
- establish a consistent interface across the various Web pages
- evaluate whether the content can justify a subscription-based service
- provide a 'hook' encouraging users to return.

Note that WWW server software can provide information useful to the review process in the form of number of visitors ('hits'), type of domain (e.g. **ac**, **uk**, **edu**, etc.), and which files are accessed most frequently. If registration is required, even more information can be gained about who is using what and why.

Promotion

There are a number of guides on the WWW that assist in announcing a new WWW service to ensure it reaches as wide an audience as possible. These are listed at:

<URL:http://www.yahoo.com/Computers_and_Internet/Internet/World_Wide_Web/Announcement_Services>

To see how many links there are to your site, use **+link:url** as the search term at AltaVista search engine (p.225), where **url** is the uniform resource locator of your site.

Human-resource overheads

Bear in mind that even a simple e-mail link for enquiries on a Web page can demand a lot of your time. Provision must be made to deal with this.

Legal issues

A medical information provider needs to consider issues of confidentiality, copyright, and disclaimers. All patient-sourced non-anonymized material requires explicit consent for it to appear on the WWW (p.59). Every effort should thus be made to conceal identifying features. Most Web pages contain a copyright statement, but the nature of electronic information means it is easy for users to obtain exact copies of your material, and to duplicate or even manipulate it as they see fit. A disclaimer is an advisable addition to a medical Web site, indicating that your information is correct as of a specified date, and that drug doses should be verified by the prescriber. If your pages include hypertext links to external sites, you may wish to disclaim responsibility for 'publishing' links to information over which you have no control.

A series of papers on copyright issues surrounding electronic information has been collated by the Joint Information Systems Committee (JISC) at:

<URL:http://www.niss.ac.uk/education/jisc/pub/copyright/start.htm>

Accreditation by professional bodies

Application forms and guidelines for PGEA approval (p.122) for Internet-based material can be obtained from the UK National Accreditation Panel Administrator, Royal College of General Practitioners, 14 Princes Gate, Hyde Park, London SW7 1PU, tel. 0171 581 3232. Application forms and guidelines for CME approval (p.122) can be obtained from the most appropriate Royal College. Where material is relevant to several specialties (e.g. physicians, surgeons, radiologists, etc.) approval by only one College is necessary.

References

LaPorte, R.E., Marler, E., Akazawa, S., Sauer, F., Gamboa, C., Shenton, C., Glosser, *et al.* (1995). The death of biomedical journals. *BMJ*, **310**, 1387–90.

Pallen, M. (1995). The world wide web. *BMJ*, **311**, 1552–6.

Pitchford, D. (1995). Microsoft continues its Internet assault (News). *Internet*, **13** (Dec), 9.

CHAPTER THIRTY ONE
Creating a Web page

Rather than maintain an ungainly list of Bookmarks or Favourites (p.202), or sift through other people's pages, an alternative providing far more flexibility is to create your own WWW page to store favourite URLs (p.102) and associated annotations. This chapter is designed to serve as a reference for those wishing to create a relatively straightforward personal or departmental Web page; be warned however—it isn't bedtime reading! Using brief examples, the focus is on providing explanations for the more common HTML tags (p.199) in the hope that the reader will be able to study the make-up of their favourite Web pages and understand how each effect was produced. Those who have a complex multimedia-rich interactive site in mind will need to refer to one of the many verbose tomes available on this subject. For more information about HTML, the following may be useful:

Yahoo HTML information:

<URL:http://www.yahoo.com/Computers_and_Internet/Software/Data_Formats/HTML/>

The bare bones guide to HTML:

<URL:http://werback.com/barebones/>

HTML specification information:

<URL:http://www.w3.org/pub/WWW/MarkUp/>

Tools for page creation

Any word processor or text editor can be used to write HTML files from scratch, provided you have some basic knowledge of HTML. Alternatively, many word processors have an option to export files as HTML without your really needing to know anything of the syntax at all. However, these simple conversions may not be able to cope with anything too complicated, and often the resultant HTML file requires some modification. There are many dedicated shareware applications that offer more options, and a range of competing commercial products designed to simplify the creation of Web pages. Commercial examples include PageMill (Adobe), Netscape Navigator Gold (Netscape), and Microsoft's FrontPage and Internet Studio. More information about shareware HTML editors can be obtained at:

<URL:http://www.yahoo.com/Computers/World_Wide_Web/HTML_Editors>

Aside from an HTML editor, a Web browser is needed to view the results of your efforts. Most graphics programs are capable of handling the creation of images and their conversion into the GIF format used on the WWW. Special graphics utilities may be required to produce transparent, interlaced, or animated GIFs (see *Inserting graphics and other media types*, below). If your site is to include multimedia, you will need a program to create movie and/or sound files and save them in common formats. Many of the above programs can be downloaded from software archives on the Internet.

Anatomy of a WWW page

As discussed on p.199, hypertext markup language (HTML) uses tags to assign a meaning to various textual elements in a Web page. At a very basic level, a Web page consists of a *head* and a *body*. Both of these elements are 'contained' within the **<HTML>** tag, like this:

```
<HTML>
<HEAD>
<TITLE>Medical links</TITLE>
</HEAD>
<BODY>This text is the body.</BODY>
</HTML>
```

Notice several things. All of the other tags are inside of the **<HTML>** and the **</HTML>** tags; the forward slash (i.e. '/') indicates the end of the effect of the opening **<HTML>** tag—in this case, the end of the HTML document. Likewise, notice how the text 'Medical links' is contained between the **<TITLE>** and **</TITLE>** tags. Many HTML tags work as a pair like this—so-called **containers**, with an opening tag and a closing tag. Note that the head must always contain the title tags (the contained text will be displayed in the title bar by the Web browser), and sits on top of the body. We have already built a basic Web page!

Many tags can be modified using **attributes**. An attribute is an additional syntax that can be included within a tag to modify the effect that it has. Sometimes an attribute must be specified; often it is optional. Common attributes are explained in the relevant section below, and common tags are listed in Table 14 (p.268). Note that all tags are spelt using American English, i.e. center, color, etc.

The head

The head, defined by the **<HEAD>...</HEAD>** containers, need only contain the title of the document for display in the title window of Web browsers. The title, which can be short or long, is contained within the **<TITLE>** and **</TITLE>** tags, and should describe the page contents as accurately as possible. Sometimes information about the document (such as the author, or original URL) is included within comment tags so it is not displayed by the browser. For example:

<!-- This page was written by Dr Joe Bloggs -->

These comments can in fact be included throughout an HTML document. The head can also contain 'meta information' which serves the same purpose, except that Internet search engines (p.225) can retrieve this information specifically. For example:

<META NAME="description**" CONTENT="**Complimentary WWW pages associated with Medicine and the Internet from Oxford University Press. Includes the original Online Updates service.**">**

Other tags that may appear within the head include the **<SCRIPT>**...**</SCRIPT>** container, used to define JavaScripts (p.208), and client-side image map definitions (see *Inserting graphics and other media types*, below).

Body elements

Everything below the head forms the body of a Web page—the text, images, links, forms, tables, etc. The **<BODY>**...**</BODY>** container can be modified by attributes specifying a background image (see *Inserting graphics and other media types*, below), and the colour of the background, text, and hyperlinks (see *Using colour*, below). It is most helpful to consider the tags used within the body under the headings of basic formatting, fonts and type style, anchors, graphics and other media, tables, forms, colour, and frames. These are discussed individually below.

Basic formatting

Most Web pages consist largely of text. Tags can be used to shape blocks of text into features common to the printed page—headings, paragraphs, lists, etc.

Headings

The heading tag is used to indicate the relative importance of a block of text through the use of different sized headings. The top-level heading, within the **<H1>**...**</H1>** containers, is rendered larger than the bottom-level heading, **<H6>**...**</H6>**. There are six levels in all.

Paragraphs

The paragraph tag, **<P>**, causes following text to move two lines down and to the left margin. This tag is necessary to prevent blocks of text from being run together, as the blank lines common to word-processed files are not recognized by Web browsers. Note that the closing tag, **</P>**, is optional. Paragraph tags can be used to create 'white space', an area devoid of text.

TABLE 14 Commonly used HTML mark-up tags

Tag	Use
Structural tags	
<HTML>...</HTML>	Marks the beginning and end of an HTML file.
<HEAD>...</HEAD>	Includes descriptive information, such as the title, creator, keywords, client-side image map definitions, etc.
<TITLE>...</TITLE>	The name of the page (appears in browser title bar).
<BODY *>...</BODY>	The main page content, including text, images, links, etc.
Basic formatting tags	
<Hn>...</Hn>	Determines the size of the heading; n=1 is largest, n=6 the smallest.
<P>...</P>	Paragraph. Following text moves two lines down and to the left margin. The closing tag is optional.
 	Line break. Following text moves one line down and to the left margin.
<BLOCKQUOTE>...</BLOCKQUOTE>	Indents contain text at both page margins, with a space above and below.
<HR *>	Horizontal rule. Produces a horizontal line across the page.
<UL>...</UL>	Unordered list.
<LI>	A list item, indicated with a bullet point.
<CENTER>...</CENTER>	Used to centre text, images, etc. within the page.
<PRE>...</PRE>	Pre-formatted text. Displays text entered in a monospaced font exactly as typed (retaining any columns).
Type style tags	
<FONT *>...</FONT>	Commonly used to change the size of text e.g. <FONT SIZE=5>...</FONT>.
<B>...</B>	Produces bold text.
<I>...</I>	Produces italic text.
<TT>...</TT>	Teletype monospaced font (all characters are the same horizontal width).
Anchor tags	
<A HREF="url">...</A>	Hyper-reference linking the enclosed text or image to another file.
<A NAME="target">...</A>	Defines a target with a Web page (see text).
Image tag	
<IMG SRC="url" *>	Inserts an image, the source URL of which is represented by "url".
Tables	
<TABLE *>...</TABLE>	Defines a table.
<TR>...</TR>	Table row.
<TD *>...</TD>	Table column (within a row).

* Denotes attribute may apply (see text).

Line breaks

The line break tag **
** operates without a closing tag. Text following this tag moves one line down and to the left margin of the page. Note that the tags for 'block quotes', horizontal lines, lists, and pre-formatted text (see below) create line breaks automatically.

'Blockquotes'

Sometimes it is desirable to indent a block of text to draw attention to it. The blockquote tag, **<BLOCKQUOTE>**...**</BLOCKQUOTE>**, is used for this purpose. This tag indents the contained text at both the left and right page margins, with a space above and below. Many Web pages make use of this effect to narrow a column of text for improved on-screen readability.

Horizontal rules

Horizontal rules (dividing lines) are created with the **<HR>** tag. Attributes specify line thickness, width, alignment, and turn off the shading feature. For example:

```
<HR SIZE=4 WIDTH="50%" ALIGN=CENTER NOSHADE>
```

This will create a horizontal rule that is four pixels thick, occupies 50 percent of the page width, is centred, and has a solid rather than a shaded fill. Any or all of these attributes can be left out to create the default horizontal rule. Note that there are two ways to specify dimensions under HTML—and this applies to the dimensions of images and tables as well. One way is to specify an absolute size in pixels; the other is a relative size, expressed as a percentage.

Lists

Although several types of list are defined in the HTML specification, the most commonly used type is the unordered list, defined by the **<UL>**...**</UL>** containers. Each list item, **<LI>**, is indicated by a bullet point (without a closing tag).

Centre

Text, images, tables, and other content can be centred within a Web page using the **<CENTER>**...**</CENTER>** container. Note the American spelling.

Pre-formatted text

Text typed between the **<PRE>**...**</PRE>** containers is displayed by the browser in a monospaced font (each character has the same horizontal width) exactly as typed, retaining any text columns, line breaks, and spaces.

Fonts and type style

The font tag is often used as an alternative to the heading tag (see above) to control the size of text, although it can do so more precisely. For example:

M**<FONT SIZE=-1>**EDICINE**</FONT>**

In this example, the word 'medicine' (in capitals) is rendered with the 'm' at the default size (i.e. 3), and the remainder of the word one size below (i.e. 2); a plus sign instead of a minus would have the opposite effect. When the attribute specifies no plus or minus sign—just a number from one to seven—instead of a relative change in size, the font size is fixed, much like a heading. In addition to size, other attributes specify colour (see *Using colour*, below) and, less commonly, type face.

There are only three commonly used type styles on the WWW; **<B>**...**</B>** produces bold text; **<I>**...**</I>** produces italic text, and **<TT>**...**</TT>** produces the teletype monospaced font. Medical authors are likely to want to include superscripts and subscripts; these are produced by the **^{**...**}** and **_{**...**}** containers, respectively. There are other type styles, but they are either not widely understood by the majority of browsers, or have less predictable effects.

Anchors are for linking

The anchor **<A HREF="url">**...**</A>** describes a 'hyper-reference' (hypertext link) from the enclosed text or image to another file. The uniform resource locator (URL, p.102) can be any URL—a Web site, FTP archive, e-mail address, newsgroup, etc. The URL may be an *absolute* or *relative* link. For example:

Absolute (full) link:

<A HREF="http://www.cybertas.demon.co.uk/palliative_care.html">Palliative care</A>

Relative link:

<A HREF="palliative_care.html">Palliative care</A>

The opening anchor tag includes the URL and the closing one indicates that the text between the containers is the hypertext link. In either case in this example you would see only the words 'Palliative care' displayed on the WWW page; clicking on these words with the mouse will activate the hypertext link. Note that you can put additional text after (or before) the link which will also be visible on your page. The main advantage of relative links is that if a set of Web pages is moved to another site (for example), the links between all the files that make up the set will still work. This would not be the case if the full URL including the server domain name had been given.

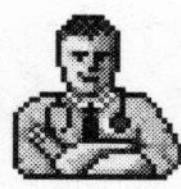

A set of Web pages that uses relative linking can be browsed offline, and all the hyperlinks should still work. Most users who create their own Web pages use this fact to test links before the pages are placed on a WWW server. Any links made to another site will, of course, not work without a live TCP/IP connection.

Getting relative links to work can sometimes be tricky if your files are in several nested folders (i.e. one inside the other). Linking to a file in a lower level should not cause problems. For example:

<A HREF="here/below/bottom.html">To the bottom**</A>**

Creating a relative link to a file higher up in the directory structure of your site may involve some trial and error! Remember that you direct the browser to a higher level using the UNIX '../' directory notation, as in:

<A HREF="../top.html">To the top**</A>**

A hyper-reference can also be made to a specific 'target' within a page. If the target is within another page, use the syntax **<A HREF="url#target">...</A>**, where **"target"** is the target name. If the target is in the same page, use the syntax **<A HREF="#target">...</A>**. The syntax **<A NAME="target">...</A>** defines the target name. For example:

Link to target in another page:

<A HREF="palliative_care.html#symptom">Symptom control</A>

Link to target in the same page:

<A HREF="#symptom">Symptom control</A>

Here, the target would be named thus:

<A NAME="symptom">...</A>

Inserting graphics and other media types

After text, graphics are the most common feature of Web pages. They make pages visually appealing, and help break large chunks of text into manageable sections. Medicine makes heavy use of imaging modalities and visualization is critical to most specialties. Luckily, medical images can be readily incorporated into WWW pages. Images such as X-rays, echocardiographs, tomographic scans, etc., can easily be digitized (although they may already be stored digitally, requiring only conversion to an appropriate format).

The basic tag to include an image takes the form **<IMG SRC="url">**, where **"url"** is the URL for the image source (which again, may be the full URL or a relative link). Attributes include image height, width, alignment, client-side image maps, border width, and a text alternative. Images can also be links to other files in the same way that text can. For example:

```
<A HREF="surgery_links.html"><IMG SRC="images/scalpel.gif"
ALIGN=MIDDLE WIDTH=64 HEIGHT=32 BORDER=1 ALT="Scalpel [6K]"></A>
```

In this example, the graphic, **scalpel.gif** (inside an images folder) is linked to a Web page named **surgery_links.html**. It is aligned to the middle of the adjacent text (not shown). Specifying the dimensions improves page loading time, telling the browser how much space to leave where the image will load. The dimensions (64 by 32 pixels) are indicated with a border one pixel wide; this enables users to see how big the graphic is if they have chosen not to automatically display images (see p.202). Users can get an idea of what the graphic shows via the alternative text attribute, which is displayed under these circumstances (it is not seen when the image is loaded). Here, text-only readers are told there is a picture of a scalpel with a file size of only six kilobytes, should they wish to load it. Note that the border around a hyperlinked image is blue (by default); around unlinked images it is black. The border can be made to disappxear by setting **BORDER=0**.

A choice of graphics format

The two common image formats on the Internet are **GIF** and **JPEG** (see Table 6, p.45). GIF files are limited to 256 colours, and consequently are ideal where photo-quality images are not required. Most medical illustrations could be adequately represented by GIF files. There are also several types of GIF that have particular uses (see below). The alternative, JPEG, enables more photo-realistic images with thousands or even millions of colours. However, as a consequence of the extra data needed to describe these colours, uncompressed JPEG files are on the large side. Compression, although effective in reducing file size, degrades image quality. JPEG is commonly used to publish X-ray images on the WWW.

Types of GIF

A good image-manipulation program will have the option to save images as **interlaced GIFs**. Interlaced GIFs are the same as ordinary GIFs, except that Web browsers begin showing the image as a crude rendering that sharpens progressively as the remaining file information is processed by the browser. Often a partially rendered GIF gives you enough information to decide whether to click on it or not (if it is hyperlinked or an image map—see opposite).

Web pages would be boring if all the images had straight edges. Some image-manipulation programs (and leading Web browsers) support **transparent GIFs**. The whole image isn't transparent (although it can be), but rather one colour. The nominated colour will match the background colour of the Web page—similar to the 'blue screen' trick used in film making. In this way, images appear to be irregular and blend into the page.

So-called **animated GIFs** are becoming popular on the WWW following their support by leading browsers. Animated GIFs contain a number of images encoded into a single file; each image is displayed at set intervals, giving the appearance of an animation. They do this without the overhead in computer memory or processing power required by some plug-ins (p.204) or Java (p.207).

Image maps

An **image map** is a common navigational aid on the Web. Just an ordinary graphics file, certain zones of the image can be pre-defined as 'hot spots', so that a mouse-click in each zone has some effect. 'Server-side' image maps rely on the presence of a Web server to work. Anyone can create 'client-side' image maps, however, as all the information needed to make the map work is contained within the HTML page. This type of image map is supported by Netscape Navigator and Internet Explorer.

In the body, the image map is positioned using the following syntax (where **map.gif** is your image, and **mapname** is the name assigned to your map):

```
<IMG SRC="map.gif" USEMAP="#mapname">
```

In the head, the image map is described as in this example:

```
<MAP NAME="mapname">
<AREA SHAPE="RECT" COORDS="w,x,y,z" HREF="url">
</MAP>
```

Here, the container tags simply identify which map you are referring to (as there may be several in a page). The middle line is the important one; it defines the shape of the hot spot and the coordinates (in pixels) that it covers. A single hot spot is obviously pointless (as simple hyperlink would do), so most image maps contain several such 'middle' lines (all specifying different coordinates). The **HREF="url"** part associated with each hot spot determines where one is taken following a mouse click in these coordinates.

Other media types, applets, and the future

The WWW is no longer just text and static images, thanks largely to plug-ins (p.204), Java, and ActiveX (p.207). As of this writing other media types (movies, sounds, etc.) can be embedded into an HTML page using Netscape's **<EMBED SRC="url">** tag. MIME types (p.160) determine which plug-in should handle the file. The following example describes an embedded Macromind Director movie:

```
<EMBED SRC="movies/medic.dcr" TYPE="application/x-director" WIDTH=500
HEIGHT=200>
```

Sun's **<APPLET>...</APPLET>** containers likewise currently allow the embedding of Java applets (p.207). For example:

```
<APPLET CODE="name.class" WIDTH=200 HEIGHT=100>
<PARAM NAME="text" VALUE="something">
</APPLET>
```

Ready-made Java applets, together with the HTML needed to embed them, can be downloaded from several repositories including:

<URL:http://www.gamelan.com/>

Note, however, that both the **EMBED** and **APPLET** tags are likely to be superseded by a new container, **<OBJECT>...</OBJECT>**. This tag will also replace the image tag and redefine client-side image maps, creating a standard syntax for embedding all types of media. In addition, the Portable Network Graphics (PNG) format, using the suffix **.png**, is expected to replace GIF (partly for legal reasons). PNG offers more colours, most of the benefits of GIF, and better compression without loss of image quality. For more information about these and other developments, see the W3C (World-Wide Web Consortium) pages:

<URL:http://www.w3.org/pub/WWW/>

Note also that before any media type can be loaded into a Web page, the server must be configured to recognize its corresponding MIME type. If you are using someone else's Web server to host your site, you may need to enquire about server configuration.

Using tables

Tables are defined by the **<TABLE>...</TABLE>** containers. Aside from simply presenting data in table form, tables are often used to provide more control over the layout of WWW pages. Optional attributes specify border and table width, cell spacing, and cell padding (see the examples below). The **BORDER** attribute draws a border *n* pixels wide around each table 'cell' (as in a spreadsheet). The **WIDTH** of the entire table can be fixed as an absolute value (in pixels), or as a percentage of the width of the page. Cell spacing (**CELLSPACING**) specifies the number of pixels between individual cells; cell padding (**CELLPADDING**) specifies the number of pixels between the cell border and the data in the cell.

Tables are, of course, made up using rows and columns. Rows and columns are added using the **<TR>...</TR>** and **<TD>...</TD>** containers, respectively. '**TD**' signifies a table data cell—a column within a row. **<TD>** has its own attributes, including **WIDTH** (see examples), **ROWSPAN** (how many rows the cell should span), and **COLSPAN** (how many columns the cell should span). The example table opposite illustrates the use of these tags and attributes.

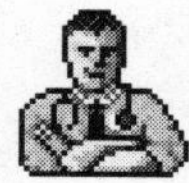

Note that a table cell containing no data appears filled in. You can counter this effect by inserting the non-breaking space 'special character ' (see below) into the cell (i.e. ** **—see example). This will create an empty cell.

```
<TABLE BORDER=4 CELLSPACING=2 CELLPADDING=4 WIDTH="80%">
<TR>
    <TD> </TD>
    <TD><B>Myoglobin</B></TD>
    <TD><B>Creatine kinase</B> </TD>
    <TD><B>Aspartate aminotransferase</B></TD>
    <TD><B>Lactate dehydrogenase</B></TD>
</TR>
<TR>
    <TD><I>Start to rise (h)</I></TD>
    <TD>3-6</TD>
    <TD>4-8</TD>
    <TD>6-8</TD>
    <TD>12-24</TD>
</TR>
<TR>
    <TD><I>Peak (h)</I></TD>
    <TD>8-12</TD>
    <TD>24</TD>
    <TD>24-48</TD>
    <TD>48-72</TD>
</TR>
<TR>
    <TD><I>Duration of rise (days)</I></TD>
    <TD>1-2</TD>
    <TD>3-5</TD>
    <TD>4-6</TD>
    <TD>7-12</TD></TR>
</TABLE>
```

The above example produces the table illustrated in Fig. 37 (p.276). The table data are from Hope and Longmore (1987), with kind permission.

Aside from presenting tabulated data, tables can be made 'invisible' and used to fix the width of a page, or to shorten the line length of blocks of text for better on-screen readability. To fix the width of a page (in pixels) with a table that is not displayed by the browser, set the table **BORDER** to zero and the **WIDTH** to an absolute number of pixels (rather than a percentage). For example:

```
<TABLE BORDER=0 WIDTH=500>...</TABLE>
```

To confine a block of text to the right two thirds of a page, say, divide the row using fixed-width columns as follows:

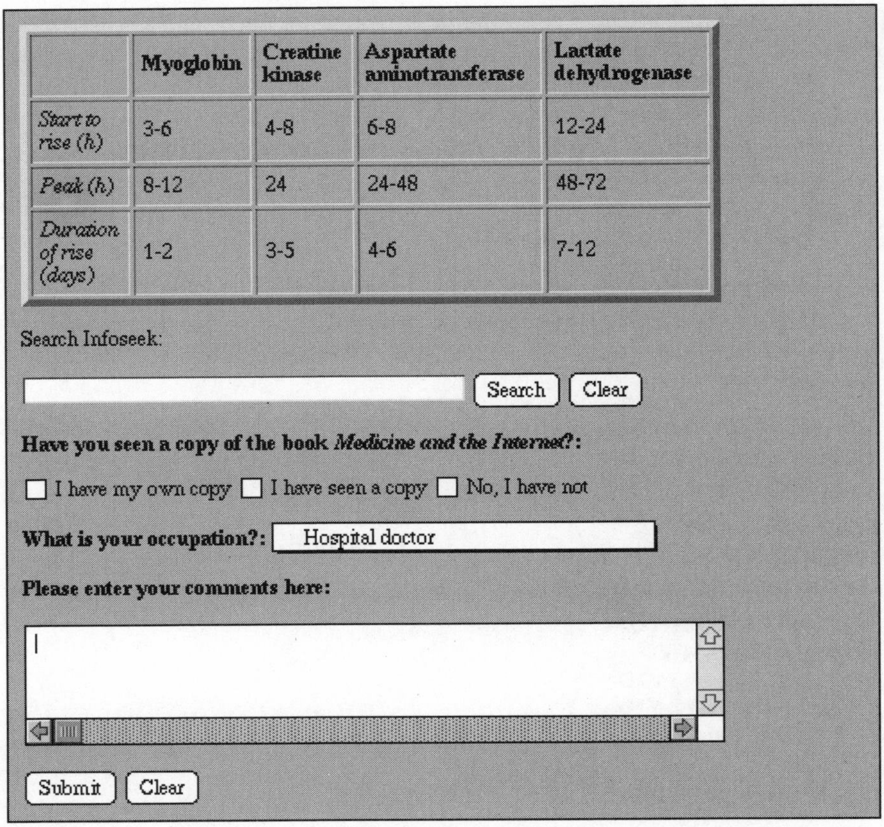

	Myoglobin	Creatine kinase	Aspartate aminotransferase	Lactate dehydrogenase
Start to rise (h)	3-6	4-8	6-8	12-24
Peak (h)	8-12	24	24-48	48-72
Duration of rise (days)	1-2	3-5	4-6	7-12

Search Infoseek:

Search Clear

Have you seen a copy of the book *Medicine and the Internet*?:

☐ I have my own copy ☐ I have seen a copy ☐ No, I have not

What is your occupation?: Hospital doctor

Please enter your comments here:

Submit Clear

Fig. 37 Tables and forms. The HTML markup used to create these elements is given within the text.

```
<TABLE BORDER=0 WIDTH=600>
<TR>
<TD WIDTH=200>Left margin content goes here.</TD>
<TD WIDTH=400>Right margin content goes here.</TD>
</TR>
</TABLE>
```

Alternatively, percentages can be substituted for absolute values. Each cell in a table can contain anything from text to graphics, or forms to Java applets. It is also possible to 'nest' tables (that is, to put one inside another).

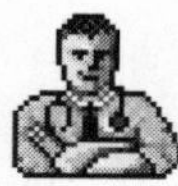

When using 'invisible tables' to lay out a page, set the border width to zero at the last minute. Using a visible border during page development helps position table contents.

Tables can be much more complicated than this, but the above guidelines should offer enough flexibility to tackle most tasks.

Fill-out forms

Forms are commonly used to search databases, supply registration details, gain access to password-protected sites, and in making online purchases, etc. Forms can contain a number of assorted elements: check boxes, radio buttons, pull-down menus, buttons, and fields for free-text entry. Most of these are illustrated in Fig. 25 (p.201). In HTML, a form is defined by the **<FORM>...</FORM>** container tags. The following example (the result of which is shown in Fig. 37) creates a very simple form for searching the Infoseek site (p.225):

```
Search Infoseek:
<P>
<FORM METHOD="GET" ACTION="http://www2.infoseek.com/IS/Titles">
<INPUT TYPE="text" VALUE="" NAME="qt" SIZE=40 >
<INPUT TYPE="submit" VALUE="Search">
<INPUT TYPE="reset" VALUE="Clear">
</FORM>
```

Information entered into a form is sent to the Web server to be acted upon—hence the **ACTION** attribute, which specifies the URL where the data should be sent. The **METHOD** attribute will be either **GET** or **POST** (a technical, but valid difference). Each part of a form (i.e. button, pull-down menu, etc.) is created using one of three tags; **<INPUT>**, **<SELECT>**, or **<TEXTAREA>**. All three must appear within the **<FORM>...</FORM>** containers.

The INPUT tag

In the above example, there are three types of **<INPUT>**. **TYPE** can take the following values:

- **TYPE="checkbox"**; a box that can be checked or unchecked
- **TYPE="hidden"**; a way of giving other unseen parameters to the server
- **TYPE="password"**; a line for text entry, but characters are disguised
- **TYPE="radio"**; a circular 'radio button' that can be filled or unfilled
- **TYPE="reset"**; a button that resets a filled-out form to its original state
- **TYPE="submit"**; a button that sends the data in the form to the server
- **TYPE="text"**; a line for text entry.

The attributes **VALUE**, **NAME**, and **SIZE** are used in association with **<INPUT>**. **VALUE** is used to give a **TYPE** of **<INPUT>** a preset value (e.g. whether a checkbox is pre-checked). In general, each element of a form containing **TYPE** must have a **NAME** attribute so that the server can make an association between each type of **<INPUT>** and its **VALUE**. If, for example, 'subcutaneous ketamine' was typed into the text field and submitted to Infoseek as above, the client would send a 'query URL' to the server like this:

```
<URL:http://www2.infoseek.com/IS/Titles?qt=subcutaneous+ketamine>
```

This tells the server that the value of the input type named '**qt**' (query text) is equal to subcutaneous plus ketamine. The importance of names becomes obvious when values for several input types are sent to the server in the same query URL. The association between **NAME** and **VALUE** is maintained where more than one **VALUE** is assigned to a given **NAME**. For example:

```
<B>Have you seen a copy of the book <I>Medicine and the Internet</I>?:</B>
<P>
<INPUT TYPE="checkbox" NAME="Seen" VALUE="own">I have my own copy
<INPUT TYPE="checkbox" NAME="Seen" VALUE="copy">I have seen a copy
<INPUT TYPE="checkbox" NAME="Seen" VALUE="not">No, I have not
```

Note that reset and submit buttons are a special case; here **VALUE** supplies the visible name of the button (see Fig. 37), and the **NAME** attribute is not required. **SIZE** is used to change the displayed length of text/password fields.

Pull-down menus and scrolling lists

Pull-down menus and scrolling lists are created using the **<SELECT>**...**</SELECT>** container and one or more **<OPTION>** tags. The following example generates a pull-down menu (see Fig. 37) of occupations:

```
<B>What is your occupation?:</B>
<SELECT NAME="Occupation" SIZE=1>
<OPTION SELECTED>Hospital doctor
<OPTION>General Practitioner
<OPTION>Medical student
<OPTION>Nurse/nursing student
<OPTION>Other health professional
<OPTION>Information technologist
<OPTION>Administrator
<OPTION>Other
</SELECT>
```

The **NAME** attribute is compulsory. In this example, setting **SIZE=4** would render a scrolling list instead of a pull-down menu, displaying four options at a time. Scrolling lists are produced whenever **SIZE** is set to any value greater than one (the actual value determines the number of options visible at once), or when the **MULTIPLE** attribute is used. **MULTIPLE** has no value, but allows multiple options to be selected at the same time from a scrolling list.

The **SELECTED** attribute to **<OPTION>** is used to specify the default selection in either a pull-down menu or scrolling list; several options can be **SELECTED** by default if the **MULTIPLE** attribute is used.

Text areas

Although **TYPE="text"** can be used to produce a single-line text entry field,the **<TEXTAREA>...</TEXTAREA>** containers define a multi-line text field with vertical and horizontal scroll bars (see Fig. 37). The **NAME** attribute is once again used to associate submitted content with this particular form element. The height and width of the text field are determined by the **ROWS** and **COLS** attributes, respectively. A simple example follows (any default textual content would appear between the containers):

```
<B>Please enter your comments here:</B>
<P>
<TEXTAREA NAME="Comments" ROWS=4 COLS=60>
</TEXTAREA>
```

Using forms in practice

Web pages containing forms can be used to access various types of database. This interaction is usually managed by a small application or script that sits between the Web server program and the database being accessed—in a 'virtual space', if you like, called the **Common Gateway Interface** (CGI). CGIs are sometimes indicated by the file suffix **.cgi** and are commonly found on Web servers in a folder named **cgi-bin**. Specifying a CGI in a URL (or clicking on the Submit button in a form) runs the CGI and directs the server to send the output resulting from the CGI back to the client.

Specialist knowledge is required to author CGIs (e.g. familiarity with the Perl scripting language), although many 'ready made' CGIs are freely available. For more information about CGIs see:

<URL:http://www.boutell.com/faq/cgi.htm>

Thus, you may need to create custom CGIs for use with your own custom forms, or use existing CGIs written specifically for the particular database hosted on your server. The easiest alternative is to modify forms that work with CGIs on someone else's server—usually a matter of studying the relevant source files (p.202).

Not everybody needs to create a forms-based interface to a database, however. If your goal is to create a simple form for the purpose of giving feedback or requesting further information, any easy route is to use a GCI that will take any data submitted via a form, and e-mail it to your e-mail address. Ask the administrator of the server hosting your pages whether this facility is available.

For more details about writing forms, see the tutorial at:

<URL:http://www.ncsa.uiuc.edu/SDG/Software/Mosaic/Docs/fill-out-forms/overview.html>

Using colour

Attributes associated with the <BODY> container tags have a role in determining the use of colour in a Web page. There are attributes to describe a background colour and the colours of ordinary text, hyperlinks, visited links (links you have already followed), and active links (for a colour change during the mouse click). The default colours in Netscape are a grey background, black text, blue hyperlinks, purple visited links, and red for active links (during the mouse click). Colours can be customized (thus overriding the defaults) using a 'hexadecimal code' or one of sixteen 'standard' colour names. For example:

```
<BODY BGCOLOR="#FFFFFF" TEXT="#000000" LINK="#0000FF"
VLINK="#000066" ALINK="#FF0000">
```

The 'standard' colour names which can be used in place of hexadecimal values are aqua; black; blue; fuchsia; grey; green; lime; maroon; navy; olive; purple; red; silver; teal; white; and yellow. Individual blocks of text can also be coloured in the same way. For example:

```
<FONT COLOR="#FF0000">Here is some red text</FONT>
```

Another attribute can specify a textured background image rather than a plain colour—usually a small JPEG file. For example:

```
<BODY BACKGROUND="texture.jpg">
```

Frames

Frames are separate divisions within the browser window that contain unique content and behave independently. To create a page with two frames, for example, replace everything within (and including) the <BODY>...</BODY> containers with the following <FRAMESET>...</FRAMESET> container:

```
<FRAMESET ROWS="*,60">
<NOFRAMES>This page uses Frames.</NOFRAMES>
<FRAME SRC="home.html">
<FRAME SRC="nav.html" SCROLLING="no">
</FRAMESET>
```

This example will create two 'rows' of frames. The frame at the bottom of the page will be 60 pixels in height, while the '*' indicates that the top frame is not of a fixed size but rather uses the remaining space. The top frame will display the contents of a scrolling file called **home.html**, perhaps containing a hypertext index page. The bottom one will load a file called **nav.html** which might contain navigation buttons (and does not display a scroll bar). Thus in this example, the user moves around the site in the top frame; the bottom frame keeps the navigation buttons constantly to hand.

The text between the **<NOFRAMES>** tags is displayed by browsers that do not support frames. Columns are made using the **COLS** attribute in place of **ROWS**. Frames can be quite challenging—and of debatable usefulness. For information about additional attributes, their values, and idiosyncrasies, see:

> **<URL:http://home.netscape.com/comprod/products/navigator/version_2.0/frames/index.html>**

Special character entities

Chapter Four stressed that ASCII text files (which includes HTML pages) could not contain special characters. The ISO 8859-1 (Latin-1) standard was also mentioned (p.30). ASCII character combinations demarcated by '&' and a semicolon, known as '**entities**', can be used to display Latin-1 (non-ASCII) characters within Web pages. For example, **é** produces a small 'e' with an acute accent; **ü** produces a small 'u' with an umlaut, 'ü'.

Note that these character entities are case sensitive. Entities can also be described using the numeric code equivalent of Latin-1 characters, this time demarcated by '&#' and a semicolon. For example, **£** produces the '£' sign, while **ü** is an alternative way of producing a small 'u' with an umlaut, 'ü'.

Patients and doctors are more likely to respond to medical information in their native tongue. Since Latin-1 characters appear in many European languages, this facility enables us to create Web pages in languages other than just English, for example. A list of Latin-1 character entities is at:

> **<URL:http://www.w3.org/pub/WWW/MarkUp/Wilbur/ISOlat1.sgml>**

A table of Latin-1 8-bit (numeric) codes is at:

> **<URL:http://www.w3.org/pub/WWW/MarkUp/Wilbur/latin1.gif>**

Design tips

When planning a set of Web pages it is helpful to create a template upon which all the pages will be based, and to set down some guidelines to follow. Miscellaneous tips include the following:

- Set a maximum size limit for each page (text and images)—30 KB is often quoted. This has two principal benefits; it avoids users having to wait for large pages to load, and it avoids the effort of scrolling through large blocks of text.

- A mechanism for peer or editorial review prior to publication will avoid embarrassing errors.
- Typing all HTML tags in upper case distinguishes them from textual content within the page when editing your markup.
- Some computers (namely UNIX) are case sensitive, so standardizing all file names (HTML files, images, etc.) in lower case letters has merit and is easier to type. Use meaningful names e.g. **medical_links.html** versus **MedLink.HTML**.
- Consider using comment tags to break your markup into easily recognizable sections; this will aid subsequent editing greatly.

Structural issues

Employing a common structure throughout a set of pages helps the user become familiar with the site as a whole. For example, the user can place similar importance on information if it appears under headings of equal weight, or know where to find a link back to the home page. Many well-designed and simple pages can be broken into three principal sections; the header, content, and footer (see Fig. 38).

- The header typically includes a banner image, a page title, and perhaps a subtitle.
- The content will be unique to each page, whereas the header and footer will be similar across most pages making up the collection.
- The footer may contain an 'official seal' in the form of a logo, the author's details and contact information, the location of the document (in case the user wishes to save the page and reconnect at a later date), and an indication of currency. A statement of copyright is also common.
- These sections can be demarcated using a graphic bar or the **<HR>** tag.

Navigational aids

There are a number of techniques to ensure that users are able to navigate your pages with ease, some of which follow:

- Work out on paper before going to the keyboard what structure a set of pages should take, whether associated files should be grouped together in sub-directories, and where the important hypertext links should be.
- Create a highly visual navigation bar using small graphics or text menus (perhaps within a table), or an image map.
- Include a link to your home page from all pages.
- Include a table of contents, index page, or main menu.
- When information is to be presented in a prescribed sequence of linked pages,

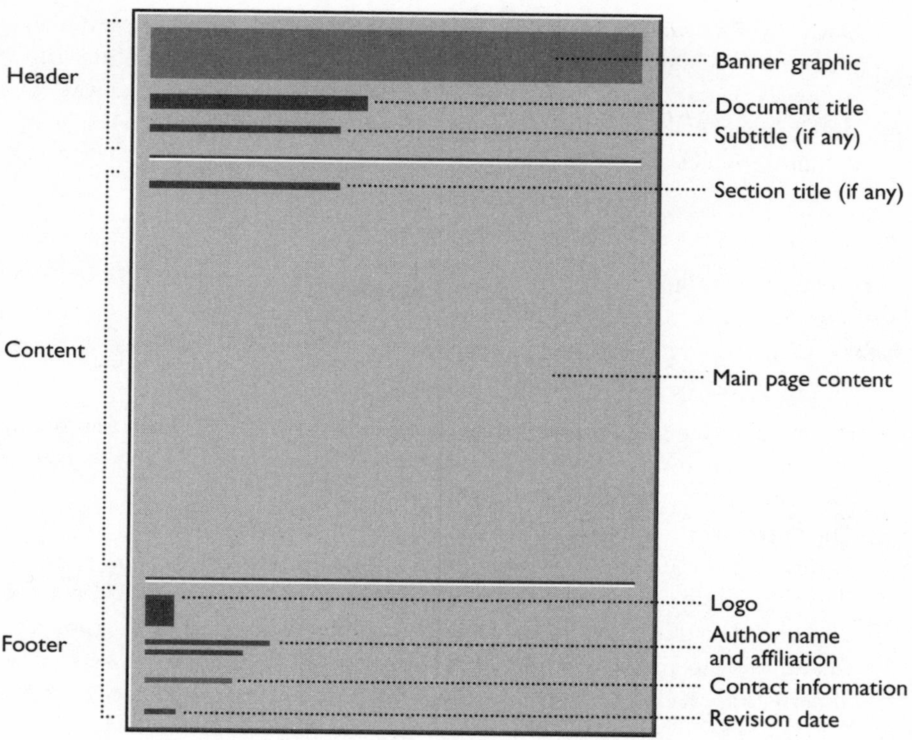

Fig. 38 The structure of a generic Web page. [Adapted from Lynch, with kind permission.]

provide 'Previous page' and 'Next page' text links or buttons.

- For longer pages, consider a 'Return to top' link at appropriate points within the text.
- Consider indicating changes from an earlier version of a document with a small 'New' graphic if they are few, or with a 'What's new' section if they are many.

HTML specification and 'browser wars'

Three things—the choice of browser (p.199); the version of the software; and the users customization of browser preferences—will determine how other people see the pages you design. In truth there is no 'standard' HTML universally subscribed to, no universal way of interpreting and displaying HTML, and no way to override the preferences set by the user. The WWW is a mix of ratified, draft, and proprietary 'extensions' to HTML from Netscape and Microsoft. The main browsers—Netscape Navigator and Microsoft Internet Explorer—battle to win market share through the regular release of new and 'improved' software. Each release brings with it a flurry of 'This page best viewed with...' messages.

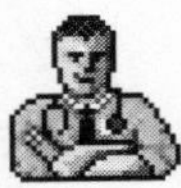

Design your pages to look good when viewed using the most prevalent versions of Navigator and Internet Explorer, and the majority of users will see pages that are visually pleasing and rendered in much the same way as the designer sees them. Thus, only use markup that is interpreted similarly by both products.

Using graphics wisely

If graphics merely consume Internet bandwidth, the apparent sparsity of text-only pages would seem to indicate a different reality. Graphics do much to relieve boredom, especially when breaking up large blocks of text. However, there is a happy medium. Remember that:

- High-resolution graphics take up more bandwidth as a larger file size is required to describe them; a graphic saved at screen resolution will look just as good as a high-resolution graphic when viewed on the Web.
- The greater the number of colours in a graphic, the greater the file size required to describe the image. Levels of colour correspond to '**bit depth**', with more colours needing more bits (p.21). Eight-bit images correspond to 256 colours—the limitation of the GIF format. If, for example, your graphics program allows you to save an image as either a 16-bit or 8-bit JPEG graphic and you can discern no appreciable difference in quality, the 8-bit image will have the smaller file size.
- Using the ALT attribute (p.226) is of immense value to the many users who turn off the automatic display of images.
- Most computer screens display at least 640 by 480 pixels (p.12), therefore an image that fits comfortably within these dimensions (e.g. a banner 500 pixels wide) will not force viewers to use the horizontal scroll bar (p.205).
- Reusing a small number of images improves page loading times as these can be reloaded from a local disk cache rather than fetched from the server.
- Some image manipulation programs can create 'anti-aliased' graphics. This is a technique for smoothing the jagged edges of bitmapped graphics (low-resolution pictures made up of pixels). Anti-aliased images have a more professional look, although introducing more colours (and thus size) to image files.
- Be wary of using background images (or colours) that obscure hypertext links by being of a similar colour.

For more advanced design tips, see the online supplement to *Creating killer Web sites* by David Siegel:

<URL:http://www.killersites.com/>

Concluding remarks

Creating a Web page or set of pages can be as simple or as complex as you want it to be.

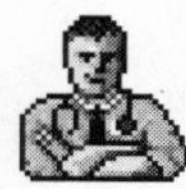

The best way to get experience in writing WWW pages is to dissect existing pages to discover how each effect was produced. Open an appealing WWW page that you have saved as an HTML file in your word processor (or choose the 'View source...' option in your browser). By studying for a few moments how the page is structured, several patterns will emerge. With a little experimentation you will soon be able to associate particular HTML tags and their attributes with a particular effect when the file is viewed in a WWW browser.

Once happy with your pages, they can be published on the Web or on an intranet (p.113), reside on your own machine for your personal use, or both. Publishing your pages if you don't have your own server typically involves using FTP to upload them to an incoming directory at the site that will host your pages.

To view your pages on your own machine (or when you connect to the Web), set your home page to the default home page (p.202) used by your browser. The documentation available with your browser will tell you how to do this. Setting a local page to your home page means you can work with your pages without the browser trying to open a PPP/SLIP connection.

References

Hope, R.A. and Longmore, J.M. (1987). *Oxford handbook of clinical medicine*. OUP, Oxford.

HTML Editorial Review Board. (1996, Apr). *Introducing HTML 3.2*, [Online]. <URL:http://www.w3.org/pub/WWW/MarkUp/Wilbur/>. World-Wide Web Consortium.

Lynch, P.J. (1995, Sep 6). *Yale C/AIM WWW style manual*, [Online]. <URL:http://info.med.yale.edu/caim/StyleManual_Top.HTML>. Yale Center for Advanced Instructional Media.

CHAPTER THIRTY TWO
Running a medical mailing list

GP-UK: A CASE STUDY

by Ian Purves, Mike Bainbridge, and Ian Trimble

Background

The practice of medicine in the UK is led by general practitioners (GPs) working together with other health professionals. Such 'group working' requires good communication, collaboration, and coordination. This process absorbs a vast amount of energy and is often conducted inefficiently. The Internet may provide a solution: e-mail can be read at a time convenient to the doctor, rather than demanding an immediate response (like a telephone call), enabling busy GPs to fulfil their communication requirements while managing their time more efficiently.

GPs experience considerable stress through their interactions with patients, and in making decisions on their patients' behalf. Sharing and relieving assimilated stress usually takes the form of discussion with other doctors. Advice sought from colleagues is often by telephone or at local postgraduate meetings, since there are only four GPs (on average) working out of the same building. An Internet mailing list offers GPs a chance to communicate, collaborate, and (occasionally) coordinate activity efficiently, on a much wider scale.

Information needs in general practice are also met inefficiently. They are served predominantly by books, academic journals, commercial magazines, and discussion with colleagues. It is said, in fact, that UK GPs need to read 17 journals a day to keep up-to-date. There is so much information available that GPs can at times feel overwhelmed.

Paper-based journals are presented in a 'one-to-many format': it is possible to respond to articles and news items via letters to the Editor, but publication can take many weeks (Robinson 1993). This, again, is inefficient. Messages to an Internet mailing list, on the other hand, are distributed in a 'many-to-many' format, allowing list members to discuss and debate issues as they arise. In effect, list members join a 'virtual conference' which is perpetual and ubiquitous.

The general aspects of mailing lists were discussed in Chapter Nineteen. This chapter describes how we set up the first mailing list for UK general practice, GP-UK. The steps involved in establishing the list and other operational issues are presented as case study.

Setting up a mailing list

There are three ways of setting up a mailing list.

Create a distribution list in your e-mail package

This can work well for small moderated lists, especially in the absence of a permanent Internet connection. E-mail sent to the list address can be forwarded manually to those on the distribution list (or rarely, automatically, using mail filters). Subscription and unsubscription must also be handled manually. Consequently the list owner must be able to devote considerable time to maintaining the list (and refrain from holidays!). Response time will invariably be slower than with a fully automated list, since it depends how often the list owner dials in to receive and redistribute messages.

Set up a list on someone else's list server

If your purpose is 'not for profit' then approaching Mailbase (see below) might be a solution, as may your campus computing centre or equivalent. Alternatively, there are several commercial sites that will be happy to take your money!

Set up your own list server

Dedicated list server software will automatically receive mail sent to the list, forward such messages to the list subscribers, compile digests of discussions, and allow users to subscribe/ unsubscribe or receive file archives/FAQs (using commands sent in the subject line or body of an e-mail message). Most lists are run on UNIX computers (and require a good knowledge of that operating system), but 'friendlier' list server software is also available for Windows NT and the Macintosh. Although list server software is not particularly demanding on system resources, it may still be demanding on your time. Solving problems such as 'mail loops' can be tricky, and automated 'I'm on holiday' e-mail messages can soon build up! For further information, see the *Mailing list management software FAQ* from N. Aleks at:

<URL:ftp://ftp.uu.net/usenet/news.answers/mail/list-admin/software-faq>

Mailbase

As our list was intended primarily for the UK, and for academic purposes, we approached Mailbase. Mailbase is the foremost academic list-server resource in the UK, funded by Joint Information Systems Committee of the Higher Education Funding Councils (JISC). Use of its lists must conform to the JANET Acceptable Use Policy, and this precludes NHS clinical and administrative use. However, individual users can apply to create new lists providing they are seen to be of benefit to the UK higher education and research community. The list owner (the person setting up a mailing list) and a significant portion of the membership should be part of this community (which in practice means they have an e-mail address ending in **.ac.uk.**). For further information, use the following URLs:

<URL:mailto:mailbase@mailbase.ac.uk> Send: send mailbase policy

<URL:mailto:mailbase@mailbase.ac.uk> Send: send mailbase new-list-template

<URL:http:/www.mailbase.ac.uk/docs/mbdocs.html>

Mailbase can also be contacted at the University Computing Service, University of Newcastle Upon Tyne, Newcastle Upon Tyne NE1 7RU, UK. Telephone 0191 222 8080, or e-mail mailbase-helpline@mailbase.ac.uk.

List ownership

The list owner requires a number of additional attributes. He or she needs to understand the politics and technical issues involved in establishing a list, and be able to invest a considerable amount of time to ensure its continuing success.

For a large list with consistently high levels of message traffic it may prove difficult to maintain continuity with a single list owner. On the other hand, it may be harder to maintain a consistent list etiquette with multiple list owners, and moderation may prove impossible (see below).

The GP-UK project involves three co-owners and Mailbase provides the facility for administrative messages to be posted to all the co-owners concurrently. We approached Mailbase early in 1994 with our proposals for GP-UK. We convinced them of our academic credentials and, after considerable discussion, the list became operational in October 1994.

Getting going

Having established list ownership and a suitable provider, we had to let the world know who we were and how to join us. We published articles in the commercial and academic medical press (Purves *et al.* 1995), and produced a printed summary for distribution at medical meetings. As membership of the list has grown we have maintained our links with the press (indeed, whole pages of the national medical press have recently been given over to correspondence from GP-UK).

Membership of a mailing list requires active subscription by its members and, unlike joining newsgroups, the act of subscription engenders a strong feeling of community amongst its members. The list owners keep a keen eye on the membership and content of the list and act accordingly (see below). For the medical fraternity this has the advantage of discouraging casual public enquiries about friends or relatives with obscure medical diagnoses, and it focuses the discussion on an agenda which is driven by active members of the list.

Cross-fertilization with other mailing lists, particularly **fam-med** in the United States, has resulted in significant recruitment from around the globe. GP-UK now boasts members from as far afield as Argentina and Iceland. One of the most successful Mailbase lists, membership has grown to over 400 in just 18 months. This does not include several hundred GPs who participate via linked bulletin boards.

The **fam-med** mailing list Web site:

<URL:http://apollo.gac.edu>

Maintaining the list

All new members are invited to submit a registration questionnaire on a voluntary basis and their details are added to a constantly updated database (which is accessible by FTP). It would be impossible to confirm professional status but all members are expected to conform to the group etiquette which is closely monitored. The list owner would remove any transgressor, but this has not yet proved necessary.

Every message sent to GP-UK is distributed: currently 20 to 30 messages a day. Unfortunately, Mailbase does not provide a facility which would sort and condense mailings into a single weekly 'digest', thus reducing the amount of e-mail each subscriber has to deal with. However, a monthly review of the list is prepared and distributed to all list members and issues of etiquette are constantly reviewed and discussed.

In addition to these tasks the list owners must keep in touch with developments at Mailbase and remove inactive members' addresses to minimize unnecessary traffic. We estimate that each list owner spends over ten hours per month on the promotion and administration of GP-UK.

Moderation

In a moderated list all messages pass through the list owner, who acts as a *de facto* editor. Moderation offers the advantage of tight editorial control, focusing discussion, and preventing abuse of the list (such as repeated postings and commercial advertising). However, as every message has to be reviewed, moderation is time consuming and inevitably imposes the agenda of the list owner, thus restricting freedom of discussion.

For a list with multiple list owners, reviewing each message would make the list unwieldy. We therefore made a conscious decision not to moderate contributions to GP-UK. Our decision has been vindicated by the consistently high quality of postings to GP-UK. Instances of abuse have been dealt with by a brisk exchange of messages between active contributors and the list has, in effect, been self-policing. In the rare event of a recurrent offender a brief personal exchange between the owners and the perpetrator has been sufficient.

Content

Discussions on the list have covered topics such as NHS-wide networking, clinical coding, security issues, evidence-based medicine, and the future of electronic publishing. GP-UK is an academic list and we are pleased to report that the quality of articles posted has been consistently high. A number of clinical issues have also been raised, and members report that each article attracts several personal e-mail responses in addition to any posted directly to the list.

Integration with other Internet services

Archived correspondence can be accessed by FTP from the Mailbase server. Some packages such as Forte's Agent can take these archives (once downloaded) and 'thread' them (p.173) in a similar way to newsgroup messages. Software is also available that will automatically thread messages posted to a mailing list, and publish these dynamically on the Web ('Hypermail').

From the appropriate Mailbase Web page, clicking on a list name (such as GP-UK) brings up a hypertext menu offering information about list members, the list owners, searchable and Hypermail message archives (so you can sample the discussion on a list without actually subscribing), and information on how to subscribe/unsubscribe.

<URL:http://www.mailbase.ac.uk/other/medi-class.html>

We have established our own GP-UK Web home page, linking to various files and other Web sites of medical interest. This page describes the function of the mailing list and is linked to the home pages of the Primary Health Care Specialist Group of the British Computer Society and their journal, *Informatics*. Web pages can be used to simplify subscription to a list by incorporating a 'Click here to subscribe' (or similar) button.

<URL:http://www.ncl.ac.uk/~nphcare/GPUK/gpukhome.html>

The Web site and the mailing list are complementary. By analogy to paper-based journals, the Web site displays editorial content while the mailing list functions as the correspondence section. The Web site remains topical only if it is regularly updated, but the mailing list is spontaneous and instantaneous, which makes it more compelling to regular participants.

What can a list achieve?

Although the brief of GP-UK is to discuss topical and academic issues a feeling of community has gradually developed, enhanced by a sprinkling of humour and mild cynicism.

As well as offering a forum for GPs to share experiences, a number of important issues have been raised. For example, recent concerns about third-generation contraceptive pills were discussed in detail. There is a constant exchange about the provision of out-of-hours services, and there has been a detailed discussion concerning the security of patient's medical records. The latter discussion has contributed to the BMA Security Guidelines (Anderson 1996) and the implementation of a pilot scheme.

Through contacts established on the list, members have collaborated in each others' research, and meetings and conferences have been announced and coordinated.

Problems

Because we have decided not to moderate the list a number of rogue messages appear from time to time—usually inadvertent subscribe/unsubscribe messages, and misdirected personal e-mail. As described above, abuse of the list has been minimal. There have been occasional instances of advertising and inappropriate uuencoded graphics (p.158), but these have been summarily dealt with by members of the list. There have been only two instances of significant downtime of the Mailbase server over the first 18 months of operation.

Although archives of the list provide a valuable record of the discussions on GP-UK and are readily available, they are seldom accessed. It is possible that this resource could be promoted by linking it more effectively to our home page.

Our decision as owners to stay 'hands-off' and let GP-UK develop in its own way has run into a political barrier between the UK Departments of Health and Education over funding. Despite being one of the most consistently successful Mailbase lists, general practice in the form of GP-UK is not regarded as being sufficiently academic to justify ongoing support from JISC, and Mailbase has reluctantly asked us to look for a new home or funding. Those interested in JISC policy on NHS use of its services and its implications for academic departments wishing to set up a mailing list (that may invariably carry some 'clinical' traffic) are advised to read *Network News 43*:

<URL:http://www.ja.net/>

The future

We believe the principal advantage the Internet offers over and above the paper medium is the ease of timely participation in debates on topical medical issues. This may best be achieved through a properly established and monitored mailing list.

A broader contention is whether an Internet Web site and mailing list could ever supplant a paper-based publication (Coiera 1995). It will be several years before Internet access achieves universality in the way that the telephone network does now. Even then there will be a proportion of any potential readership with an inherent distrust of the electronic medium—'techno-phobes'. Eventually, however, the advantages will overcome such reservation and we predict an increasing presence of academic journals on the Internet (Delamonte 1995).

List traffic has increased as membership of our list has grown. It has already reached the point where some members decide it is no longer worth their while to read every message. The list owners can either allow the list to find its own equilibrium or elect to further develop the list.

We are actively considering dividing the list into a 'superlist' (which would act as the administrative focus of GP-UK) and several dependent 'daughter lists', each focusing on a major area of discussion. We have held talks with major academic publishers about the possibility of linking the correspondence sections of their journals directly with GP-UK, via their own WWW pages. This would promote interest in their publications and extend the 'virtual conference' concept discussed above. We have also discussed these issues with those involved in developing the new UK National Health Service wide-area network (NHSnet, p.137). We shall continue to seek new sponsorship and, possibly, a new Internet host.

It is likely that GP-UK will eventually be hosted by one or more of the following resources:

- Mailbase (for UK academically focused lists)
- The NHS wide-area network (for clinically focused lists)
- A private Internet resource (run by professionals under the direction of a steering group).

Although GP-UK is really several lists rolled into one we would not like to see GP-UK lose its lack of focus or 'fuzziness' which is appreciated by many of its members. We receive frequent messages from GPs who already feel GP-UK has become part of their life, and that its variety adds to the spice. However, it will be important to develop new, tightly focused lists (and probably newsgroups) where community is not required. It is for us as list owners, in conjunction with our members, to face the challenge of overlap with the current GP-UK list, to find solutions to keep our community alive—and more importantly, make it grow into an information resource for the future which is still fun to use.

At the time of writing we cannot be certain about the future of GP-UK, but we are convinced that mailing lists are part of the future for UK general practice.

References

Anderson, R. (1996). Clinical system security: interim guidelines. *BMJ*, **312**, 109–11.

Coiera, E. (1995). Medical informatics. *BMJ*, **310**, 1381–7.

Delamonte, T. (1995). BMJ on the Internet. *BMJ*, **310**, 1343–4.

Robinson, G.J. (1993). Journal publication times. *British Journal of General Practice*, **43**, 261. [Letter.]

Purves, I., Bainbridge, M., and Trimble, I. (1995). Ongoing electronic conference is available for general practitioners. *BMJ*, **311**, 512–13.

CHAPTER THIRTY THREE
Developing for the WWW

BIOMEDNET: A CASE STUDY

by Richard Charkin and Paul Lynas

BioMedNet is presently (in July 1996) the leading world-wide club for the biological and medical communities.

<URL:http://BioMedNet.com>

The club has 18 000 members to date and new members are joining at the rate of 1000 each week. The total targeted market is 150 000 members. Members range from undergraduate students to full professors, from cell biologists to rheumatologists, and from 18 to 85 year-olds. Half the membership is in North America, with the rest divided by country approximately in proportion to national research budgets. Members from the medical community come mainly from research institutions rather than clinical practice—a reflection partly of different levels of access to the Internet, and partly of BioMedNet's initial focus on scientific information.

On joining the club, members are asked to complete a detailed registration form—the rationale being that a complex registration process would 'filter' membership (so that only those with a genuine interest from the biological and medical community would take the time and effort to register). A further practical benefit of having such a detailed registration form is the creation of a powerful marketing database—something a simple registration process could not provide.

New members are asked to provide personal and professional details which can be made available to other members (only with their approval). Once a new member has registered they can be supplied with information which is specific to their needs. In addition, they can search the profiles of other members and communicate with those who have similar interests using IRC (p.229), meeting rooms (pre-booked private IRC channels), and discussion groups (utilizing HyperNews, a program developed by the NCSA). See Fig. 39.

Members can seek or advertise jobs, purchase software, instrumentation, reagents, or books in the shopping mall, and keep up to date with scientific gossip from John Maddox (the distinguished former editor of *Nature*). They can also search or browse through the full-text and image library. Most of these activities are free, the costs being supported by advertising and sponsorship. Members pay for information only where copyright is held

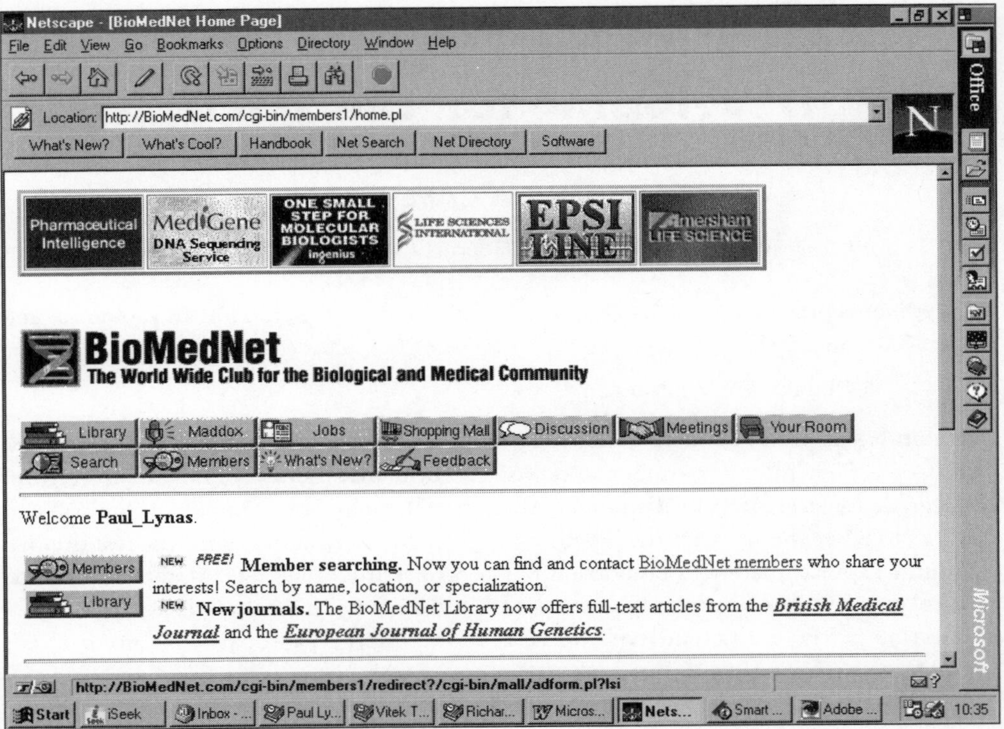

Fig.39 The BioMedNet home page provides members with access to a full-text and image library, scientific gossip, employment opportunities, discussion and conferencing forums, and a way to contact other members with like interests.

by other scientists and their publishers. A typical price is as little as $US1.00 per journal article which allows for downloading and printing as well as reading on-screen. Abstracts are usually free, so members can check the relevance of an article before they buy.

BioMedNet is a distributor of information, not a publisher in its own right. From the outset BioMedNet resolved not to interfere with the pricing policies of publishers, allowing them to set their own fees, whether this was on a 'pay-as-you-go' basis or a fixed-fee subscription (the former being preferred).

The costs are charged to the member's credit card using a secure online transaction system we developed in-house. However, a fax hotline was also introduced so that members who fear such online transactions could have an alternative for providing their details and, of course, 'snail mail' still plays a role (albeit a lesser one).

While advertisers and sponsors are important to BioMedNet, their role has yet to be clearly defined and it may be too early to tell how dependent on them we will become. At present membership of the club is free, and in order to maintain this we hope to recover our costs through the sponsorship of some content. As the club develops and as more publishers, advertisers, and members join, the prospects for sponsorship from pharmaceutical companies (for example) would naturally increase.

Beginnings

The concept of BioMedNet originated in 1994. From the start the intention was to create a forum for collaboration between scientists—not simply a distribution channel for information. The idea was originally developed by Vitek Tracz (Chairman of the Current Science Group) in 1990. It crystallized into the club concept after he and his senior programmer, Andrew Witbrock, first realized the importance of communication between individuals as shown by the chat, library, shopping, and job exchange facilities used heavily in consumer-orientated services such as America OnLine.

In the area of scientific collaboration, early work on a virtual environment for biologists, pioneered by the 'BioMOO' project at the Weitzman Institute (p.231), was another source of inspiration. However, these ideas had not yet developed into a fully realized online community of scientists.

The first years were devoted to developing the software required for BioMedNet to function. During most of this period very little reliable software had been developed for the Internet—and waiting for developments would have slowed progress unacceptably. Indeed, we even developed our own viewer for BioMedNet which was ditched when the World-Wide Web took the Internet by storm in early 1995. This is still the most popular information system on the Internet, and as in the case of most things, the majority rules, so we developed further with the World-Wide Web in mind. Several versions of the search engine, BiblioteK, were developed. A fully integrated transaction and billing system had to be created, and the design of every sub-function and every page was an invention in its own right.

In parallel with this a programme of publisher relations was put in place in order to acquire significant volumes of appropriate material for the club Library. Beta testing began in autumn 1995 and BioMedNet officially went live in April 1996.

Issues

BioMedNet's development has identified a number of issues, many of which will be applicable to other groups seeking to develop an Internet-based information service. These are as follows:

Financial

The up-front costs have exceeded £10 million and we need more than 50 staff to run the club on a continuing basis.

Human

From the outset we have insisted on the highest standards of software, design, and content. These require rare talents. Finding, retaining, and nurturing these people has been a major challenge, particularly given the huge demand for 'Web-literate' editors and engineers.

Structure

BioMedNet is neither publisher, wholesaler, nor retailer. No paradigms existed (nor exist) for the management of a 'cyberspace club' for professionals. The closest model we have found is the learned society, and many of our structures are similar. For example, we have a Membership Secretary, Advisory Boards, Executive Committee, etc.

Suppliers

Our biggest problem has been that few scientific and medical publishers (including those in our own Group) have the resources to convert their existing data into a useable format. Conversion of data to SGML and HTML (p.199) can involve complex programming and as this facility is so recent, there is a deficiency in both qualified personnel and suitable software for the task. Not even the software companies have managed to address this issue. Although scientific journals have been at the forefront of the information revolution, constant pressure on costs has slowed full implementation of the electronic capture of data. This is improving daily—but we had expected more rapid development.

Linked to this technological problem is a more telling psychological issue: publishers fear the Web. We have had to spend enormous amounts of time persuading publishers that BioMedNet presents a way of increasing the penetration of their materials among biologists and medical scientists. BioMedNet is not 'stealing' business, but creating it. Most publishers now understand this, but some are still distrustful of any collaboration and are insisting on creating exclusive single publisher or single journal sites which are great for egos but do little for science or commerce.

Members

The biggest issue is the expectation among the early users that everything should be free. We have tried to keep charges as low as possible in the belief that high quality and low prices will lead to high volume, but there is still resistance to paying even $US1.00 for a paper in some quarters. As the Web becomes more commercial, and as members realize that without payment there will be little quality publishing, this should diminish. The other side of this coin is the enormous support we have had from working scientists in terms of feedback and encouragement.

Access and speed

While the performance of Internet access providers is beyond our control, we have focused on our own service as information providers. Scientists do not want to spend a lot of time waiting for information to be downloaded. In order to ensure that we deliver a faster, more efficient service, a series of maintenance checks are performed regularly on the server (and if necessary, the server hardware is upgraded to cope with the demand from members). This has yet to cause any major headaches as we anticipated large usage and prepared ourselves accordingly. However, this area will need to be readdressed as the amount of data available through BioMedNet increases.

The future

By the time this book is published BioMedNet will have changed. Exactly how, we do not know. Certainly the Library will be bigger and will contain not just journals but a wide range of databases including MEDLINE. The shopping mall will contain many bookshops, subscription agents, and even record stores. Members will be able to charge the costs of purchase against their BioMedNet account. The News section will be extended to link to other databases such as Reuters for financial information and to the latest information about conferences—and travel agents for getting there. Members will be able to communicate with each other via an internal BioMedNet e-mail system. We are developing a current awareness program for linking a member's profile with selected news and research items within the club. Another program is creating the technology to link all medical and biological intellectual resources allowing members to find relevant information, even where the relevant paper is not held in the Library. We are working with learned societies and pharmaceutical companies to create subsets of BioMedNet (relating to sub-disciplines or to single diseases) serving smaller communities of interest. We are working with librarians to establish ways of allowing their users to charge all or part of their purchases to institutional budgets, and to use the enormous expertise of librarians to help users get the best out of the new technologies.

Most importantly, we recognize that BioMedNet in July 1996 is only the beginning of an idea. It will develop—and the direction of development will be driven by its members not its executive. Our most important asset is our network of members, and in particular those who give us constant feedback (even the negative feedback which usually relates to speed of connection). As we develop the medical side of the club we particularly need clinical input—simply join the club and hit the feedback button.

Medicine and the Internet on the World-Wide Web

Do you want to visit the resources mentioned in this book? Would you like to keep up-to-date with relevant developments? You can do both as *Medicine and the Internet* has its own home page on the World-Wide Web. From this page you can browse our Bookmarks and Online Updates.

Bookmarks: one-click access

Throughout this book many Internet resources have been mentioned—and some have had rather complex Internet addresses (URLs). To save you the effort of typing them in, we have listed all the resources in the 'Bookmarks' section of the Web site. They are organized by chapter, heading, and subheading just as in the book, making it exceptionally easy to locate resources you have been reading about—just click on them! Furthermore, because these Bookmarks are accessed directly from the Web and the links are periodically checked, we can keep them up-to-date to reflect any changes.

Online Updates: what's new?

The dynamic nature of the Internet means that new developments and medical applications generate a steady stream of information. Current information is disseminated very effectively by electronic means, and these Web pages provide readers of *Medicine and the Internet* with just that. They acknowledge the portability and other advantages of the paper-based text, yet add a new dimension to medical publishing through the complementary provision of 'Online Updates'. Readers can even register to receive notification of new Updates by e-mail! We believe that this service offers an exceptionally useful marriage between traditional and electronic information access. As the contents of these free Online Updates reflect future editions of this book, you can be sure that your investment in this printed edition is protected.

There's more?

We have also provided an 'e-Profile' of the book featuring the table of contents, extracts, and ordering details enabling colleagues to obtain the book on your recommendation. A Feedback page offers you the chance to influence future editions of the book or contact the author directly. The Search page links to major search tools, medical catalogues, and MEDLINE facilities. To see these pages at their best, we recommend that you use a current version of either the Navigator or Internet Explorer WWW browser. Just point it at:

<URL:http://www.oup.co.uk/scimed/medint/>

APPENDIX
Medical specialty resources

by Eric Rumsey

The following collection of World-Wide Web sites has been supplied by Eric Rumsey at the Hardin Library for the Health Sciences, University of Iowa. Under each specialty is listed the address (universal resource locator, or URL) of three Web pages boasting large indexes of relevant resources, taken from the Hardin Meta Directory—a 'list of lists'. The Hardin Meta Directory (MD) contains further listings arranged according to the approximate size of each index:

<URL:http://www.arcade.uiowa.edu/hardin-www/md.html>

By indicating list size, the Hardin Library for the Health Sciences believe that their directory makes it easier for specialists to locate the most comprehensive resource collections. Furthermore, it conveniently links directly to the relevant page within multi-subject catalogues such as MedWeb and Yahoo, in addition to incorporating independent discipline-specific lists.

Allergy resources

MedWeb: Immunology (Health Sciences Library, Emory University):

<URL:http://www.gen.emory.edu/medweb/medweb.immunology.html>

WWW Virtual Library: Immunology (Keith Robinson, Harvard University):

<URL:http://golgi.harvard.edu/biopages/immuno.html>

MIC-KIBIC MeSH Index: Immunologic Diseases (Karolinska Institute):

<URL:http://www.mic.ki.se/Diseases/c20.html>

See also Hardin Meta Directory Allergy:

<URL:http://www.arcade.uiowa.edu/hardin-www/md-allergy.html>

Anaesthesiology resources

Anesthesia and Critical Care Resources on the Internet (A. J. Wright and Dr. Frank O'Connor):

<URL:http://www.eur.nl/FGG/ANEST/wright/contents.html>

Virtual library: Anesthesiology (Keith J. Ruskin, Yale University):

<URL:http://gasnet.med.yale.edu/index.html>

MedWeb: Anesthesiology (Health Sciences Library, Emory University):
<URL:http://www.gen.emory.edu/medweb/medweb.anesthesiology.html>

See also Hardin Meta Directory Anesthesiology:
<URL:http://www.arcade.uiowa.edu/hardin-www/md-anesth.html>

Biotechnology resources

MedWeb: Biotechnology (Health Sciences Library, Emory University):
<URL:http://www.gen.emory.edu/medweb/medweb.biotechnology.html>

BioTech: Professional Resources (Indiana University):
<URL:http://biotech.chem.indiana.edu/pages/prores.html>

WWW Virtual Library: Biotechnology (D. Hopp, Cato Research):
<URL:http://www.cato.com/interweb/cato/biotech/>

See also Hardin Meta Directory Biotechnology:
<URL:http://www.arcade.uiowa.edu/hardin-www/md-biotech.html>

Cardiology resources

Hot Heart Links: Cardiology on the World Wide Web (Cleveland Clinic):
<URL:http://www.heartcenter.ccf.org:8080/www_eps/hot_hart/heart.htm>

Cardiology Compass (Washington University):
<URL:http://osler.wustl.edu/~murphy/cardiology/compass.html>

MedWeb: Cardiology (Health Sciences Library, Emory University):
<URL:http://www.gen.emory.edu/medweb/medweb.cardiology.html>

See also Hardin Meta Directory Cardiology:
<URL:http://www.arcade.uiowa.edu/hardin-www/md-cardio.html>

Dentistry resources

Dental Related Internet Resources (New York University):
<URL:http://www.nyu.edu:80/Dental/intres.html>

Highlander Index of Dental Resources (Art Brown, DMD):
<URL:http://www.mindspring.com/~cmcleod/cmcleod.html>

Internet Dentistry Resources (Janice Quinn, University of Iowa):
<URL:http://indy.radiology.uiowa.edu/Beyond/Dentistry/sites.html>

See also Hardin Meta Directory Dentistry:

<URL:http://www.arcade.uiowa.edu/hardin-www/md-dent.html>

Dermatology resources:

HealthWeb: Dermatology (CIC/Indiana Univerisity):

<URL:http://www.medlib.iupui.edu/cicnet/derma/derma.html>

MIC-KIBIC MeSH Index: Skin and Connective Tissue Diseases (Karolinska Institute):

<URL:http://www.mic.ki.se/Diseases/c17.html>

Dermatology Resources (Tom Ray M.D., University of Iowa):

<URL:http://tray.dermatology.uiowa.edu/home.html#Dermatology>

See also Hardin Meta Directory Dermatology:

<URL:http://www.arcade.uiowa.edu/hardin-www/md-derm.html>

Emergency medicine resources:

MedWeb: Emergency Medicine (Health Sciences Library, Emory University):

<URL:http://www.gen.emory.edu/medweb/medweb.emergency.html>

Emergency Services WWW Site List (Dean Tabor, Fairbanks, Alaska):

<URL:http://gilligan.uafadm.alaska.edu/www-911.htm>

World Wide Web of Emergency Services (Rochester Institute of Technology):

<URL:http://dumbo.isc.rit.edu/ems/>

See also Hardin Meta Directory Emergency Medicine:

<URL:http://www.arcade.uiowa.edu/hardin-www/md-emerg.html>

Endocrinology and diabetes resources:

Diabetes Monitor (Midwest Diabetes Care Center, Kansas City):

<URL:http://www.castleweb.com/~monitor/index.html>

MedWeb: Endocrinology (Health Sciences Library, Emory University):

<URL:http://www.gen.emory.edu/medweb/medweb.endocrinology.html>

MIC-KIBIC MeSH Index: Endocrine Diseases (Karolinska Institute):

<URL:http://www.mic.ki.se/Diseases/c19.html>

See also Hardin Meta Directory Endocrinology and Diabetes:

<URL:http://www.arcade.uiowa.edu/hardin-www/md-endocrin.html>

Family medicine/general practice resources:

Medical Resources on the World Wide Web (Journal of Family Practice, Mark Ebell):

<URL:http://www.phymac.med.wayne.edu/jfp/fammed.htm>

MedWeb: Family Medicine (Health Sciences Library, Emory University):

<URL:http://www.gen.emory.edu/medweb/medweb.family.html>

Family Medicine Related Internet Resources (V. Olchanski, Medical College of Virginia):

<URL:http://views.vcu.edu/views/fap/volc-r.html>

See also Hardin Meta Directory Family Medicine:

<URL:http://www.arcade.uiowa.edu/hardin-www/md-fam.html>

Gastroenterology resources:

Gastroenterology Resources (Columbia University):

<URL:http://cpmcnet.columbia.edu/dept/gi/elsewhere.html>

MIC-KIBIC MeSH Index: Digestive System Diseases (Karolinska Institute):

<URL:http://www.mic.ki.se/Diseases/c6.html>

Diseases of the Liver (Howard J. Worman M.D., Columbia University):

<URL:http://cpmcnet.columbia.edu/dept/gi/disliv.html>

See also Hardin Meta Directory Gastroenterology:

<URL:http://www.arcade.uiowa.edu/hardin-www/md-gastro.html>

Geriatrics/care of the elderly resources:

Internet and E-Mail Resources on Aging (Joyce A. Post):

<URL:http://www.aoa.dhhs.gov/aoa/pages/jpostlst.html>

MedWeb: Geriatrics (Health Sciences Library, Emory University):

<URL:http://www.gen.emory.edu/medweb/medweb.geriatrics.html>

Directory of Aging Directories (DHHS/University of North Texas):

<URL:http://www.aoa.dhhs.gov/aoa/webres/direct.htm>

See also Hardin Meta Directory Geriatrics:

<URL:http://www.arcade.uiowa.edu/hardin-www/md-ger.html>

Haematology resources:

MIC-KIBIC MeSH Index: Hemic and Lymphatic Diseases (Karolinska Institute):

<URL:http://www.mic.ki.se/Diseases/c15.html>

Medical Matrix: Hematology (American Medical Informatics Association):

<URL:http://www.slackinc.com/matrix/SPECIALT/HEMATOLO.HTML>

Hematology Resources (University of Pittsburgh Health Sciences Library):

<URL:http://www.falk.med.pitt.edu/subjects/hemat.html>

See also Hardin Meta Directory Hematology:

<URL:http://www.arcade.uiowa.edu/hardin-www/md-hem.html>

Medical informatics resources:

Medical Informatics and Medicine: some useful links (Dr. Jeremy Rogers, Manchester UK):

<URL:http://www.cs.man.ac.uk/mig/people/medicine/medicine.html>

MedWeb: Informatics (Health Sciences Library, Emory University):

<URL:http://www.gen.emory.edu/medweb/medweb.informatics.html>

Veterinary Informatics Home Page (Ken Boschert, Washington University):

<URL:http://netvet.wustl.edu/info.htm>

See also Hardin Meta Directory Medical Informatics:

<URL:http://www.arcade.uiowa.edu/hardin-www/md-inform.html>

Microbiology and infectious diseases resources:

All the Virology Servers in the World (David M. Sander, Tulane University):

<URL:http://www.tulane.edu/~dmsander/garryfavweb.html>

WWW Virtual Library: Microbiology and Virology (Keith Robison, Harvard University):

<URL:http://golgi.harvard.edu/biopages/micro.html>

MedWeb: Infectious Diseases (Health Sciences Library, Emory University):

<URL:http://www.gen.emory.edu/medweb/medweb.id.html>

See also Hardin Meta Directory Microbiology and Infectious Diseases:

<URL:http://www.arcade.uiowa.edu/hardin-www/md-micro.html>

Nephrology/urology resources:

RenalNet (Gamewood Data Systems):

<URL:http://ns.gamewood.net/renalnet.html>

NephroNet (StanNet WWWeb Site Designing & Publishing Co):

<URL:http://www.nephronet.com/stannet/nephro/welcome.html>

MIC-KIBIC MeSH Index: Urologic and Male Genital Diseases (Karolinska Institute):

<URL:http://www.mic.ki.se/Diseases/c12.html>

See also Hardin Meta Directory Nephrology/Urology:

<URL:http://www.arcade.uiowa.edu/hardin-www/md-nephrol.html>

Neurology/neurosciences resources:

Neurosciences on the Internet (Neil A. Busis M.D., Pittsburgh):

<URL:http://ivory.lm.com:80/~nab/index.html>

MedWeb: Neurology (Health Sciences Library, Emory University):

<URL:http://www.gen.emory.edu/medweb/medweb.neurology.html>

MIC-KIBIC MeSH Index: Nervous System Diseases (Karolinska Institute):

<URL:http://www.mic.ki.se/Diseases/c10.html>

See also Hardin Meta Directory Neurology/Neurosciences:

<URL:http://www.arcade.uiowa.edu/hardin-www/md-neuro.html>

Nursing resources:

MedWeb: Nursing (Health Sciences Library, Emory University):

<URL:http://www.gen.emory.edu/medweb/medweb.nursing.html>

NursingNet (Mark and Mary Carraway):

<URL:http://www.communique.net/~nursgnt/>

HealthWeb: Nursing (CIC/University of Michigan):

<URL:http://www.lib.umich.edu/tml/nursing.html>

See also Hardin Meta Directory Nursing:

<URL:http://www.arcade.uiowa.edu/hardin-www/md-nurs.html>

Nutrition resources:

Arbor Communications Nutrition Pages (Tony Helman, Royal Australian College of General Practice):

<URL:http://netspace.net.au/%7Ehelmant/nutid.htm>

MedWeb: Nutrition (Health Sciences Library, Emory University):

<URL:http://www.gen.emory.edu/medweb/medweb.nutrition.html>

Food Science Sites (David MacKinnon, University of Prince Edward Island, Canada):

<URL:http://www.upei.ca/~dkmackin/food.html>

See also Hardin Meta Directory Nutrition:

<URL:http://www.arcade.uiowa.edu/hardin-www/md-nutr.html>

Obstetrics, gynaecology, and women's health resources:

Obstetrics and Gynecology links (Armando G. Amador, M.D., Southern Illinois University):

<URL:http://www.siumed.edu/ob/oblink.html>

MedWeb: Gynecology and Women's Health (Health Sciences Library, Emory University):

<URL:http://www.gen.emory.edu/medweb/medweb.gynecology.html>

MIC-KIBIC MeSH Index: Female Genital Diseases and Pregnancy Complications (Karolinska Institute):

<URL:http://www.mic.ki.se/Diseases/c13.html>

See also Hardin Meta Directory Obstetrics, Gynecology, and Women's Health:

<URL:http://www.arcade.uiowa.edu/hardin-www/md-obgyn.html>

Oncology resources:

Oncolink (University of Pennsylvania College of Medicine):

<URL:http://oncolink.upenn.edu/>

HealthWeb: Oncology (CIC/Indiana University):

<URL:http://www.medlib.iupui.edu/cicnet/onco/onco.html>

MedWeb: Oncology (Health Sciences Library, Emory University):

<URL:http://www.gen.emory.edu/medweb/medweb.oncology.html>

See also Hardin Meta Directory Oncology:

<URL:http://www.arcade.uiowa.edu/hardin-www/md-oncol.html>

Ophthalmology resources:

MedWeb: Ophthalmology and Optometry (Health Sciences Library, Emory University):

<URL:http://www.gen.emory.edu/medweb/medweb.optometry.html>

Eye Care Links (American Academy of Ophthalmology):

<URL:http://www.eyenet.org/eyelinks.html>

Ophthalmology Sites (*Digital Journal of Ophthalmology*):

<URL:http://netope.harvard.edu:80/meei/OtherSites.html>

See also Hardin Meta Directory Ophthalmology:

<URL:http://www.arcade.uiowa.edu/hardin-www/md-ophth.html>

Orthopaedics resources:

Orthopaedic Links (Myles Clough, in association with the **sci.med.orthopedics** newsgroup):

<URL:http://www.netshop.net/~cloughs/orthlink.html>

Biomechanics World Wide (J. Pierre Baudin/Biomch-l listserv):

<URL:http://dragon.acadiau.ca/~pbaudin/biomch.html>

LinkOrthopaedics (University of Dundee, UK):

<URL:http://www.dundee.ac.uk/orthopaedics/link/welcome.htm>

See also Hardin Meta Directory Orthopedics:

<URL:http://www.arcade.uiowa.edu/hardin-www/md-ortho.html>

Otolaryngology resources:

Otolaryngology Resources on the Internet (Baylor College of Medicine):

<URL:http://www.bcm.tmc.edu/oto/others.html>

WWW Virtual Library: Otolaryngology (Gerald R. Popelka, Association for Research in Otolaryngology):

<URL:http://www.aro.org/showcase/aro/library/sites.html>

MedWeb: Hearing (Health Sciences Library, Emory University):

<URL:http://www.gen.emory.edu/medweb/medweb.hearing.html>

See also Hardin Meta Directory Otolaryngology:

<URL:http://www.arcade.uiowa.edu/hardin-www/md-oto.html>

Pathology and laboratory medicine resources:

Internet Resources for Pathology (Anthony A. Killeen, Frances Pitlick, University of Michigan):

<URL:http://www.pds.med.umich.edu/users/amp/path_resources.html>

MedWeb: Pathology and Laboratory Medicine (Health Sciences Library, Emory University):

<URL:http://www.gen.emory.edu/medweb/medweb.pathology.html>

Pathology Internet Resource page (Leon A. Metlay M.D., University of Rochester):

<URL:http://wwwminer.lib.rochester.edu/wwwml/Leon/URPLM.html>

See also Hardin Meta Directory Pathology and Laboratory Medicine:

<URL:http://www.arcade.uiowa.edu/hardin-www/md-path.html>

Paediatrics resources:

MedWeb: Pediatrics (Health Sciences Library, Emory University):

<URL:http://www.gen.emory.edu/medweb/medweb.pediatrics.html>

PedInfo: Pediatrics WebServer (Andy Spooner M.D., University of Alabama):

<URL:http://www.lhl.uab.edu:80/pedinfo/>

Points of Pediatric Interest (Johns Hopkins/Marshall University):

<URL:http://www.med.jhu.edu/peds/neonatology/poi.html>

See also Hardin Meta Directory Pediatrics:

<URL:http://www.arcade.uiowa.edu/hardin-www/md-ped.html>

Pharmacy and pharmacology resources:

WWW Virtual Library: Pharmacy (David Bourne, University of Oklahoma):

<URL:http://www.cpb.uokhsc.edu/pharmacy/pharmint.html>

PharmWeb (A. D'Emanuele, University of Manchester, UK):

<URL:http://www.mcc.ac.uk/pharmweb/>

PharmInfoNet (VirSci Corporation):

<URL:http://pharminfo.com/>

See also Hardin Meta Directory Pharmacy and Pharmacology:

<URL:http://www.arcade.uiowa.edu/hardin-www/md-pharm.html>

Psychiatry and mental health resources:

Mental Health Resources (Western Psychiatric and Clinic Library, University of Pittsburgh):

<URL:http://wpic.library.pitt.edu/psychiat.htm>

MedWeb: Mental Health, Psychiatry, Psychology (Health Sciences Library, Emory University):

<URL:http://www.gen.emory.edu/medweb/medweb.mentalhealth.html>

Internet Mental Health Resources (Herb Stockley):

<URL:http://freenet.msp.mn.us/ip/stockley/mental_health.html>

See also Hardin Meta Directory Psychiatry/Mental Health:

<URL:http://www.arcade.uiowa.edu/hardin-www/md-psych.html>

Public, occupational, and environmental health resources:

MedWeb: Public Health (Health Sciences Library, Emory University):

<URL:http://www.gen.emory.edu/medweb/medweb.ph.html>

Health Services and Public Health Sites (Laura Larsson, University of Washington):

<URL:http://weber.u.washington.edu/~larsson/hsic94/resource/hsr-ph.html>

Global Health Network (University of Pittsburgh):

<URL:http://www.pitt.edu/HOME/GHNet/GHNet.html>

See also Hardin Meta Directory Public, Occupational and Environmental Health:

<URL:http://www.arcade.uiowa.edu/hardin-www/md-publ.html>

Radiology and medical imaging resources:

HealthWeb: Radiology (CIC/Indiana University):

<URL:http://www.medlib.iupui.edu/cicnet/rad/radnetho.html>

MedWeb: Radiology and Imaging (Health Sciences Library, Emory University):

<URL:http://www.gen.emory.edu/medweb/medweb.radiology.html>

The Medical Radiography Home Page (Richard Terrass, RT(R)):

<URL:http://web.wn.net/~usr/ricter/web/medradhome.html>

See also Hardin Meta Directory Radiology and Imaging:

<URL:http://www.arcade.uiowa.edu/hardin-www/md-rad.html>

Respiration medicine resources:

Respiratory on the Web (Steve Grenard):

<URL:http://www.xmission.com/~gastown/herpmed/respi.htm>

MedWeb: Respiration Medicine (Health Sciences Library, Emory University):

<URL:http://www.gen.emory.edu/medweb/medweb.respmed.html>

MIC-KIBIC MeSH Index: Respiratory Tract Diseases (Karolinska Institute):

<URL:http://www.mic.ki.se/Diseases/c8.html>

See also Hardin Meta Directory Respiration Medicine:

<URL:http://www.arcade.uiowa.edu/hardin-www/md-resp.html>

Rheumatology resources:

The Rheumatology Page (Fred Tempereau):

<URL:http://www.serve.com/~fredt/rheum.html>

MedWeb: Rheumatology (Health Sciences Library, Emory University):

<URL:http://www.gen.emory.edu/medweb/medweb.rheumatology.html>

Medical Matrix: Rheumatology (American Medical Informatics Association):

<URL:http://www.slackinc.com/matrix/SPECIALT/RHEUMAT.HTML>

See also Hardin Meta Directory Rheumatology:

<URL:http://www.arcade.uiowa.edu/hardin-www/md-rheum.html>

Speech pathology/audiology resources:

Homepage on Communication Disorders (Judith Kuster):

<URL:http://www.mankato.msus.edu/dept/comdis/kuster2/welcome.html>

Net Connections for Communication Disorders and Sciences (Judith Kuster, hypertext version by Judith Anderson):

<URL:http://www.jmu.edu/libliaison/andersjl/commdis/cd-intro.html>

FAQ from comp.speech newsgroup:

<URL:http://www.speech.cs.cmu.edu/comp.speech/>

See also Hardin Meta Directory Speech Pathology/Audiology:

<URL:http://www.arcade.uiowa.edu/hardin-www/md-speech.html>

Surgery resources:

MedWeb: Surgery (Health Sciences Library, Emory University):

<URL:http://www.gen.emory.edu/medweb/medweb.surgery.html>

MIC-KIBIC MeSH Index: Surgery, Operative (Karolinska Institute):

<URL:http://www.mic.ki.se/Diseases/e4.html>

Health Science Guide: Surgery (Jim Martindale):

<URL:http://www-sci.lib.uci.edu/HSG/MedicalSurgery.html#SU>

See also Hardin Meta Directory Surgery:

<URL:http://www.arcade.uiowa.edu/hardin-www/md-surg.html>

Telemedicine resources:

MedWeb: Telemedicine (Health Sciences Library, Emory University):

<URL:http://www.gen.emory.edu/medweb/medweb.telemed.html>

Telemedicine Resources and Services (University of Texas):

<URL:http://naftalab.bus.utexas.edu/nafta-7/tmpage.html>

Telemedicine Projects (University of Arizona):

<URL:http://zax.radiology.arizona.edu/umc.html>

See also Hardin Meta Directory Telemedicine:

<URL:http://www.arcade.uiowa.edu/hardin-www/md-telemed.html>

Toxicology resources:

MedWeb: Toxicology (Health Sciences Library, Emory University):

<http://www.gen.emory.edu/medweb/medweb.toxicology.html>

Toxicology Internet Resources (University of Pittsburgh):

<URL:http://www.pitt.edu/~martint/pages/toxres.htm>

Useful Web Sites for Chemical Safety Information (Global Information Network on Chemicals, NIHS, Japan):

<URL:http://www.nihs.go.jp:80/GINC/useful.html>

See also Hardin Meta Directory Toxicology:

<URL:http://www.arcade.uiowa.edu/hardin-www/md-tox.html>

Glossary

The terms highlighted in **bold** within the text of the book appear in this Glossary. Where an explaination includes terms appearing elsewhere within the Glossary, those terms are indicated by the use of *italics*.

486 An abbreviation for the Intel 80486 *microprocessor*, predecessor of the *Pentium*. Provides the performance necessary to run *Microsoft Windows* adequately. There are several design variations.

ActiveX A technology from Microsoft that enables designers to embed small *applications* (ActiveX controls) into a *WWW* page that are run by the *browser*, similar to *Java applets*.

American National Standards Institute (ANSI) A standards organization responsible for the **ANSI.SYS** file used under *DOS* to control various attributes of the display of *characters* on the screen. This can be mimicked by other *computers* using ANSI *terminal emulation* to enhance the interface of PC-based *bulletin boards*.

American Standard Code for Information Interchange (ASCII) See *ASCII character set*, *ASCII encoding*, *ASCII file transfers*.

animated GIF A special type of the *GIF* graphics format that incorporates several distinct images into the one file. *WWW browsers* capable of handling this format display each image in sequence after a specified delay, producing the appearance of an animation.

anonymous FTP Retrieval of a file from a public *FTP* archive using 'anonymous' as a *user name*, and an *e-mail* address as a password.

ANSI See *American National Standards Institute*.

applet A small *application* (applet), written in the *Java* programming language, embedded into a *WWW* page and run by the *browser*. Similar to *ActiveX controls*.

application A *program* belonging to a class of *software* designed to manage a particular computing task. Thus, Microsoft Word is a 'word-processing application'. Applications perform these tasks with the help of another type of software—an *operating system*. Can also refer to a computing task itself, such as *telemedicine*, rather than a specific program.

Archie An *Internet service* which assists in locating files available from public *FTP* sites, providing you know the name of the file.

ASCII character set American Standard Code for Information Interchange allows different *computer* types to share information. Each of the 128 ASCII *characters* are described by a 7-*bit* code, most of which are represented by a key on the computer *keyboard*. In practice, ASCII is synonymous with 'text'. See *ASCII file*, *binary file*, *text file*, *extended character set*.

ASCII encoding The process of converting *binary files* into *ASCII files* so that they can be transmitted as *e-mail*. The common types of encoding are *BinHex*, *MIME*, and *uuencode*.

ASCII file A *computer* file that contains *characters* from the *ASCII character set* only. Synonymous with *text file*. See *binary file*.

ASCII file-transfer protocol The transfer of a file containing 7-*bit* data. Although the term is in common use, *ASCII* is a set of codes/*characters* and not a standard for file transfers.

asynchronous In telecommunications, this term is commonly used to indicate that an exchange of information involves a significant delay between the sending and receiving of that information (the alternative is *real-time* communication). In a more technical context, it refers to the transmission of information at a variable rate through a *serial communications port*.

Asynchronous Transfer Mode (ATM) A type of *network* that uses 'virtual channels' within a shared physical link to distribute data to several sites simultaneously (a technique called 'multiplexing'). ATM does not operate over *TCP/IP* networks such as the *Internet*, although ATM networks can carry TCP/IP traffic and host Internet *servers*.

ATM See *Asynchronous Transfer Mode*.

attributes In *HTML*, the language used to create *WWW* pages, the effect of many mark-up tags can be altered by specifying an attribute. For example, the horizontal rule **<HR>** can be widened with the **SIZE** attribute, as in **<HR SIZE=4>**.

authenticity In terms of data security, an authentic message is one where the identity of the sender can be verified, often by means of a *digital signature*.

avatar An *online* persona graphically depicting the 'character' of an *Internet Relay Chat* user in a virtual environment. For example, one may choose to appear with the head of a fish, although doing so may present a somewhat ambiguous message to fellow users.

bandwidth In common usage, the capacity of a communications channel to transmit information. *Modem* connections to the *Internet* are 'low' bandwidth relative to a *SuperJANET* connection, for example. Bandwidth is said to be 'congested' when many *users* are sharing the same communications channel, using up the available bandwidth.

baud An outdated term used to measure the speed of a *modem* connection. See *bits per second*, *modulation protocols*.

BBS See *bulletin-board service*.

binary code A string of *bits* is known as binary code: code strings that are 7 bits in length define the *ASCII character set* whilst 8-bit codes define various *extended character sets*. All information stored on and used by a *computer* is ultimately binary code.

binary files Binary files include any *program* or data file used by the *computer* that contains non-*ASCII characters*. Because the *extended characters* found in binary files may be unique to a particular computer *platform*, most binary files cannot be used on more than one type of computer. See *binary file transfer*.

binary file-transfer protocol The transfer of a file containing 8-*bit* data, as opposed to 7-bit *ASCII characters*. See *file-transfer protocol*.

BinHex A standard method on the *Macintosh* of converting *binary files* into *text files* by *ASCII encoding*. This allows *software* etc. to be transferred on the *Internet* by *e-mail*. BinHexed files have the *file suffix* **.hqx**.

bit Information is processed and stored on *computers* using a variation in electrical current between two states. This variation can be represented by using the digits 0 and 1. 'Bit' is derived from 'binary digit', and thus represents the smallest unit of information used by computers. See *binary code*.

bit depth A measure of how many colours can be displayed on a *computer monitor*. For example, an 8-*bit* display corresponds to 256 colours.

BITNET A *network* primarily linking North American and European academic institutions. Similar to the former EARN (European Academic Research Network). See *LISTSERV*.

bits per second (bps) A measure of the number of *bits* transferred per second over a communications channel. *Modem* speeds, measured in bps, are defined by *modulation protocols*. See *characters per second*.

Bookmark A facility present in most *WWW browsers* allowing users to store and manage the *URLs* of Web sites they have visited. In the Internet Explorer *client*, Microsoft has renamed them 'Favourites'.

Boolean operator Also called a logical operator, used to define search criteria when using databases such as those indexed by *WAIS* or *MEDLINE*. AND, NOT, and OR are Boolean operators, used in the form 'Find asthma NOT occupational'.

bps See *bits per second*.

browser A synonym for a *World-Wide Web client*. Refers to the casual ease that these clients bring to navigating the *Internet*.

bulletin-board service (BBS) A *computer* running *communications software* that is set up to allow callers to connect with it using a *modem*. It provides a shared forum for the exchange of messages and files. See *online service*.

byte A sequence of 8 *bits* used to describe a *character*. Also the basic unit of *computer* memory. See *hard disk*, *gigabyte*, *kilobyte*, *megabyte*, *RAM*.

cable modem A device that fulfils the role of a conventional *modem*, but instead of using telephone lines to transfer data, it uses cable television *networks*.

cache A reserved memory space on a *computer* for storing frequently required instructions, speeding its operation. This memory space is usually in the form of dedicated circuitry (a *hardware* cache), or part of *RAM* memory (a *software* cache). Web *browsers* use a *hard disk* cache to store *WWW* pages so they do not have to be repeatedly retrieved by the *modem*. See *proxy server*.

CD-ROM See *compact disk read-only memory*.

central processing unit (CPU) Synonymous with *microprocessor*.

CGI See *common gateway interface*.

channel In a similar fashion to CB radio, *Internet Relay Chat users* hold conversations on particular channels. Instead of changing frequencies, however, an IRC channel is joined by typing its name into your IRC *client*.

character A symbol encoded into one byte of data, corresponding to *keyboard* equivalents such as **A**, **a**, and **ESC** (the 'escape character'), for example. Commonly encountered sets of characters are the *ASCII character set*, *extended character sets*, and ISO Latin 1.

characters per second (cps) A measure of the speed of a file transfer, estimated from the *bits per second* and length of the transmitted *character* (typically 10 bits for each *byte* after the addition of stop *bits*).

chat A facility present on many *bulletin boards* and *online services*, as well as the *Internet* (as *Internet Relay Chat*). Provides for the two-way exchange of messages as they are typed in *real time*, as opposed to *e-mail* which involves a lag between the sending and receiving of the message.

client A *program* that makes requests for the services of another *computer*, called a *server*. Each client works with a specific type of server or, as in the case of *WWW* clients, several types of server.

clock speed Also called clock frequency, this is the speed (in megahertz) at which a *microprocessor* is able to process information.

command-line interface The alternative to a *graphical user interface*, a command-line interface is presented by an *operating system* such as *DOS* and *UNIX*, requiring the *user* to type in sometimes unintuitive commands to instruct the *computer*.

common gateway interface (CGI) In simple terms, a 'virtual space' that sits between a *WWW server* and another *program* or database. A small 'CGI script' in this space mediates *client* access to the program/database.

communications software Any *application* directly involved in exchanging information with other *computers*. Communications programs include *terminal emulators* and dedicated *clients*, and may offer support for various *file-transfer protocols*.

compact disk read-only memory (CD-ROM) A plastic disk just like an audio CD, containing files that can be read but not altered by a **computer**. Many CD-ROMs contain *multimedia*. Requires a special CD-ROM disk drive.

compression protocol In relation to data transmission, a set of rules for reducing the size of a file so it can be transmitted in less time. Examples of protocols are *MNP5* and *V.42bis*. See *file compression*.

computer An electronic device that uses coded instructions to manage information and efficiently automate the manipulation of data. See *desktop computer*, *notebook computer*, *personal computer*.

conference An *online* discussion area, synonymous with forum or special interest group (SIG), where *users* can hold 'virtual meetings', or read and post messages relating to a particular topic.

confidentiality In terms of data security, confidentiality implies that the contents of a message are visable only to the authorized recipient(s), and not by unauthorized persons who may intercept the message intentionally or inadvertently at any point in transit. Confidentiality is often preserved using *encryption* techniques.

container tags In *HTML*, the language used to create *WWW* pages, many mark-up tags work together as a pair. The effect of the tag is applied to any text between the opening tag and the closing tag. For example, **<B>**this**</B>** creates bold text.

coprocessor Also known as a floating point unit, a specialized *microprocessor* used to perform calculations that are mathematically intensive, such as complicated graphics.

cps See *characters per second*.

CPU See *central processing unit*.

crash An interruption in the normal operations of a *computer*, often resulting in the inability to give commands via the *keyboard* and a 'frozen' screen.

cross-platform See *platform*.

cursor A blinking vertical bar used to indicate where the next line of typing will appear on a *computer* screen.

data bits A connection setting encountered when configuring *communications software*. Because 8 *bits* make up a *character*, 'character bits' is used synonymously.

data integrity In terms of data security, the retention of integrity implies that a message will pass unaltered over a communications channel, and that all attempts to breach *confidentiality* will be unsucessful. When this is not the case, the data has lost its integrity.

desktop computer A *personal computer* that can be comfortably placed on a desktop, operating as a self-contained unit. See *notebook computer*, *terminal*.

digital signature authentication In terms of data security, a common means of ensuring the *authenticity* of data. A unique digital signature appended to a data transmission is used to verify that the message is indeed from the stated sender.

disk cache See *cache*.

domain name The unique name of a *computer* on the *Internet*, comprised of several sub-domains that are used to group computers together. For example, all computers with **uk** in their domain name are located in the UK, but some of these will be located at academic sites (...**ac.uk**), and others on commercial premises (...**co.uk**), etc. See *Internet Protocol address*.

DOS An common abbreviation for the Microsoft Disk Operating System, an operating system with a *command-line interface*. There are other types of DOS.

dot pitch A measure of the proximity of the holes through which coloured beams of light project an image on a *computer* display. A small dot pitch produces a sharp image. See *monitor*.

download The process of retrieving a file from a remote *host* to your own *computer* over a communications link. See *file-transfer protocol*, *upload*.

driver Instructions in the form of a small file sometimes needed to make an *operating system* aware of *hardware* such as a video card, *modem*, *printer*, or *CD-ROM* drive.

dual scan display A type of 'passive matrix' technology used in low-end *notebook computer* screens to display an image. See *thin film transistor*.

duplex A *terminal emulation* setting encountered when configuring *communications software*. In a full duplex link, data can be sent and received simultaneously: half duplex links are less common and alternate between sending and receiving data.

electronic mail (e-mail) Messages delivered over an electronic *network* (such as the *Internet*) to an electronic mailbox where they can be read, saved to disk, and/or replied to. See *mailing list*.

e-mail See *electronic mail*.

emulation Using one device to mimic the operation of another. For example, the *Macintosh* can run special *software* to 'emulate' a *PC* running *Microsoft Windows*. See *terminal emulation*.

encryption See *public-key cryptography*.

entities In *HTML*, the language used to create *WWW* pages, some non-*ASCII characters* can be included in a Web page using special codes composed of ASCII characters. For example, '**é**' is produced by the entity '**é**'.

error-correction protocol In relation to data transmission, a set of rules negotiated by *modems* to ensure that a transmitted file is received intact (i.e. without error). Example protocols are *MNP4* and *V.42*. Error correction is also performed by most *file-transfer protocols*.

extended character set A collective term for several *platform*-specific *character* sets describing 128 characters additional to the original 128 of the *ASCII character set*. Mostly used for lines and graphics symbols. See *binary file*.

FAQ See *frequently-asked questions*.

FidoNet A large world-wide amateur *network* of *bulletin boards* allowing the exchange of *e-mail*, *conference* messages, and files. See *OneNet*.

file compression Using special compression software, most *computer* files can be made smaller so that they take less time to transfer and occupy less storage space. Compressed files are denoted by a characteristic *file suffix*, and must be expanded before they can be used. See *compression protocol*.

file name The name of a file stored on a *computer*, with or without its *file suffix*.

file suffix An acronym forming part of the *file name*, often comprising three *characters*, which indicates the type of file or *program* necessary to expand or decode it (e.g. **.ZIP**). See *ASCII encoding*, *file compression*.

file-transfer protocol In relation to data transmission, a set of rules describing how a file is to be transmitted. So-called *ASCII file-transfer protocol* can transfer only *ASCII characters* (i.e. *text files*), whereas several *binary file-transfer protocols* can transmit *binary files*. Binary protocols include *Xmodem*, *Ymodem*, *Zmodem*, and *Kermit*. See *File Transfer Protocol*.

File Transfer Protocol (FTP) Part of the *TCP/IP* protocol suite used on the *Internet* for transferring files across TCP/IP connections. Files that are available by FTP are commonly held in public archives on FTP sites. See *anonymous FTP*.

firewall A secure *gateway* protecting an internal *network*, such as an *intranet*, from unauthorized access. Firewalls can be crossed by way of an ultra-secure *proxy server*.

flame A harmful or derogatory, sometimes deserved and sometimes uncalled-for, response to an *e-mail* message or *Usenet* news item that the 'recipient' considers offensive. A 'flame war' is the online equivalent of a heated argument.

floppy disk A 3.5 inch flexible disk used by modern *personal computers* to install new *software* and exchange files. Requires a floppy-disk drive, although alternative higher-capacity removable disk drives are now popular.

freeware *Software* that is copyrighted by the author but made available to *users* without charge.

frequently-asked questions (FAQ) Originating in *Usenet newsgroups*, an FAQ is a file serving to answer questions commonly asked by new *users*, or merely to record information about a particular subject that has been collated for the benefit of others. Many FAQs are now available on the *World-Wide Web*.

FTP See *File Transfer Protocol*.

gateway A communications link between two different kinds of *network*. Serves to convert information into a compatible format before it can be passed on to an adjoining network. Many networks which are not connected directly to the *Internet* use a gateway to enable *e-mail* exchange with Internet *users*.

GB See *gigabyte*.

GIF A common graphics file format used extensively in *WWW* pages. See *animated GIF*, *interlaced GIF*, *transparent GIF*, *JPEG*, *PNG*.

gigabyte (GB) A measure of *RAM* memory and *hard disk* space, equal to 1 073 741 824 *bytes* (i.e. 2 to the power of 30)—roughly a thousand *megabytes*.

Gopher An easy-to-use but dated *Internet service* that organizes information on the *Internet* into a series of hierarchical menus. See *Veronica*.

graphical user interface The presentation of information using visual features such as point-and-click, *icons*, drag and drop, *pull-down menus*, and *windows*. Popularized by the *Macintosh*, *Microsoft Windows* brings similar features to the *PC*. See *command-line interface.*

greyscale A video capability allowing a *monitor* to display shades of grey, or a *printer* capable of producing output in shades of grey.

GUI See *graphical user interface.*

handshaking Also known as flow control, handshaking is a method of regulating the flow of data between two *modems* and between modem and *computer*. This ensures that neither device must wait for or be swamped by too much information at once. Handshaking can take place using *hardware* or *software* (XON/XOFF).

hard disk Not commonly removable from the *system unit*, an internal hard disk is used by modern *personal computers* to store *programs* and files in a memory space that is permanent until deliberately changed by the *user*. Storage capacity is measured in *megabytes*. See *floppy disk*, *RAM*.

hardware All the components of a *computer* and its accessories which are made of plastics and metals, etc. See *software.*

hardware handshake See *handshaking*.

Hayes AT command set A set of commands devised by Hayes that have become the *de facto* standard for issuing commands to *modems*. A modem which is Hayes-compatible can be connected to any *computer* and controlled by issuing these commands using *communications software*.

helper application On the *Internet*, an external *application* needed by a *client* (such as a *WWW browser*) to provide functionality not contained within the client, such as the ability to play a sound file or act as a *Telnet* client. See *plug-in*.

home page The default *hypertext* page to be loaded by a *WWW client* when it is first launched or when the *user* clicks the '**Home**' button. Also the top-level page of any WWW site. Most home pages function as a combined 'cover' and index page.

host Refers to a *computer* on a *network* that provides services to many *users*. Dial-up users connect to the *Internet* via a host computer maintained by their *service provider*. Host computers often run server *software* with which users interact by means of a *client*.

HTML See *Hypertext Markup Language.*

HTTP See *Hypertext Transport Protocol.*

hypertext A document containing links to other documents. The reader is not forced to read a hypertext document from beginning to end, but can freely follow any one of several marked links to associated material. Hypermedia, a superset of hypertext, implies other media such as graphics, sounds, and animations can lead to or be the result of clicking on a link. The *WWW* uses the metaphor of a hypertext 'page'.

Hypertext Markup Language (HTML) A format used by the *WWW* to structure *hypertext* documents.

Hypertext Transport Protocol (HTTP) The protocol used to transfer *hypertext* pages between a *World-Wide Web server* and *client.*

IBM-compatible A *PC* designed to be compatible with an original design by IBM, whether it is made by IBM or one of many 'clone' manufacturers. The *Macintosh* is not IBM-compatible. Sometimes called 'industry standard compatible' by clone manufacturers.

icon A small on-screen picture used to represent *programs* and documents under a *graphical user interface.*

image map A graphic within a *WWW* page that contains a number of 'hot spots'. Clicking on one of these spots with the *mouse* causes a new page to be displayed, as happens when clicking on a text-based *hypertext* link.

initialization In communications, the preparation of a *modem* to send and receive data using an initialization string composed of *Hayes AT commands*. Also refers to the formatting of a *floppy disk* or *hard disk* in preparation for putting data on the disk.

installation The process of *loading* new *software* on to a *computer.*

Integrated Services Digital Network (ISDN) A high-speed digital telephone line that achieves data transmission rates over 64 000 *bps* by sending the data as a stream of *bits*, rather than converting it to sound for transmission as does a *modem.*

interface Refers to the *hardware* and *software* components of a connection between two elements of a *computer* or its *peripheral* devices. *Operating systems* and *applications* have a 'user interface', described in terms of the characteristics of their presentation of information to the *user*. See *graphical user interface*, *command-line interface*.

interlaced GIF A special type of the *GIF* graphics format. *WWW browsers* initially display a rough-looking image that is progressively sharpened as the remainder of the image file is *downloaded* and processed. *Users* can decide whether to view the fully-rendered page on the basis of the 'sketch', or move on.

Internet Strictly, a world-wide *network* of networks that communicate using the *TCP/IP* protocol suite. Informally, being a part of the Internet has come to mean the ability to exchange *e-mail* with other Internet *users*.

Internet dialer *Software* supplied by a *service provider* or as an *operating system* add-on that is used to manage *SLIP* or *PPP* configuration, other dial-up settings, connection/ disconnection, and sometimes provides menu access to a range of *Internet clients*.

Internet Protocol (IP) address A unique identifying number assigned to every *computer* directly connected to the *Internet*. Comprised of a group of four numbers separated by full stops, it corresponds to an easier-to-remember *domain name*.

Internet Relay Chat (IRC) A *chat* facility on the *Internet* allowing *users* to communicate with each other on various topic-based *channels* via *real-time* typing. Newer IRC clients provide graphical 'virtual environments' in which users are represented by an *avatar*.

Internet services A collective term for applications available over the *Internet*. Primary tools are *electronic mail*, *File Transfer Protocol*, and *Telnet*. Later generation tools, such as *Archie*, *Gopher*, *Wide Area Information Servers*, and the *World-Wide Web*, build on these basic applications. *Usenet* is not strictly an Internet service. See *newsgroups*.

Internet telephony With special *software*, a microphone, speakers, and a *sound card* for digitizing speach, *Internet users* can converse with each other while *online*. Although sound quality is less than that of an ordinary telephone, the system provides intercontinental communications for the cost of a local call to your *service provider*.

intranet A private, internal *network* based on the same *TCP/IP* protocols and *applications* (e.g. *WWW browsers*) as the *Internet*. The *NHSnet* is an example of an intranet. An intranet provides its users with a more controlled and secure network environment, and may be connected to the Internet by way of a *firewall*.

IP address See *Internet Protocol (IP) address*.

IRC See *Internet Relay Chat*.

ISDN See *Integrated Services Digital Network*.

JANET See *Joint Academic Network*.

Java A programming language from Sun Microsystems that can be used to write small applications (*applets*) that are *downloaded* and run by Java-aware *WWW browsers*. See *ActiveX*, *JavaScript*.

JavaScript A scripting language from Netscape based on *Java* that is simpler to learn than the full Java programming language. JavaScripts are embedded directly within *HTML* and primarily used to make *WWW* pages more interactive.

Joint Academic Network (JANET) A *network* linking UK universities, colleges, and research establishments. Originally using the *X.25* protocol, it is now based on *TCP/IP*. See *SuperJANET*.

JPEG A graphics file format in common use on the *Internet*. Although JPEG files can contain more colours than *GIF* files, the *file compression* technique used to keep the file size down causes some loss of data and therefore degrades the sharpness of the image. See *PNG*.

KB See *kilobyte*.

Kermit A *file-transfer protocol* that incorporates *error checking*, now little used but most *platforms* support it. Can transfer *binary files* over 7-*bit* communication links.

keyboard A device used to enter data into a *computer* containing many keys similar to those on a typewriter, while others are specific to the operation of computers (such as *cursor* control keys, arrow keys, etc.).

kilobyte (KB) A measure of *RAM* memory and *hard disk* space, equal to 1024 *bytes* (i.e. 2 to the power of 10).

LAN See *local-area network*.

leased line An expensive, typically high-speed, constant connection to the *Internet* that is leased from an Internet *service provider* or telephone company.

line feed An *ASCII* control code used on some *platforms* to indicate the beginning of a new line of typing.

list owner A person responsible for maintaining, and perhaps *moderating*, a *mailing list*.

LISTSERV A *mail server* used on *BITNET* to manage discussion groups, the equivalent of *mailing lists* on the *Internet*.

loading Copying an *application* or file into *RAM* memory from storage on a *hard disk*, *floppy disk*, *CD-ROM*, etc.

local-area network (LAN) A *network* of *computers* physically located on the same premises, or within a relatively small geographic area. See *WAN*.

local echo A *modem* setting causing it to send every *keyboard character* that is typed to the screen of the local *computer*, i.e. an 'echo' of the characters being sent to the remote *host*.

log-off Synonymous with log-out, in *telecommunications* the act of ending a session with a *host*.

log-on Synonymous with 'log-in' or 'login', in *telecommunications* refers to the act of accessing a *host*. May require a 'login' name (*user name*) and/or password.

MacBinary A file format that combines *Macintosh* Finder information with the data and resource forks unique to Mac files, forming a single *binary file*. This prevents the loss of *icons*, file type, and other vital information when Mac files are transferred through non-Macintosh *computers*.

Macintosh An innovative range of *personal computers* introduced by Apple Computer in 1984. The Mac uses *icons*, folders, *windows*, *pull-down menus*, point-and-click, plug-and-play, and many other features as standard, which have been gradually borrowed by operating systems for the *PC*. See *IBM-compatible*, *Microsoft Windows*.

Mac OS The *operating system* used by the Apple *Macintosh* and its clones.

Mailbase The National Mailbase Service operates *mailing lists* and other *Internet services* for the benefit of the UK academic and research community.

mailing list A list of *e-mail* addresses used by a *mail server* to automatically distribute messages relating to a particular topic to persons on the list. Some lists are *moderated*. See *LISTSERV*.

mail server A *program* that manages *e-mail* messages. Some mail servers, also known as list servers, are used primarily to manage *mailing lists* (e.g. *LISTSERV*) whereas others have a role in sending files from *FTP* archives by e-mail (e.g. ftpmail). Mail servers are used by *Internet service providers* to manage e-mail for dial-up users.

MB See *megabyte*.

Mbone See *Multicast Backbone of the Internet*.

Medical Subject Headings (MeSH) A hierarchical classification system developed by the US National Library of Medicine, used to map a *user's* search terms to those indexed in *MEDLINE*.

megabyte (MB) A measure of *RAM* memory and *hard disk* space, equal to 1 048 576 bytes (i.e. 2 to the power of 20)—roughly a thousand *kilobytes*.

MeSH See *Medical Subject Headings*.

microprocessor Also known as the *CPU* or a 'chip', the electronic circuitry that interprets instructions within a *program*, and directs other systems within the *computer* to perform operations upon the data.

Microsoft Windows A family of *operating systems* from Microsoft that brings a *Macintosh*-like graphical user interface to the *PC*. The family includes Windows 3.1, Windows for Workgroups 3.11 (Windows 3.1 optimized for *networked users*), Windows NT (a robust product for multi-user *computers*), and Windows 95 (an improved *interface* borrowing features from other operating systems). See *DOS*.

MIME See *Multi-purpose Internet Mail Extensions*.

mirror A mirror site replicates the directory structure and file content of another site, such as an *FTP* archive or set of *WWW* pages. Mirrors serve to increase the number of *users* that can have simultaneous access to particular resources, and help reduce *bandwidth* congestion on certain parts of the *Internet*.

MNP4 An *error-correction protocol* devised by Microcom.

MNP5 As *MNP4*, but also functioning as a *compression protocol*, theoretically halving transmission time.

mode *FTP clients* can be configured to transfer files in either *ASCII* mode or binary mode. This corresponds to the transfer of 7-*bit* or 8-bit data, respectively. *Binary files* are corrupted if they are inadvertently transfered in ASCII mode.

modem A device allowing *computers* to communicate using telephone lines. A modem works by converting digital information into analogue sound for transmission (MOdulation), which is converted back into digital information by the receiving modem (DEModulation).

moderation The role of a person who screens postings to *mailing lists* and *online* forums, including *newsgroups*, to ensure that they are appropriate to the stated aims of the discussion.

modulation protocol A protocol that is agreed upon by both *modems* in a communications link that governs the basic speed of the connection. These protocols include *V.22bis*, *V.32*, *V.32bis*, and *V.34*. See *baud*, *bits per second*.

monitor The unit comprised of the display screen, housing, and controls used to adjust the characteristics of the screen image. See *bit depth*, *dot pitch*, *resolution*.

MOO A abbreviation for 'Multi-User Dungeons, Object-Oriented'. MOOs are virtual environments in which *users* interact with each other and with various virtual objects by way of typed instructions (e.g. 'Look article' or 'Go lobby'). MOOs can be accessed via *Telnet*, although integration with a *WWW* page enables point-and-click navigation under a graphical *interface*; here Telnet (perhaps implemented as a *Java applet*) remains necessary only for *real-time chat* with other users of the system.

mouse A mechanical device used in conjunction with the *keyboard* to operate the *computer*. The movement of the mouse on a flat space corresponds to the movement of an on-screen 'pointer'.

Multicast Backbone of the Internet (Mbone) Mbone is a 'virtual *network*' running over the *Internet* using its own *routers* and a special class of *IP address* to 'tunnel' data from one *computer* to many simultaneously—a technique known as '*multicasting*'. Mbone can also run over *ATM* networks (on top of *TCP/IP*), but is seen as a temporary solution until such time as the majority of Internet routers support multicasting directly.

multicasting Sending data to more than one *network* simultaneously is called 'multicasting' (one-to-many), as opposed to 'broadcasting' (one-to-all) or unicasting (one-to-one). Most *Internet routers* unicast only, which may involve the inefficient tranmission of the same data several times over seperate connections. Multicasting is possible on the Internet using *Mbone*.

multimedia A *computer*-based *application* (or video, etc.) that delivers information or entertainment to the *user* in the form of several types of media, including sound, text, graphics, animation, and video. Such applications are often based on *CD-ROM* or on the *World-Wide Web*.

Multipurpose Internet Mail Extensions (MIME) A standard for the *ASCII encoding* of *binary files* so that they can be sent by *e-mail* on the *Internet*. MIME content types, a special line of text within MIME files, tell *programs* that recognize MIME about the type of encoded file (e.g. movie, graphic).

multiscan A category of *monitor* that can adapt to more than one video signal frequency, as happens when screen *resolution* is altered.

netiquette A code of appropriate behaviour, or 'network etiquette', expected of all *users* when posting messages to *Usenet newsgroups*.

network The linking together of *computers* and/or their *peripherals* (such as *printers*) to enable resources to be shared, or to foster communication between the users of those computers. There are many types of network, such as *FidoNet*, the *Internet*, *JANET*, *LANs*, *OneNet*, and *WANs*.

network computer In essence, a stripped-down *PC* designed to use *network*-based resources (such as *Java applets*) without the need for the *programs*, *hard disk*, *floppy disk* drive, or memory requirements of more familiar *desktop computers*. Promoted as a cheap alternative for *Internet* access, it may become established in the home entertainment and corporate *intranet* markets.

network news A collective term for *Internet newsgroups* propagated using the *Network News Transfer Protocol*. Although *Usenet* newsgroups are propagated in this way on the Internet, they are propagated using different protocols over other networks making up Usenet.

Network News Transfer Protocol (NNTP) The protocol used on the *Internet* to exchange *network news*.

newsgroup A collection of messages relating to a certain topic or topics on the *Internet* and *Usenet*, arranged into a hierarchical naming system. An example of a newsgroup is **sci.med**.

news reader A *client* used on the *Internet* to read and post *newsgroup* articles via *NNTP*.

news server A *computer* running *software* that enables a *news reader* to retrieve *newsgroup* articles using *NNTP*.

NHSnet A *wide-area network* for the UK's National Health Service. Among other services, a one-way *gateway* enables NHS *users* to explore the *WWW* and exchange *e-mail* with *Internet* users. The *intranet* also has its own NHS-specific WWW pages (NHSweb), protected from outside access by a *firewall*.

NNTP See *Network News Transfer Protocol*.

notebook computer A portable *computer* about the size of a notebook that unfolds to reveal the *keyboard* and display screen. See *desktop computer*, *dual scan display*, *TFT display*.

offline In the context of *telecommunications*, the state of being disconnected from an *online service*, *bulletin board*, or the *Internet*.

offline reader A *client* that can automatically gather *e-mail*, *conference* messages, or *newsgroup* messages upon connection to an *online service*, and then disconnect from the service. The *user* reads the collected messages *offline* and composes any replies which are stored on his or her *computer* until the next time that user goes *online*.

OneNet A loose *network* of *bulletin boards* running the proprietary FirstClass server, set up to exchange messages in a similar way to *FidoNet* and *Usenet*. OneNet includes several medical *conferences*.

online In the context of *telecommunications*, the act of connecting to (going online) or being connected to an *online service*, *bulletin board*, or other *network* such as the *Internet*. See *offline*.

online service Incorporating similar facilities to a *BBS*, an online service is typically a large commercial *network* offering many additional resources and services to a greater number of people. Several traditional online services have moved their content from proprietary systems to subscriber-only sites on the *World-Wide Web*. The exact definition of an online service is thus no longer clear.

operating system A set of special *programs* and routines a *computer* uses to perform basic tasks like starting up the computer and managing files. *DOS*, the *Mac OS*, *Microsoft Windows*, *OS/2*, and *UNIX* are operating systems. See *application*.

OS/2 An *operating system* marketed by IBM in competition with *Microsoft Windows*.

parity An infrequently used technique for *error correction* in a *telecommunications* setting. A parity *bit* can be added to each transmitted *character*, instructing the receiving *modem* to expect either an even or odd number of bits. If the actual sum of bits does not match, the data is resent.

path name A description of the location of a file on a storage device such as an *FTP* archive, *hard disk*, or *floppy disk*. On the *Internet*, *uniform resource locators* use a path name to specify the directory location and/or *file name* of a particular resource.

PC An abbreviation for a *personal computer* that is (generally) *IBM-compatible*.

PC card The size of a credit card, a device that can be inserted into many *notebooks* and *PDAs* to provide extra storage space, *networking*, or *telecommunications* capabilities. Formerly known as PCMCIA devices (from Personal Computer Memory Card International Association).

PDA See *personal digital assistant*.

Pentium A *microprocessor* designed by Intel as the successor to the *486*.

peripherals A collective term for external *hardware* (such as *printers*, *modems*, etc.) connected to a *computer*.

personal computer A collective term for all types of *computer* designed to meet the computing needs of an individual *user*. Includes *IBM-compatibles* (*PCs*) and *Macintosh*. The main components are the *system unit*, *monitor*, *keyboard*, and *mouse*. See *desktop computer*, *notebook computer*.

personal digital assistant A small hand-held *computer*, often using an electronic stylus, used to organize information (e.g. appointments, addresses, case notes, patient billing details, etc.)

pixel Derived from 'picture element', the individual dots of light that make up the image on the screen of a *monitor*.

platform A category of *computer hardware*, such as *Macintosh* or *IBM-compatible*. Hardware and *software* engineered for one platform do not commonly operate in association with one another. When they *are* compatible, this hardware or software is said to provide 'cross-platform' compatibility.

plug-in Extra files that, although not critical to basic operation, extend the capabilities of many *programs*. Netscape's plug-in technology is used by both Navigator and Internet Explorer, the most popular *WWW browsers*, enabling various file formats to be handled by the browser without the need for external *helper applications*.

PNG The Portable Network Graphics format is being developed to replace *GIF* and *JPEG* as the graphic file format of choice on the *World-Wide Web*.

Point of Presence (PoP) A bank of *modems* supplied by an *Internet service provider*, often permitting access to their high-speed *TCP/IP network* by way of a local call.

Point to Point Protocol (PPP) A *network interface* that allows dial-up users to temporarily connect their *computers* to the *Internet* and use *TCP/IP*-based *clients*. It is generally preferred to the alternative, *SLIP*.

PoP See *Point of Presence*.

POP See *Post Office Protocol*.

port A *hardware interface* at the back of the *system unit* for connecting *peripherals*, such as a *printer* port or *serial-communications port*. See *port number*.

port number In *networking*, a port number is used to indicate a 'contact address' for the *server* on a *host computer*. Certain *Internet services* have a default port. For example, *Gopher clients* expect to find the Gopher server at 'port 70' on a given host. See *port*.

Post Office Protocol (POP) A protocol used on the *Internet* for storing and retrieving *e-mail*. See *SMTP*.

PowerPC A high-performance *microprocessor* developed jointly by Apple, IBM, and Motorola to compete with Intel's *Pentium* and its successor, the P6.

PPP See *Point to Point Protocol*.

printer A *hardware* device capable of printing output from a *computer*, including both text and graphics, on paper. There are several categories of printer, including dot matrix, ink jets, and laser printers.

program Synonymous with *software*.

proxy server Refers to a *server* acting as a secure *gateway* between an internal *network* and the wider *Internet*. Incoming and outgoing requests made by *clients* must pass through the server. Alternatively, it refers to a *disk cache* on the Internet for storing frequently-accessed *WWW* pages. Specifying a proxy in this instance usually helps conserve *bandwidth* on intercontinental communications links, and can result in a quicker response to client requests.

public domain A category of *software* where the author does not exercise copyright, permitting use of the item without the necessity of permission or payment.

public-key cryptography A common method of encryption—the encoding or enciphering of data to preserve its *confidentiality* and *integrity*. The public-key system uses two software 'keys'—one public, used to encrypt a message, and one private, used by the receipient to decode it. A *digital signature* is often included as part of an encrypted message to indicate *authenticity*.

pull-down menu A system for organizing options and commands under a *graphical user interface*. Clicking on a menu item (e.g. '**Edit**') reveals a list of related options (e.g. '**Cut**' or '**Paste**').

RAM See *random-access memory*.

random-access memory (RAM) All *software*, including *applications* and the *operating system*, must be loaded into RAM—a working space that can be accessed at high-speed by the *microprocessor*. The contents of RAM are erased when the *computer* is turned off. RAM is measured in *megabytes*. See *hard disk*.

read-only memory (ROM) A memory space containing instructions which can be read by a *computer* but are unchangeable. Sometimes parts of the *operating system* or *modem* settings are stored in ROM. See *CD-ROM*.

real time In *telecommunications*, interaction between two or more *computers/users* occuring without a significant time lag. For example, users of *Internet Relay Chat* communicate in real-time typing—a line of text is visible to the recipient virtually the moment it is sent. See *asynchronous*.

refresh rate The frequency with which each line on a display screen is redrawn by the electron gun in a *monitor*. Measured in hertz, a low refresh rate causes the display to flicker.

Remote Imaging Protocol (RIP) A type of *terminal emulation* using graphical elements stored on the caller's computer to rapidly draw colour screens. Also permits *mouse* input.

Request for comments (RFC) A collection of documents used on the *Internet* to record descriptions of evolving protocols and standards. An authoritative source of information about the workings of the Internet.

resolution The resolution of a *monitor* refers to the horizontal and vertical number of *pixels* that make up the display on a screen. Similarly, the resolution of a *printer* is measured in dots per inch (dpi).

RFC See *Request for comments*.

RIP See *Remote Imaging Protocol*.

ROM See *read-only memory*.

routers Devices on the *Internet* that send information from one *network* to another (known as 'unicasting'). *Mbone* allows *multicasting* on the Internet.

scroll bar An area at the vertical and/or horizontal edge of an *application window* under a *graphical user interface*. Clicking on an arrow or dragging a scroll box in this area reveals part of a document otherwise hidden from view.

search engine A collective term applied to the various *programs* that look for information in response to a query made by a *user*. A number of search engines have been developed for the *WWW* to help locate files on the *Internet*.

serial communications port A *hardware interface* used to connect a device such as a *modem* or *printer* to the *computer*. 'Serial' refers to the sending and receiving of data one *bit* at a time. Serial ports use *handshaking* to regulate the flow of data.

Serial Line Internet Protocol (SLIP) A *network interface* that allows dial-up users to temporarily connect their *computer* to the *Internet* and use *TCP/IP*-based *clients*. It is an older standard than the alternative, *PPP*.

server Refers to either a *host* running 'server' *software* (as in 'servant'), or to the software itself. A server directs the sharing of resources among many *users* on a multi-user host, and fulfils requests made by *client* software (or, in some cases, by *e-mail*). See *mail server*.

service provider In relation to the *Internet*, a collective term for the companies and organizations that offer *Internet* access. Many companies specialize in providing access to dial-up *modem* users, supplying much of the *software* needed to get *online*, along with *Points of Presence* providing connections at local telephone call rates.

shareware A category of *software* that users can try out for a specified evaluation period before buying. An extremely popular method of distributing software via *bulletin boards*, *online services*, and the *Internet*.

Simple Mail Transport Protocol (SMTP) The main protocol used on the *Internet* for sending and receiving *e-mail*.

SLIP See *Serial Line Internet Protocol*.

SMTP See *Simple Mail Transport Protocol*.

software Synonymous with *program*. Software is a term describing a set of instructions for performing a computing task involving the manipulation of data. The two broad categories of software are *applications* and *operating systems*. See *hardware*.

sound card A circuit board inside the *system unit* that enables a *computer* to playback sounds (requiring speakers) and to record sound (requiring a microphone).

source A small file describing the location of a *WAIS* database (i.e. the name of the *host*, the *path name*, and the name of the database), usually with a brief synopsis of the database contents. Also, the original file used to generate a *WWW* page, containing the *HTML* tags.

startup Synonymous with 'booting', the act of powering on a *computer*, *loading* the *operating system* into *RAM*, and the self-checking process it goes through in preparation for use.

stop bits Extra *bits* placed at either end of a *character* by *communications software* to mark its beginning and end.

streaming audio The playback of sound files during *downloading* as a stream of data, as oppossed to waiting until the entire file has been retrieved before playback.

SuperJANET A project replacing the original *JANET network* in the UK with high-speed fibre optic cabling. SuperJANET is a *TCP/IP*-based network, although it currently also supports *X.25*-based traffic.

Super VGA (SVGA) A graphics standard for *PCs* requiring compliant systems to be capable of displaying a screen *resolution* of 800 x 600 or 1024 x 768 *pixels*. More than 256 colours at these resolutions may be supported. See *Video Graphics Array*.

SVGA See *Super VGA*.

sysop See *system operator*.

system operator (sysop) Some times called the 'administrator', a sysop is a person who runs, or is responsible for, a *bulletin board*.

system unit The plastic or metal box containing the main *hardware* components of a desktop *personal computer*, such as the *microprocessor*, *hard disk*, etc.

tags In *HTML*, the language used to create *WWW* pages, codes enclosed in angle brackets that give meaning the elements of the page. For example, the first-level heading tags are used to specify a main heading, as in **<H1>**Medicine**</H1>**. See *containers*, *attributes*.

TCP/IP See *Transmission Control Protocol/Internet Protocol*.

telecommunications Communications over telephone lines, whether a conversation between people or the exchange of digital information between *computers*, fax machines, or other devices.

telemedicine The use of telecommunications technologies and *computers* to overcome barriers in health care posed by the factor of physical distance. In practice, this can enable doctors to provide a 'virtual presence' in locations previously deprived of such contact.

Telnet The name of a protocol forming part of the *TCP/IP* protocol suite used on the *Internet*. Also an *Internet service*, where a Telnet *client emulates* a 'virtual Internet *terminal*' allowing remote access to a *host computer*.

terminal A reference usually to a 'dumb' terminal, a *monitor* and *keyboard* providing access to a central *host computer*, but without its own *microprocessor* (a 'smart' terminal does have a microprocessor). See *terminal emulation*.

terminal emulation The imitation (*emulation*) of a physical terminal by *communications software*. A terminal emulator can be used over a *telecommunications* link to interact with a *host* that might be thousands of miles away. Popular terminal types to emulate include *TTY*, *ANSI*, *VT100*, and *RIP*.

text file A *computer* file that contains *characters* from the *ASCII character set* only. Synonymous with *ASCII file*. See *binary file*.

TFT See *thin film transistor display*.

thin film transistor display (TFT) A type of 'active matrix' technology used in high-end *notebook computer* screens to display an image. See *dual scan display*.

threading Message threading refers to the ability of a *conference* message reader or *news reader* to automate a *user's* ability to 'follow a thread'. That is, to read all the messages in a particular conversation in the sequence in which they were posted, rather than a chronological sequence of individual messages pertaining to many conversations posted to the conference or *newsgroup*.

toolbar Under a *graphical user interface*, a row of distinctive buttons across the top of the *browser* (or other *application*) *window*. Pictures on the buttons depict their function.

Transmission Control Protocol/Internet Protocol (TCP/IP) A protocol suite including Transmission Control Protocol, Internet Protocol, *SMTP*, *FTP*, *Telnet*, and many other protocols operating on the *Internet*.

transparent GIF A special type of the *GIF* graphics format that allows one colour within the image to become 'invisible'. Similar to the blue-screen effect used in cinematography, the 'invisible' parts of the image appear transparent against the background colour of the *WWW* page.

TTY An acronym for 'teletype', a very basic type of *terminal*. See *terminal emulation*.

UMLS See *Unified Medical Language System*.

Unified Medical Language System (UMLS) A classification system developed by the US National Library of Medicine. The UMLS Metathesaurus contains information about medical terms and their co-occurrence in *MeSH* and other thesauri, enabling *MEDLINE* searches to be conducted using the vocabulary most familiar to the searcher.

uniform resource locator (URL) A standardized syntax used on the *Internet* describing the location and method of accessing Internet resources. Each URL is composed of several elements: the type of *Internet service*, the *domain name* of the *host*, the *port address*, and the *path name*.

UNIX A robust *operating system* designed to support multiple simultaneous *users*. Versions exist for virtually all computing *platforms*, and *hosts* running UNIX are predominant on the *Internet*. UNIX shells providing a *graphical user interface* are sometimes employed to isolate users from a *command-line interface*—similar to the way *Microsoft Windows* acted as a front-end to *DOS* (pre-Windows 95).

UNIX-to-UNIX CoPy (UUCP) UUCP refers to both a file-transfer *program* used by *UNIX computers*, and to a particular *network* of UNIX computers. The UUCP network maintains *e-mail gateways* to the *Internet*, providing many *bulletin boards* with a cost-effective way to receive e-mail and *Usenet* news via UUCP.

upgrade card Also called an expansion card, a board containing circuitry that improves the specification of a *computer*. It may add more *RAM*, increase video capabilities (more colours, higher *resolution*), or add an internal *modem*, etc.

upload The process of sending a file from your own *computer* to a remote *host* over a communications link. See *file-transfer protocol*, *download*.

URL See *uniform resource locator*.

user A generic term for anybody who operates a *computer* for any purpose.

user name Many *bulletin boards*, *online services*, and some *Internet hosts* require each *user* to identify him or herself with a user name (or user ID) on that system. This is often used in association with a password.

Usenet A kind of global *conferencing* system where messages pertaining to particular subjects are distributed in the form of *newsgroups* over the *Internet* and many other *networks*. Although it is most often described as one, Usenet is not strictly an *Internet service* because it doesn't rely on *TCP/IP*-based networks for message distribution.

UUCP See *UNIX-to-UNIX CoPy*.

uuencode The name of a *program* originating on *UNIX* machines, now a standard for the *ASCII encoding* of *binary files* so that they can be sent by *e-mail* on the *Internet*.

V.22bis A *modulation protocol* enabling compliant *modems* to transfer data at speeds up to 2400 *bps* prior to the application of *compression protocols*.

V.32 A *modulation protocol* enabling compliant *modems* to transfer data at speeds up to 9600 *bps* prior to the application of *compression protocols*.

V.32bis A *modulation protocol* enabling compliant *modems* to transfer data at speeds up to 14 400 *bps* prior to the application of *compression protocols*.

V.34 A *modulation protocol* enabling compliant *modems* to transfer data at speeds up to 28 800 *bps* prior to the application of *compression protocols*.

V.42 An *error-correction protocol* standardized by the UN agency, International Telecommunication Union (ITU-T).

V.42bis A *compression protocol*, theoretically quartering transmission time.

VBScript A scripting language used to make *WWW* pages more interactive, based on the Visual Basic programming language. Microsoft's answer to Netscape's *JavaScript*.

Veronica The name of a *search engine* which locates objects indexed by *Gopher*, such as a keyword in a menu or document title.

VGA See *Video Graphics Array*.

videoconferencing *Telecommunications* between two or more people using a video signal to transmit images and audio in *real time*. Can be achieved over direct *ISDN* lines, *ATM networks*, or the *Internet* (often, but not always, using *Mbone*).

Video Graphics Array (VGA) A *PC* graphics standard requiring compliant systems to be capable of displaying 256 colours with a screen *resolution* of 640 x 480 *pixels*.

video RAM (VRAM) Memory chips used by a *computer*, in combination with other video circuitry, to produce the image on the screen of a *monitor*. The amount of VRAM relates to the number of colours that can simultaneously be displayed (the *bit depth*) and the *resolution* of the image. See *random-access memory*, *Super VGA*, *Video Graphics Array*.

Viewdata A type of *terminal* which can display text and basic colour graphics. See *terminal emulation*.

Virtual Reality Modelling Language A graphics file format describing the *computer*-generated simulation of a physical environment that permits interaction with the 'virtual' objects within it. *Plug-ins* are available to allow VRML files to be viewed with a *WWW* browser, but significant computing power is required for realistic 3D renderings.

virus A small segment of *software* code created by a malicious prankster that 'infects' files on a *hard disk*, causing the *computer* to behave strangely or to lose data. Virus-detection software can scan for unusual activity that might be caused by a virus. Viruses cannot be transmitted by *e-mail* unless they are contained within a *binary file* attachment (which must then be run on the recipient's computer to cause damage). *Downloading Java applets* does not pose a threat since applets cannot write files to your hard disk.

VRAM See *video RAM*.

VRML See *Virtual Reality Modelling Language*.

VT100 The most universal type of *terminal*. See *terminal emulation*.

WAIS See *Wide Area Information Servers*.

WAN See *wide-area network*.

Wide Area Information Servers (WAIS) A *server* that supports *client* access to a database indexing the full contents of documents pertaining to a certain topic. Searches are composed in plain English, and 'relevance feedback' is used to identify documents that best fit the search criteria. See *source*.

wide-area network (WAN) A *network* of *computers*, or a network of networks, not physically located in the same small geographic area. See *LAN*.

wild card A *character* such as an asterisk used to 'stand in' for an uncertain or variable character or characters in a search string. For example, 'Find cardio*' would include cardiology, cardiopathy, cardiogram, etc.

window A key element of a *graphical user interface*, rectangular windows are drawn on the screen of a *monitor* by some *operating systems* and *applications* to simplify using a *computer*. Such windows frequently incorporate features such as *scroll bars*, title bars, and *pull-down menus*, etc.

Windows See *Microsoft Windows*.

World-Wide Web (WWW) An extremely popular *Internet service* using the metaphor of a page, each associated via *hypertext* links with other pages widely distributed over the *Internet*. Readers of WWW pages—which may include graphics and other *multimedia* elements—use a WWW *browser* to navigate this 'web' of links in any order that they choose. See *HTML*, *HTTP*.

WWW See *World-Wide Web*.

X.25 A *networking* protocol, used on *JANET* prior to the adoption of *TCP/IP*. X.400 (*e-mail*) and X.29 (the equivalent of *Telnet*) are examples of X.25-based services.

Xmodem A widely-supported *file-transfer protocol*, able to transfer *binary files* and incorporating *error correction*. See *communications software*.

XON/XOFF See *handshaking*.

Ymodem A *file-transfer protocol*, able to transfer *binary files* and incorporating *error correction*. See *communications software*.

Zmodem An efficient, good all-round *file-transfer protocol*, able to transfer *binary files* and incorporating *error correction*. See *communications software*.

INDEX

Bold numbers denote reference to illustrations; italic numbers denote reference to tables.

MEDICINE AND THE INTERNET

Quick Reference Card

Personal Internet info

E-mail address: ....

Domain name: ....

IP number: ....

Mail-server domain name: ....

News-server domain name: ....

Support e-mail address: ....

Support telephone number: ....

Support Web page: ....

Home page: ....

Important addresses

Name:	E-mail address:
....	....
....	....
....	....
....	....
....	....
....	....
....	....

Mail server (commands):	List address (to all):
....	....
....	....
....	....
....	....
....	....
....	....
....	....

MEDICINE AND THE INTERNET

Quick Reference Card

Binary files by e-mail

Archie by e-mail—find a file:

To: archie@archie.doc.ic.ac.uk
find *filename* (e.g. *meddoc.zip*)
quit

FTP by e-mail—retrieve a file:

To: ftpmail@doc.ic.ac.uk
open *site* (e.g. *ftp.elsewhere.com*)
cd *directory* (e.g. */pub/med/*)
ascii
get *filename* (e.g. *meddoc.zip*)
quit

Downloading files

Check: Is your FTP software in ASCII or binary mode?

File suffix:	Expander program:
....	....
....	....
....	....
....	....

Preferred search engines

http:// ....

http:// ....

Favourite Web sites

http:// www.oup.co.uk/scimed/medint/

http:// ....

http:// ....

http:// ....

http:// ....

© 1997 Oxford University Press